MW01166407

Instructor's Manual to Accompany

The Professional Cosmetologist

FOURTH EDITION

John W. Dalton

West Publishing Company
St. Paul New York Los Angeles San Francisco

WEST'S COMMITMENT TO THE ENVIRONMENT

In 1906, West Publishing Company began recycling materials left over from the production of books. This began a tradition of efficient and responsible use of resources. Today, up to 95% of our legal books and 70% of our college texts are printed on recycled, acid-free stock. West also recycles nearly 22 million pounds of scrap paper annually—the equivalent of 181,717 trees. Since the 1960s, West has devised ways to capture and recycle waste inks, solvents, oils, and vapors created in the printing process. We also recycle plastics of all kinds, wood, glass, corrugated cardboard, and batteries, and have eliminated the use of styrofoam book packaging. We at West are proud of the longevity and the scope of our commitment to our environment.

Production, Prepress, Printing and Binding by West Publishing Company.

COPYRIGHT © 1992 by WEST PUBLISHING CO.
610 Opperman Drive
P.O. Box 64526
St. Paul, MN 55164–0526

All rights reserved
Printed in the United States of America
99 98 97 96 95 94 93 92 8 7 6 5 4 3 2 1 0

ISBN 0–314–00787–3

Acknowledgements

The author wishes to acknowledge Bridget Neumayr, Hugh Johnson, and Frank Jacobi: Ms. Neumayr for her invaluable editorial assistance, support, and patience in the preparation of the manuscript; Mr. Johnson for his design and layout skills, and his ingenuity with the various computer programs involved; Mr. Jacobi for his expert advice on the Final Test questions.

Table of Contents

Introduction – Instructor Lesson Plans

Lesson Overview and Motivation:	The Lesson Overview and Motivation describes the general chapter topic and supplies some "hints", or "trouble-shooting tips that may prove helpful for the beginning classroom teacher.
Acceptable Level:	The level of acceptance reflects the criteria used in The Professional Cosmetologist , 4th Edition. The actual level used should be determined by your school administrator.
Location:	The cosmetology course is typically taught in one of the following areas: Theory classroom_____ Lab classroom_____ Clinic_____. This area of the Lesson Plans allows instructors to identify the location for their class according to the subject that will be taught. You should also consider whether the room has adequate ventilation, heating/cooling, seating, workstations, etc., to create a learning environment that is comfortable for the students.
Time for Lecture/ Demonstration:	This section of the Instructor's Manual provides a space for instructors to indicate how long a particular lecture will take, or how long the demonstration/practice room will be needed, so as to avoid any scheduling conflicts with other instructors or course offerings. 30 min._____ 60 min._____ 90 min._____
Student Level:	Since resources need to be selected for each class, it is important to determine in advance the learning level of the audience in the class to be taught. Resources selected for students with 1000 hours of instruction and practice would normally have a different comprehension level and level of difficulty than those for a group of students just beginning your program. Beginning_____ Intermediate_____ Advanced_____
Equipment/Models Needed:	In order to teach most classes, certain pieces of equipment are necessary. Prior to the class, the instructor should make a comprehensive list of what will be needed. For example, to give a permanent hair coloring demonstration, shampoo facilities would be required in order to remove the processed color from the model's hair. Special arrangements may need to be made for recruiting models, or for acquiring mannequins and clamps.

Supplies Needed:

General supplies are listed here. These should include supplies that the instructor or student will need to complete the demonstration or exercise requirements of the class. For a lecture class this would include basic supplies, such as chalk. A styling class may require curling irons, clippies, rollers, scissors, styling lotion, combs, brushes, etc.

Sanitation Supplies and Equipment:

Because cosmetology students work so closely with the general public and follow state licensing agency rules and regulations, it is of particular importance for the instructor to emphasize sanitation procedures. Sanitation supplies e.g., quats, alcohol, protective gloves, wet sanitizer, etc., should be carefully listed in this section, so that sanitation procedures can easily be taught.

Teaching Aids Needed:

Modern technology provides more classroom equipment than ever before. When considering the implementation of cosmetology computer software for student study and testing, better transparency masters, and videotapes of school procedures - planning ahead for the necessary equipment that will be used in the instructional process is essential. Some examples are: TPC Textbook, Theory and Practical Workbook, State Board Review Questions book, chalkboard, overhead projector, VCR and videotape(s), computer, and printer. Additionally, make sure to check for electrical outlets and extension cords for plugging in various pieces of electrical equipment, e.g., an overhead projector, etc.

Theory Objectives

This feature provides a listing of the minimum number of theory objectives that should be taught per chapter. It is not intended to indicate all the information that could be taught - just the minumum number of objectives that should be developed through instruction.

Practical Objectives

This feature provides a listing of the minimum number of practical objectives (services or exercises) that should be taught per chapter. You will have an area consisting of two lines for writing in your own supplementary student exercises.

Word Review:

This section of the Instructor's Manual is a three-column listing of terminology that will be new to the basic student. In some cases, the student will not only have trouble spelling these terms, but also pronouncing them.

Answers to End-of-Chapter Questions:

At the end of each chapter in the textbook - The Professional Cosmetologist - there are questions that should assist students in focusing their study energies. Think of these questions as "hints" to the student with respect to important terms and concepts contained within a particular chapter. For classroom discussion, this section of the Instructor's Manual contains the ***answers to those chapter-ending questions.***

Special Safety Considerations:

Most of the services taught in a cosmetology school or college require instruction in special safety considerations. This section identifies some of the essential safety considerations associated with each chapter. It is not intended to cover all safety concerns or situations, but rather to remind you to incorporate *your own* classroom safety practices into the instructional strategy process.

Transparency Master:

When one or more full color transparencies have been produced by West Publishing Company for classroom use, the exact Figure Number, or Table Number of the item from the main textbook will be listed in this section of the Instructor's Manual.

Theory Objective 1:

All of the theory and practical objectives will be listed for each chapter. The purpose is to give the instructor a panoramic view of knowledge and performances that ought to be introduced during the instruction of that chapter. It also affords an opportunity for insertion of additional objectives, which will customize the program for a particular school.

Learning Steps	Resources
When these steps have been followed and completed by the student, and complemented with instruction and practice, - the student should eventually be able to master the particular task .	These items locate the resources that will allow the student to identify the resource for the learning steps described in the previous column. Page numbers referencing the textbook, or the Theory and Practical Workbook, should be listed in this area, so students can be given accurate assignments. For instance, if you are requiring students to view a vidoetape you have selected - the title and perhaps instructions for which part of the videotape needs to be viewed, e.g., from reference number 23.34 to 78.90, should also be included.

Instructor's Resource Notes:

Considering that instructors have attended, and in most cases taught, many classes, and have also worked in a salon, this is an opportunity for you to "plug in" your own special instructor resource information. This might include a special lecturer, or demonstrator for a particular subject, a new service or hairstyle, introduction of a new transparency, or perhaps a videotape that covers a certain procedure or point of instruction better than anything else you have reviewed. Since the classroom instructor is the facilitator of learning, you should certainly be provided with space for incorporating your own resources to enhance the student learning experience.

Lesson Plan

Special Report
Ecology in the Salon

Lesson Overview and Motivation: This section of the book is devoted to making the student aware of the need to conserve energy, use products that are ecologically sound, recycle waste, protect our environment, and conserve natural resources. Develop a project for the program to recycle reusable items, such as aluminum cans. Emphasize the importance for the need to reduce any excessive waste of supplies used in the process of providing cosmetology services.

Acceptable Level: Score 85 percent or better on the questions at the end of this chapter.

Location: Theory classroom_____ Lab classroom_____ Clinic_____

Time for Lecture/ Demonstration: 30 min._____ 60 min._____ 90 min._____

Student Level: Beginning_____ Intermediate_____ Advanced_____

Supplies Needed: Videotape(s) of ecology/conservation strategies.

Teaching Aids Needed: Textbook, Theory and Practical Workbook, State Board Review Questions, chalkboard, overhead projector, VCR. (See chart at end of this section for organizing and implementing your own cosmetology resource information).

Word Review:

biodegradable	ecology	environment
nonaerosol	recyclable	recycle
MSDA	WHMIS	
Materials Safety Data Sheet	Workplace Hazard Materials Information Standards	

Answers to End-of-Chapter Questions: **1.** No. **2.** Yes. **3.** Compare your answer to the information in the text. **4.** The surroundings of living things, such as the air and water. **5.** Compare your answer to the information in the text. **6.** Compare your answer to the information in the text. **7.** High-efficiency, energy-saving water heater. **8.** Fluorescent lighting. **9.** Yes. **10.** Nonaerosol pump.

Evaluation of Instruction:

_____ A. Discussed answers to end of chapter questions.
_____ B. Collected completed workbook assignments.
_____ C. Collected student progress charts.
_____ D. State board sheets current.
_____ E. Answered written test(s), and/or computer test questions.

Student Assignments: ____

____

Instructor Planning Form Cosmetology Program

____
Instructor(s)

Date____________________

	Lect./Demo	Tranparencies	Videotape(s)	Guest-Lect./Demo	Practical Exercises	Workbook	Written/Pract. Test
Special Report: Ecology In The Salon							
1 Careers In Cosmetology							
2 Ethics In Cosmetology							
3 Sanitizing And Sterilization							
4 Describing The Hair							
5 Shampooing							
6 Conditioning							
7 Scalp Treatments							
8 Finger Waving							
9 Sculpture Curls							
10 Setting The Hair With Rollers							
11 Selecting Hairstyles							
12 Hair Shaping							
13 Air Waving And Blow-Drying							
14 Iron Curls							
15 Temporary Hair Coloring							
16 Semipermanent Hair Coloring							
17 Permanent Hair Coloring							
18 Lightening And Toning							
19 Creative Lightening & Toning							
20 Permanent Wave							
21 Chemical Hair Relaxing							
22 Thermal Pressing							
23 Ecurling The Hair							
24 Describing The Skin							
25 Facial Treatments							
26 Applying Makeup							
27 Nail Anatomy, And Disorders,							
28 Manicuring And Pedicuring							
29 Wigs And Hairpieces							
30 Shaving							
31 Planning A Salon							
32 Salon Operations							
33 Psychology Of Interpersonal Skills/ Retailing							
34 Principles Of Electricity							
35 Chemistry Of Cosmetology							
36 Anatomy And Physiology - Bones							
37 Anatomy And Physiology - Vasc./Endo. System							

1

Lesson Plan

Careers in Cosmetology

Lesson Overview and Motivation: Students will gain a familiarity with the vocational specialties they can choose from. This chapter also serves to acquaint them with some general concepts of the business, and introduces some fundamental cosmetology terms.

Acceptable Level: Score 85 percent or better on a multiple choice exam.

Location: Theory classroom_____ Lab classroom_____ Clinic_____

Time for Lecture/ Demonstration: 30 min._____ 60 min._____ 90 min._____

Student Level: Beginning_____ Intermediate_____ Advanced_____

Equipment/Models Needed: VCR

Supplies Needed: Videotape(s) of cosmetology careers.

Teaching Aids Needed: Textbook, Theory and Practical Workbook, State Board Review Questions, chalkboard, overhead projector, computer, printer, guest lecturer, e.g., salon owner.

Transparency Master: Figure 1.2.

Word Review:

personal grooming
verbal communications
percentage
barber stylist
commission
cosmetology
esthetics
guarantee
manicurist
personal grooming
research technician
personal hygiene
guarantee
nonverbal communications
body language
salon owner
electrologist
field technician
halitosis
tonsorial
personal hygiene
competition hairstylist
commission
minimum wage
allergy
color blindness
cosmetologist
esthetician
good posture
manager-operator
nutrition
platform hairstylist
verbal communication

Answers to End-of-Chapter Questions:

1. Cosmetology is the art and science of beauty care. **2.** The cosmetologist is licensed to perform services on the hair, skin and nails. **3.** Personal hygiene refers to a daily routine for maintaining one's health. **4.** Yes. **5.** Allergy, or an allergic reaction. **6.** The minimum wage. **7.** Forty hours per week. **8.** Esthetician. **9.** Electrologist. **10.** Bad breath. **11.** Cover letter. **12.** Yes. **13.** No.

Evaluation of Instruction:

_____ A. Discussed answers to end of chapter questions.
_____ B. Collected completed workbook assignments.
_____ C. Collected student progress charts.
_____ D. State board sheets current.
_____ E. Answered written test(s), and/or computer test questions.

Student Assignments:

____

____

2

Lesson Plan

Ethics in Cosmetology

Lesson Overview and Motivation: Although the need for ethical behavior should be stressed early-on, it must not be presented as a mere "beginner's class." Here the instructor can make the greatest difference by personalizing the subject with his/her own experience. You may also wish to invite a guest lecturer, such as a salon owner, or a representative from the National Cosmetology Association.

Acceptable Level: Score 85 percent or better on a multiple choice exam.

Location: Theory classroom_____ Lab classroom_____ Clinic_____

Time for Lecture/ Demonstration: 30 min._____ 60 min._____ 90 min._____

Student Level: Beginning_____ Intermediate_____ Advanced_____

Teaching Aids Needed: Textbook, Theory and Practical Workbook, State Board Review Questions, chalkboard, overhead projector, VCR and videotape(s), computer, printer.

Answers to End-of-Chapter Questions: **1.** Yes. It would be against professional ethics. **2.** Yes. **3.** Yes. **4.** Yes. It would be against professional ethics. **5.** Yes. **6.** You are acting ethically. **7.** Voluntary. **8.** A code of ethics. **9.** True. **10.** True. **11.** False. **12.** No. **13.** Yes. **14.** False.

Evaluation of Instruction:

_____ A. Discussed answers to end of chapter questions.
_____ B. Collected completed workbook assignments.
_____ C. Collected student progress charts.
_____ D. State board sheets current.
_____ E. Answered written test(s), and/or computer test questions.

Student Assignments: ______________________________

____

3

Lesson Plan

Sanitation and Sterilization

Lesson Overview and Motivation: This chapter describes bacteria, viruses, and the immune system, and stresses the importance of these matters in the practice of cosmetology. Students will learn how to sanitize setting, combing, and cutting implements within 20 minutes.

Acceptable Level: Score 85 percent or better on a multiple choice exam, and complete the performance product checklist for this task.

Location: Theory classroom_____ Lab classroom_____ Clinic_____

Time for Lecture/ Demonstration: 30 min._____ 60 min._____ 90 min._____

Student Level: Beginning_____ Intermediate_____ Advanced_____

Equipment/Models Needed: Chalkboard, shampoo bowl, shampoo chair, hydraulic chair, facial chair, steamer, manicure table, manicure implements, facial implements, hairstyling implements.

Supplies Needed: Student kit. Student kits vary from one school to the next; however, they will generally contain the following implements and supplies: styling combs, brushes, rat-tail comb, rake comb, clippies, sectioning clips, scissors, electric clipper, tweezers, shampoo cape, combout cape, manicure and facial implements and facial supplies, mannequin, holder, neutralizing bib, rollers, and hand dryer.

Sanitation Supplies and Equipment: Wet sanitizer, dry sanitizer, alcohol, astringent, peroxide, quats, formaldehyde, fumigant envelopes, disposable gloves.

Teaching Aids Needed: Textbook, Theory and Practical Workbook, State Board Review Questions, chalkboard, overhead projector, VCR and videotape(s), computer, printer. (Refer to master state listing of safety precautions at end of this section).

Theory Objectives

1. Terms used to describe and classify bacteria.
2. Viruses, the immune system, and infection control.
3. Methods of sanitation.
4. Measures used to sanitize the service area.
5. Safety measures for the use and storage of chemicals, fire safety, and first aid in schools and salons.

Practical Objectives

6. Sanitize implements and equipment.

Word Review:

public sanitation	bacilli	bacteriology
bacteria	antiseptic	staphylococci
cocci	microorganisms	general infection
microscope	spirilla	diplococci
local infection	virus	communicable
contagious	susceptible	Routes of transmission
safe sex	Hepatitis B	AIDS
immunity	life-styles	HIV
active immunity	passive immunity	epidermis
transfusion of blood	infection control procedures	toxins/Anti-toxins
routes of transmission	dry sanitizer	sterilization methods
corrosive	disinfectant	wet sanitizer
bactericides	germicides	antiseptic
fungicides	hydrogen peroxide	alcohol
dry heat	formaldehyde packets	formaldehyde
ultraviolet rays	moist heat	humidifier
electric air precipitator	dehumidifier	vacuum breaker
Neosporin	flammable products	fire extinguisher
Mycitracin	ammonia	closed waste container
1:000 quats	fumigant	
Acquired Immunodeficiency Syndrome	Human Immunodeficiency Virus	quaternary ammonium compounds

Answers to End-of-Chapter Questions:

1. Public hygiene. **2.** Matter. **3.** Cells. **4.** Microorganisms. **5.** Bacteria. **6.** Bacteriology. **7.** Yes. **8.** No. **9.** Cocci, spirilla, and bacilli; round, spiral, and rod-shaped. **10.** Heat, moisture, absence of sunlight. **11.** Sterilization kills all bacteria; sanitation kills only pathogenic bacteria. **12.** Antiseptics halt or prevent the growth of bacteria. Fumigants (fumes) and disinfectants (generally liquids) kill pathogenic bacteria. **13.** Yes, probably fatal. **14.** Quaternary ammonium ("quats") and formaldehyde. **15.** 70 percent alcohol. **16.** 3-5 percent. **17.** No, ethyl alcohol is stronger. **18.** One (1) part quats to 1,000 parts water; 2/3 ounce quats mixed with 1 gallon water. **19.** Yes. **20.** No. **21.** A closed container. **22.** Spontaneous combustion. **23.** In a cool, dry place. **24.** Mycitracin or Neosporin ointment. **25.** Absolutely not. **26.** Only cool water. **27.** False. **28.** False. **29.** True. **30.** True. **31.** True. **32.** False. **33.** True. **34.** True. **35.** False. **36.** True.

Special Safety Considerations:

Cleansing of hands before and after service; chemicals coming in contact with clients' skin (neck and hairline), eyes, or ears; cleansing of bottles etc.; and sanitation of the work area; sanitation of items that can be reused, such as combs and brushes; disposal of used items; return and proper storage of unused supplies; disposable gloves for exposure to blood or caustic chemicals; check temperature of product or electrical device. Don't inhale or smell fumes of sanitation/sterilization chemicals because they may irritate mucus membranes.

Theory Objective 1: **Define the terms used to describe and classify bacteria.**

Learning Steps

1. Read chapter in textbook.
2. Complete assignment in workbook.
3. View videotape(s).
4. Proceed to next objective.

Resources

1. *The Professional Cosmetologist,* 4th ed., ch. 3, pp. 34-37.
2. *Theory and Practical Workbook,* ch. 3, p. 11.
3. Videotape library.

Instructor's Resource Notes: ____________________

____

Theory Objective 2: **Define viruses, the immune system, and infection control.**

Learning Steps

1. Read chapter in textbook.
2. Complete assignment in workbook.
3. View videotape(s).
4. Proceed to next objective.

Resources

1. *The Professional Cosmetologist,* 4th ed., ch. 3, pp. 37-41.
2. *Theory and Practical Workbook,* ch. 3, p. 13.
3. Videotape library.

Instructor's Resource Notes: ____________________

____

Theory Objective 3: **Describe the five methods of sanitation.**

Learning Steps

1. Read chapter in textbook.
2. Complete assignment in workbook.
3. View videotape(s).
4. Proceed to next objective.

Resources

1. *The Professional Cosmetologist,* 4th ed., ch. 3, pp. 41-45.
2. *Theory and Practical Workbook,* ch. 3, p. 17.
3. Videotape library.

Instructor's Resource Notes: ______________________________

____

Theory Objective 4: **Describe the measures used to sanitize the work area.**

Learning Steps

1. Read chapter in textbook.
2. Complete assignment in workbook.
3. View videotape(s).
4. Proceed to next objective.

Resources

1. *The Professional Cosmetologist,* 4th ed., ch. 3, pp. 45-47.
2. *Theory and Practical Workbook,* ch. 3, p. 19.
3. Videotape library.

Instructor's Resource Notes: ______________________________

____

Theory Objective 5: **Describe the safety measures for the use and storage of chemicals, fire safety, and first aid in schools and salons.**

Learning Steps

1. Read chapter in textbook.
2. Complete assignment in workbook.
3. View videotape(s).
4. Proceed to next objective.

Resources

1. *The Professional Cosmetologist,* 4th ed., ch. 3, pp. 47-51.
2. *Theory and Practical Workbook,* ch. 3, p. 19.
3. Videotape library.

Instructor's Resource Notes: ______________________________

____

Practical Objective 6: **Sanitize implements and equipment.**

Learning Steps	Resources
1. Read chapter in textbook.	1. *The Professional Cosmetologist,* 4th ed., ch. 3, pp. 51-56.
2. Complete assignment in workbook.	2. *Theory and Practical Workbook,* ch. 3, p. 21.
3. View videotape(s).	3. Videotape library.
4. Proceed to next chapter.	

Instructor's Resource Notes: ______________________________

____

Evaluation of Instruction:

_____ A. Discussed answers to end of chapter questions.
_____ B. Collected completed workbook assignments.
_____ C. Collected student progress charts.
_____ D. State board sheets current.
_____ E. Answered written test(s), and/or computer test questions.
_____ F. Completed Performance/Product Checklist.

Student Assignments: ______________________________

____

STANDARD SCHOOL AND SALON SAFETY & SANITATION PRACTICES

(Consult your State Rules and Regulations)

No.	Name	Sanitation Practice
1	Alcohol, 70%	Disinfect metal instruments with cutting edges and points.
2	Animals	Dogs, birds, and cats etc. not permitted in salon.
3	Animals	(exception) Seeing/hearing dog for blind or deaf.
4	Article dropped on floor	Sanitized before reuse.
5	Clean towels	Store in clean, closed, dustproof cabinet.
6	Closed receptacles	For clean towels, and soiled towels
7	Directions of manufacturer	Followed at all times.
8	Disinfectant	Quats - 1:1000 , or sodium hypochlorite (household bleach) 10%.
9	Drinking water	Provided, but no common cups, or glasses, etc.
10	Dry sanitizer	Ultraviolet light closed cabinet, or cabinet with vapors.
11	Electrical appliances	Should be grounded to prevent electrical shock.
12	Electrolysis needle	Sanitized with 70% alcohol.
13	Equipment repair	Should be in good repair at all times.
14	First Aid kit	Complete kit on hand at all times in school or salon.
15	Floors, walls, ceilings, curtains	Kept clean and free of dirt and dust.
16	Glass electrodes	Sanitized with 70% alcohol.
17	Gloves	Sanitized after each use with alcohol, or use disposable type, use for protection from chemicals, or infection control.

18 Hair clippings .... Swept up immediately after each haircut. Clippings placed in closed container.

19 Hands .... Washed immediately before and after each client.

20 Hand washing facilities .... Provided with hot and cold water, soap, and sanitary towels, or approved dryer.

21 Headrests .... Clean paper or laundered towel headrest changed before each client.

22 Inspection report posting .... Displayed conspicuously in school or salon.

23 Labeling of bottles .... Clearly labeled to disclose contents. Important when mixing from a concentrated solution into a ready-to-use formulation.

24 Laundering, water temperature .... Some states require 140 degrees for laundering of towels.

25 Leaving client alone .... Do not leave client unattended during chemical processing service.

26 License posting .... Displayed conspicuously in school or salon.

27 Lighting .... School and salon should have adequate lighting.

28 Linens .... Clean linens (towels) should be stored in a clean, closed container.

29 Metal electric clippers .... Sanitized with 70% alcohol.

30 Metal razors .... Sanitized with 70% alcohol.

31 Metal scissors .... Sanitized with 70% alcohol.

32 Metal thinning shears .... Sanitized with 70% alcohol.

33 Metal tweezers .... Sanitized with 70% alcohol.

34 Mouth .... Don't put combs, bobby pins and hair pins in your mouth.

35 Neck dusting brushes .... Not permitted because they can't be sanitized.

36 Odors .... School and salon should be well ventilated to remove hazardous fumes.

37 Orangewood sticks, emery boards . Dispose of after each use.

38 Pencil cosmetics .... Sharpened before each use.

39 Pockets carrying supplies .... Beauty supplies and implements are not to be carried or stored in pocket.

40 Powders .... Dispensed from a clean, labeled shaker to avoid spread of disease.

41 Quaternary Ammonium .... 1:1000 strength used as disinfectant.

42 Rules & Regs, display copy of .... Displayed conspicuously in school or salon.

43 Shampoo bowls .... Sanitized with soap and water after each client.

44 Shampoo cape .... Should not touch client's neck - use laundered towel or sanitized neck strip. Cape should be routinely washed with soap and water; then, dried.

45 Soiled towels .... Placed in a closed container.

46 Spatula .... Should be used to dispense creams etc. to avoid contamination with bacteria. Discard after use.

47 Toilets/lavatories .... Clean at all times, and not used for storage. Wash hands before leaving.

48 Unsanitized items .... Shall not be stored with sanitized items, i.e., money, pens, or pencils.

49 Ventilation .... Proper flow and removal of air resulting from artificial nail supplies, etc.

50 Vermin, rodents, flies .... The school/salon premises should be free from all - including insects.

51 Vibrators .... Sanitized before each use.

52 Waste .... Placed in closed container. Should be removed daily from school or salon.

53 Wet sanitizer .... Containing enough fresh disinfectant to submerge implements for at least 10 minutes.

4

Lesson Plan

Describing the Hair

Lesson Overview and Motivation: This chapter introduces students to hair structure, function and composition. Students will learn to define, identify, describe and analyze the hair. Emphasis is placed upon hair diseases, hair disorders, and hair condition. (Microscopic slides of human hair may also be available for student viewing.)

Acceptable Level: Score 85 percent or better on a multiple choice exam.

Location: Theory classroom_____ Lab classroom_____ Clinic_____

Time for Lecture/ Demonstration: 30 min._____ 60 min._____ 90 min._____

Student Level: Beginning_____ Intermediate_____ Advanced_____

Teaching Aids Needed: Textbook, Theory and Practical Workbook, State Board Review Questions, chalkboard, overhead projector, VCR and videotape(s), computer, printer, microscope.

Transparency Master: Figures 4.2, 4.6, 4.11, and 4.13.

Theory Objectives

1. Hair function, location, composition, and types.
2. The basic histology of the hair and surrounding structures.
3. Human hair growth.
4. Factors involved in analyzing hair condition.
5. Abnormal conditions, diseases, and disorders of the hair and scalp.
6. Removal of superfluous hair.

Practical Objectives

None.

Word Review:

trichology	trichologist	lanugo hair
capilli hair	supercilia hair	cilia hair
appendage	keratin	amino acids
epidermis	cystine	polypeptide bonds
tyrosine	cystine bonds	hair histology
hair shaft	cortex	medulla
cuticle	arrector pili muscle	hair root
heredity	papilla	hair bulb
stages of hair growth	anagen, catagen, telogen	male pattern baldness
congenital	coarse hair	porosity
porous	porosity test	acid
alkaline	trichosis	hypertrichosis
alopecia	male pattern baldness	trichoptilosis
pili	epilation	depilation
hot wax	electrologist	electrolysis
electrology	lighten hair	superfluous hair

Answers to End-of-Chapter Questions:

1. Trichology. **2.** Adornment—it improves our individual appearances. **3.** Lanugo is fine, lightly pigmented hair found almost all over the body. **4.** A hair. **5.** Epidermis. **6.** Molecule. **7.** Amino acid. **8.** Disulfide bonds. **9.** Compare your answer to the information in the chapter. **10.** Compare your answer to the information in the chapter. **11.** The pocket like depression in the skin through which the hair grows. **12.** Arrector pili muscle. **13.** The base of the follicle supplies blood and nerves to the hair bulb so hair will form and grow. **14.** Cells that give hair its color. **15.** Gray hair. **16.** Keratinization. **17.** Anagen, catagen, and telogen. **18.** Capilli—scalp; supercilia—eyebrows; cilia—eyelashes; barba—beard. **19.** Summer. **20.** Alopecia areata. **21.** Tinea capitis of the scalp. **22.** Allergy test. **23.** To prevent a severe skin burn.

Theory Objective 1: **Define hair and describe its function, location, composition and types.**

Learning Steps

1. Read chapter in textbook.
2. Complete assignment in workbook.
3. View videotape(s).
4. Proceed to next objective.

Resources

1. *The Professional Cosmetologist*, 4th ed., ch. 4, pp. 63-65.
2. *Theory and Practical Workbook*, ch. 4, p. 25.
3. Videotape library.

Instructor's Resource Notes: ______________________________

____

Theory Objective 2: **Describe the basic histology of the hair and surrounding structures.**

Learning Steps

1. Read chapter in textbook.
2. Complete assignment in workbook.
3. View videotape(s).
4. Proceed to next objective.

Resources

1. *The Professional Cosmetologist*, 4th ed., ch. 4, pp. 65-70.
2. *Theory and Practical Workbook*, ch. 4, p. 28.
3. Videotape library.

Instructor's Resource Notes: ______________________________

____

Theory Objective 3: **Describe hair growth.**

Learning Steps

1. Read chapter in textbook.
2. Complete assignment in workbook.
3. View videotape(s).
4. Proceed to next objective.

Resources

1. *The Professional Cosmetologist*, 4th ed., ch. 4, pp. 71-75.
2. *Theory and Practical Workbook*, ch. 4, p. 30.
3. Videotape library.

Instructor's Resource Notes: ______________________________

____

Theory Objective 4: **Identify the factors involved in analyzing hair condition.**

Learning Steps

1. Read chapter in textbook.
2. Complete assignment in workbook.
3. View videotape(s).
4. Proceed to next objective.

Resources

1. *The Professional Cosmetologist*, 4th ed., ch. 4, pp. 75-77.
2. *Theory and Practical Workbook*, ch. 4, p. 31.
3. Videotape library.

Instructor's Resource Notes: ______________________________

____

Theory Objective 5: **Describe the abnormal conditions, diseases, and disorders of the hair and scalp.**

Learning Steps

1. Read chapter in textbook.
2. Complete assignment in workbook.
3. View videotape(s).
4. Proceed to next objective.

Resources

1. *The Professional Cosmetologist*, 4th ed., ch. 4, pp. 78-81.
2. *Theory and Practical Workbook*, ch. 4, p. 32.
3. Videotape library.

Instructor's Resource Notes: ______________________________

____

Theory Objective 6: **Describe the removal of superfluous hair.**

Learning Steps

1. Read chapter in textbook.
2. Complete assignment in workbook.
3. View videotape(s).
4. Proceed to next chapter.

Resources

1. *The Professional Cosmetologist*, 4th ed., ch. 4, pp. 81-85.
2. *Theory and Practical Workbook*, ch. 4, p. 33.
3. Videotape library.

Instructor's Resource Notes: ______________________________

____

Evaluation of Instruction:

_____ A. Discussed answers to end of chapter questions.
_____ B. Collected completed workbook assignments.
_____ C. Collected student progress charts.
_____ D. State board sheets current.
_____ E. Answered written test(s), and/or computer test questions.
_____ F. Completed Performance/Product Checklist.

Student Assignments: ______________________________

____

5

Lesson Plan
Shampooing

Lesson Overview and Motivation: Shampooing is a simple art but a complex science. Students will learn how to avoid damaging problem hair, and how to choose the correct shampoo supplies to suit the individual client. This may be a good time for you to introduce methods for testing the pH of various shampoos.

Acceptable Level: Score 85 percent or better on a multiple choice exam, and complete the performance product checklist for this task.
Perform a shampoo service within 10 to 15 minutes

Location: Theory classroom_____ Lab classroom_____ Clinic_____

Time for Lecture/ Demonstration: 30 min._____ 60 min._____ 90 min._____

Student Level: Beginning_____ Intermediate_____ Advanced_____

Equipment/Models Needed: Chalkboard, shampoo bowl, shampoo chair, hydraulic chair. Classmate or client, pH meter, litmous paper, Nitrizine Testing strips, etc

Supplies Needed: Student kit, towel(s), neck strips, client release form, shampoo, neutralizing rinse (if necessary.)

Sanitation Supplies and Equipment: Sanitized towels.

Teaching Aids Needed: Textbook, Theory and Practical Workbook, State Board Review Questions, chalkboard, overhead projector, VCR and videotape(s), computer, printer.

Transparency Master: Figures 5.2 and 5.3.

Theory Objectives	*Practical Objectives*
1. The physical and chemical actions of shampooing and the effects of alkaline shampoos and acid rinses. 2. Characteristics and contents of shampoos and products for conditioning the client's scalp and hair. 3. Scalp and hair irregularities and corrective measures.	4. Drape and preparation of scalp and hair. 5. Shampoo the hair.

Word Review:

potential Hydrogen	acid	alkaline
neutral	acetic acid	imbrications
distilled water	acid-balanced	medicated shampoo
herbal shampoo	liquid-dry shampoo	acid-balanced shampoo
powder-dry shampoo	non-stripping shampoo	de-medicating shampoo
conditioning shampoo	shampoo concentrate	hard water
soft water	minerals	permanent wave
hair color	chemical relaxer	congenital
acute	chronic	psoriasis
pityriasis	herpes simplex	cold sores
pediculosis	head lice	medicated shampoo
tinea of the scalp	vegetable fungus	sebborrhea
asteatosis	steatoma	wen
acne	comedones	milia
prickly heat	miliaria rubra	

Answers to End-of-Chapter Questions:

1. The cleansing of the hair and scalp. **2.** Potential hydrogen. **3.** 4.5 to 5.5. **4.** Nonstripping, medicated, conditioning, herbal, powder-dry, and liquid-dry. **5.** A viral infection that causes cold sores. **6.** Milia. **7.** No. **8.** Nonstripping shampoo. **9.** It is flammable. **10.** Dandruff.
11. Pityriasis. **12.** Absolutely not. **13.** Ringworm of the scalp. **14.** Yes. **15.** Seborrhea. **16.** The area around the face where makeup collects. **17.** In the drain position.

Special Safety Considerations:

Cleansing of hands before and after service; chemicals coming in contact with clients' skin (neck and hairline), eyes, or ears; cleansing of bottles etc.; and sanitation of the work area; sanitation of items that can be reused, such as combs and brushes; disposal of used items; return and proper storage of unused supplies.

Mix shampoo according to manufacturer's directions. Don't allow shampoo to run into the client's eyes or ears. Be careful not to saturate the neck area of the client's clothing.

This is a good time to introduce the pH concept.

Should shampoo enter the client's eyes, flush with cool water.

Theory Objective 1: **Describe the physical and chemical actions of shampooing, including the effects of alkaline shampoos and acid rinses.**

Learning Steps	***Resources***
1. Read chapter in textbook.	1. *The Professional Cosmetologist,* 4th ed., ch. 5, pp. 92-94.
2. Complete assignment in workbook.	2. *Theory and Practical Workbook,* ch. 5, p. 35.
3. View videotape(s).	3. Videotape library.
4. Proceed to next objective.	

Instructor's Resource Notes: ______________________________

____

Theory Objective 2: **Describe the characteristics and contents of various kinds of shampoos and identify appropriate products for conditioning the client's scalp and hair.**

Learning Steps	***Resources***
1. Read chapter in textbook.	1. *The Professional Cosmetologist,* 4th ed., ch. 5, pp. 94-96.
2. Complete assignment in workbook.	2. *Theory and Practical Workbook,* ch. 5, p. 36.
3. View videotape(s).	3. Videotape library.
4. Proceed to next objective.	

Instructor's Resource Notes: ______________________________

____

Theory Objective 3: **Recognize scalp and hair irregularities and suggest corrective measures.**

Learning Steps	***Resources***
1. Read chapter in textbook.	1. *The Professional Cosmetologist,* 4th ed., ch. 5, pp. 96-99.
2. Complete assignment in workbook.	2. *Theory and Practical Workbook,* ch. 5, p. 38.
3. View videotape(s).	3. Videotape library.
4. Proceed to next objective.	

Instructor's Resource Notes: ______________________________

____

Practical Objective 4: **Drape the client and prepare the hair and scalp for shampoo.**

Learning Steps

1. Read chapter in textbook.
2. Complete assignment in workbook.
3. View videotape(s).
4. Proceed to next objective.

Resources

1. *The Professional Cosmetologist*, 4th ed., ch. 5, pp. 99-104.
2. *Theory and Practical Workbook*, ch. 5, p. 39.
3. Videotape library.

Instructor's Resource Notes: ______________________________

____

Practical Objective 5: **Shampoo the hair.**

Learning Steps

1. Read chapter in textbook.
2. Complete assignment in workbook.
3. View videotape(s).
4. Proceed to next chapter.

Resources

1. *The Professional Cosmetologist*, 4th ed., ch. 5, pp. 104-108.
2. *Theory and Practical Workbook*, ch. 5, p. 41.
3. Videotape library.

Instructor's Resource Notes: ______________________________

____

Evaluation of Instruction:

_____ A. Discussed answers to end of chapter questions.
_____ B. Collected completed workbook assignments.
_____ C. Collected student progress charts.
_____ D. State board sheets current.
_____ E. Answered written test(s), and/or computer test questions.
_____ F. Completed Performance/Product Checklist.

Student Assignments: ______________________________

____

6

Lesson Plan
Conditioning

Lesson Overview and Motivation: Hair conditioning is more than a mere extension of shampooing. Students will learn to evaluate the individual client's hair in greater depth, and to choose the right conditioner from a broader array of options.

Acceptable Level: Score 85 percent or better on a multiple choice exam, and complete the performance product checklist for this task.

Location: Theory classroom_____ Lab classroom_____ Clinic_____

Time for Lecture/ Demonstration: 30 min._____ 60 min._____ 90 min._____

Student Level: Beginning_____ Intermediate_____ Advanced_____

Equipment/Models Needed: Shampoo bowl.

Supplies Needed: Various conditioners, towels, shampoo cape.

Sanitation Supplies and Equipment: Sanitized towels.

Teaching Aids Needed: VCR, overhead projector, computer and printer.

Transparency Master: Figure 6.3.

Theory Objectives

1. Physical and chemical actions that damage the hair and five terms that describe hair condition.
2. The use of proteins in conditioning the hair.
3. The different types of conditioners.

Practical Objectives

4. Damage assessment and application of an appropriate conditioner.

Word Review:

conditioners	elasticity	animal protein
physical damage	appearance	vegetable protein
chemical damage	manageability	reconditioning
porosity	preconditioning	texture
over-conditioning	in-process conditioning	

Answers to End-of-Chapter Questions:

1. Porosity, elasticity, texture, appearance, and manageability. **2.** Timing and effectiveness. **3.** The basic protein found in hair. **4.** The feel and diameter of hair. **5.** No. **6.** Almost 50 percent. **7.** Porosity.

Special Safety Considerations:

Cleansing of hands before and after service; chemicals coming in contact with clients' skin (neck and hairline), eyes, or ears; cleansing of bottles etc.; and sanitation of the work area; sanitation of items that can be reused, such as combs and brushes; disposal of used items; return and proper storage of unused supplies.

Some conditioners need to be carefully diluted with water, so following label directions is important. To avoid damage to the client's scalp and hair, it is necessary to determine whether there are any abnormal skin conditions or disorders. The condition of the hair should be known before proceeding with chemical services.

Any water on the floor should be mopped up immediately.

Theory Objective 1: **List the physical and chemical actions that damage the hair, and define five terms that describe hair condition.**

Learning Steps	Resources
1. Read chapter in textbook.	1. *The Professional Cosmetologist*, 4th ed., ch. 6, pp. 114-116.
2. Complete assignment in workbook.	2. *Theory and Practical Workbook*, ch. 6, p. 45.
3. View videotape(s).	3. Videotape library.
4. Proceed to next objective.	

Instructor's Resource Notes: ______________________________

____

Theory Objective 2: **Describe how proteins are used in conditioning the hair.**

Learning Steps

1. Read chapter in textbook.
2. Complete assignment in workbook.
3. View videotape(s).
4. Proceed to next objective.

Resources

1. *The Professional Cosmetologist*, 4th ed., ch. 6, pp. 116-118.
2. *Theory and Practical Workbook*, ch. 6, p. 46.
3. Videotape library.

Instructor's Resource Notes: ____

____

Theory Objective 3: **Classify and describe the different types of conditioners.**

Learning Steps

1. Read chapter in textbook.
2. Complete assignment in workbook.
3. View videotape(s).
4. Proceed to next objective.

Resources

1. *The Professional Cosmetologist*, 4th ed., ch. 6, pp. 118-121.
2. *Theory and Practical Workbook*, ch. 6, p. 47.
3. Videotape library.

Instructor's Resource Notes: ____

____

Practical Objective 4: **Assess hair damage and select and apply the appropriate conditioner.**

Learning Steps

1. Read chapter in textbook.
2. Complete assignment in workbook.
3. View videotape(s).
4. Proceed to next chapter.

Resources

1. *The Professional Cosmetologist*, 4th ed., ch. 6, pp. 121-124.
2. *Theory and Practical Workbook*, ch. 6, p. 48.
3. Videotape library.

Instructor's Resource Notes: ____

____

Evaluation of Instruction:

_____ A. Discussed answers to end of chapter questions.
_____ B. Collected completed workbook assignments.
_____ C. Collected student progress charts.
_____ D. State board sheets current.
_____ E. Answered written test(s), and/or computer test questions.
_____ F. Completed Performance/Product Checklist.

Student Assignments: ____

____

7

Lesson Plan

Scalp Treatments

Lesson Overview and Motivation: Scalp treatments extend the benefit of cleansing and conditioning to the very roots of the hair. Students will learn to give a complete scalp treatment.

Acceptable Level: Score 85 percent or better on a multiple choice exam, and complete the performance product checklist for this task.
Exercise the correct procedure for this service within a 30- to 40-minute time limit.

Location: Theory classroom_____ Lab classroom_____ Clinic_____

Time for Lecture/ Demonstration: 30 min._____ 60 min._____ 90 min._____

Student Level: Beginning_____ Intermediate_____ Advanced_____

Equipment/Models Needed: Steamer or heating cap.

Supplies Needed: Scalp conditioner and shampoo cape.

Sanitation Supplies and Equipment: Sanitized towels, combs and brushes.

Teaching Aids Needed: Textbook, Theory and Practical Workbook, State Board Review Questions, chalkboard, overhead projector, VCR and videotape(s), computer, printer.

Transparency Master: Figure 7.1 (two page spread of manipulations).

Theory Objectives

1. The benefits of scalp manipulations.
2. Basic safety precautions for a scalp treatment.

Practical Objectives

3. Give a scalp treatment.

Word Review: anterior auricular, occipital bone, trapezius muscle, cervical vertebra, posterior auricular, mastoid bone, temporal arteries

Answers to End-of-Chapter Questions: **1-5.** Compare your answer to information in the chapter (see Figure 7.2). **6.** No. **7.** Four. **8.** No. **9.** Increases the flow of blood. **10.** Neck and shoulders. **11.** Plastic undercap.

Special Safety Considerations: Cleansing of hands before and after service; chemicals coming in contact with clients' skin (neck and hairline), eyes, or ears; cleansing of bottles etc.; and sanitation of the work area; sanitation of items that can be reused, such as combs and brushes; disposal of used items; return and proper storage of unused supplies.

It is important to know whether the client will be having a chemical service, such as a permanent wave before stimulating the scalp. To avoid burning the client's scalp, monitor the temperature of any steamer or heating cap used in this service.

Theory Objective 1: **Describe the benefits of scalp manipulations.**

Learning Steps

1. Read chapter in textbook.
2. Complete assignment in workbook.
3. View videotape(s).
4. Proceed to next objective.

Resources

1. *The Professional Cosmetologist*, 4th ed., ch. 7, p. 128.
2. *Theory and Practical Workbook*, ch. 7, p. 51.
3. Videotape library.

Instructor's Resource Notes: ____

____

Theory Objective 2: **List the basic safety precautions for a scalp treatment.**

Learning Steps

1. Read chapter in textbook.
2. Complete assignment in workbook.
3. View videotape(s).
4. Proceed to next objective.

Resources

1. *The Professional Cosmetologist*, 4th ed., ch. 7, pp. 128-129.
2. *Theory and Practical Workbook*, ch. 7, p. 51.
3. Videotape library.

Instructor's Resource Notes: ____

____

Practical Objective 3: **Give a scalp treatment.**

Learning Steps	*Resources*
1. Read chapter in textbook.	1. *The Professional Cosmetologist*, 4th ed., ch. 7, pp. 129-132.
2. Complete assignment in workbook.	2. *Theory and Practical Workbook,* ch. 7, p. 52.
3. View videotape(s).	3. Videotape library.
4. Proceed to next chapter.	

Instructor's Resource Notes: ____

____

Evaluation of Instruction:

_____ A. Discussed answers to end of chapter questions.
_____ B. Collected completed workbook assignments.
_____ C. Collected student progress charts.
_____ D. State board sheets current.
_____ E. Answered written test(s), and/or computer test questions.
_____ F. Completed Performance/Product Checklist.

Student Assignments: ____

____

8

Lesson Plan

Finger Waving

Lesson Overview and Motivation: Students will learn to comb, then brush, the client's hair in even, alternating rows of finger waves. The practice of finger waving assists the development of finger strength, coordination, and general dexterity that the student will need to perform other cosmetology services.

Acceptable Level: Score 85 percent or better on a multiple choice exam, and complete the performance product checklist for this task.
Design the hair (length permitting) in finger waves within 30 minutes.

Location: Theory classroom_____ Lab classroom_____ Clinic_____

Time for Lecture/ Demonstration: 30 min._____ 60 min._____ 90 min._____

Student Level: Beginning_____ Intermediate_____ Advanced_____

Equipment/Models Needed: Mannequin, clamp, work station.

Supplies Needed: Student kit, water applicator bottle, sectioning clips, finger-waving lotion.

Sanitation Supplies and Equipment: Sanitized towels.

Teaching Aids Needed: Textbook, Workbook, State Board Review Questions, chalkboard, overhead projector, VCR and videotape(s), computer, printer.

Transparency Master: Figures 8.1, 8.2, 8.3, and 8.14.

Theory Objectives	*Practical Objectives*
1. Parts of a fingerwave and waves, shapings, sculpture curls, and base-directed hair.	2. Styling sections of the head.

Word Review:

trough	wave pattern	ridges
wave trough	parallel	"S"
base direction	nape section	hair direction
clockwise	counter-clockwise	semicircular
crown section	top section	side sections

Answers to End-of-Chapter Questions:

1. Ridge. **2.** Trough. **3.** Ridge parallel to (a). **4.** Diagonal wave. **5.** Ridge, trough, alternating direction, "C" shaping, "S" shaping. **6.** A finger wave. **7.** Hair shapings. **8.** Base direction.

Special Safety Considerations:

Cleansing of hands before and after service; and sanitation of the work area; sanitation of items that can be reused, such as combs and brushes; disposal of used items; return and proper storage of unused supplies. This includes mannequins, holders, combs, brushes, and setting lotions.

Theory Objective 1: **Describe the parts of the fingerwave, and identify waves, shapings, sculpture curls, and base-directed hair.**

Learning Steps

1. Read chapter in textbook.
2. Complete assignment in workbook.
3. View videotape(s).
4. Proceed to next objective.

Resources

1. *The Professional Cosmetologist*, 4th ed., ch. 8, pp. 136-137.
2. *Theory and Practical Workbook*, ch. 8, p. 55.
3. Videotape library.

Instructor's Resource Notes: ______________________________

____

Practical Objective 2: **Part off the five styling sections of the head.**

Learning Steps

1. Read chapter in textbook.
2. Complete assignment in workbook.
3. View videotape(s).
4. Proceed to next objective.

Resources

1. *The Professional Cosmetologist*, 4th ed., ch. 8, pp. 137-139.
2. *Theory and Practical Workbook*, ch. 8, p. 57.
3. Videotape library.

Instructor's Resource Notes: ______________________________

____

Practical Objective 3: **Set and comb three alternating rows of horizontal finger waves in the crown section of the client's head.**

Learning Steps

1. Read chapter in textbook.
2. Complete assignment in workbook.
3. View videotape(s).
4. Proceed to next chapter.

Resources

1. *The Professional Cosmetologist*, 4th ed., ch. 8, pp. 140-144.
2. Videotape library.

Instructor's Resource Notes: ______________________________

____

Evaluation of Instruction:

_____ A. Discussed answers to end of chapter questions.
_____ B. Collected completed workbook assignments.
_____ C. Collected student progress charts.
_____ D. State board sheets current.
_____ E. Answered written test(s), and/or computer test questions.
_____ F. Completed Performance/Product Checklist.

Student Assignments: ______________________________

____

9

Lesson Plan
Sculpture Curls

Lesson Overview and Motivation: Students will learn to set all the client's or mannequin's hair in sculpture curls and comb it into place. This chapter provides the student with the necessary practice to develop visual recognition of different hair formations necessary to become an accomplished hairstylist.

Acceptable Level: Score 85 percent or better on a multiple choice exam, and complete the performance product checklist for this task.
Set hair in 30 minutes, dry it; comb into place in 20 minutes.

Location: Theory classroom_____ Lab classroom_____ Clinic_____

Time for Lecture/ Demonstration: 30 min._____ 60 min._____ 90 min._____

Student Level: Beginning_____ Intermediate_____ Advanced_____

Equipment/Models Needed: Mannequin and clamp, classmate, or client.

Supplies Needed: Student kit, rat-tail comb, rake comb, styling comb, brush, hairpins, bobby pins, single-prong clips, double-prong clips, hair sectioning clips, styling lotion, creme rinse, water in spray bottle, cotton, end wraps.

Sanitation Supplies and Equipment: Sanitized towels.

Teaching Aids Needed: Textbook, Workbook, State Board Review Questions, chalkboard, overhead projector, VCR and videotape(s), computer, printer, setting and combing patterns.

Transparency Master: Figures 9.4, 9.7, and 9.8.

Theory Objectives	Practical Objectives
1. Setting and combing implements used to style the hair. 2. Hairstyling terms and parts of a sculpture curl. 3. Kinds of sculpture curls and their three strengths.	4. Set and comb sculpture curls in the crown and nape of the head.

Word Review:

barber comb	rat-tail comb	rake comb
circle end	geometric forms	stand away curls
long-stem	no-stem	half-stem
counterclockwise	base	clockwise
shaping	skip waving	stem
mobility	pickup line	pickup point
wave pattern	no-stem	long-stem
barrel curls	skip waving	stand-away curl
diagonal wave	cascade curls	skipwave
styling comb/finger waving comb	alternating rows	

Answers to End-of-Chapter Questions:

1. No-stem, half-stem, and long-stem. **2.** Compare your answer to the information in the chapter. **3.** Compare your answer to the information in the chapter. **4.** Where the curl is carved out of the shaping. **5.** Triangular-shaped curl bases. **6.** No-stem curl. **7.** Long-stem or full-stem curl. **8.** By brushing the hair. **9.** The wet hair will go straight. **10.** The hair will be stiff, sticky, or gummy. **11.** On the inside of the curl.

Special Safety Considerations:

Cleansing of hands before and after service; cleansing of bottles etc.; and sanitation of the work area; sanitation of items that can be reused, such as combs and brushes; disposal of used items; return and proper storage of unused supplies.

Equipment and supplies, such as mannequins, holders, and clippies should be properly stored.

Theory Objective 1: **List the setting and combing implements used to style the hair.**

Learning Steps	Resources
1. Read chapter in textbook. 2. Complete assignment in workbook. 3. View videotape(s). 4. Proceed to next objective.	1. *The Professional Cosmetologist*, 4th ed., ch. 9, pp. 148-149. 2. *Theory and Practical Workbook*, ch. 9, p. 59. 3. Videotape library.

Instructor's Resource Notes: ______________________________

____

Theory Objective 2: **Identify hairstyling terms and define the three parts of a sculpture curl.**

Learning Steps	*Resources*
1. Read chapter in textbook.	1. *The Professional Cosmetologist,* 4th ed., ch. 9, pp. 150-151.
2. Complete assignment in workbook.	2. *Theory and Practical Workbook,* ch. 9, p. 61.
3. View videotape(s).	3. Videotape library.
4. Proceed to next objective.	

Instructor's Resource Notes: ______________________________

____

Theory Objective 3: **Describe the basic types of sculpture curls and their variations and list the three strengths of sculpture curls.**

Learning Steps	*Resources*
1. Read chapter in textbook.	1. *The Professional Cosmetologist,* 4th ed., ch. 9, pp. 151-155.
2. Complete assignment in workbook.	2. *Theory and Practical Workbook,* ch. 9, p. 63.
3. View videotape(s).	3. Videotape library.
4. Proceed to next objective.	

Instructor's Resource Notes: ______________________________

____

Practical Objective 4: **Set and comb sculpture curls: (a) in horizontal wave patterns in the crown and nape sections of the head; (b) in one large semicircular formation in both side sections; (c) in alternating diagonal-wave formations in both side sections; and (d) in the top section to form an outside movement away from the head.**

Learning Steps	*Resources*
1. Read chapter in textbook.	1. *The Professional Cosmetologist*, 4th ed., ch. 9, pp. 155-171.
2. Complete assignment in workbook.	2. *Theory and Practical Workbook*, ch. 9, p. 64.
3. View videotape(s).	3. Videotape library.
4. Proceed to next chapter.	

Instructor's Resource Notes: ______________________________

____

Evaluation of Instruction:

_____ A. Discussed answers to end of chapter questions.
_____ B. Collected completed workbook assignments.
_____ C. Collected student progress charts.
_____ D. State board sheets current.
_____ E. Answered written test(s), and/or computer test questions.
_____ F. Completed Performance/Product Checklist.

Student Assignments: ______________________________

____

10

Lesson Plan

Setting the Hair with Rollers

Lesson Overview and Motivation: Students will learn to set all the mannequin's or client's hair in rollers and comb the style into place. Exercises associated with this chapter should provide exercises allowing the student to learn control of the height and direction of the hair in the different styling sections of the head.

Acceptable Level: Score 85 percent or better on a multiple choice exam, and complete the performance product checklist for this task.
Set the hair in rollers in 15 to 25 minutes, dry it; comb into place within 20 to 30 minutes.

Location: Theory classroom_____ Lab classroom_____ Clinic_____

Time for Lecture/ Demonstration: 30 min._____ 60 min._____ 90 min._____

Student Level: Beginning_____ Intermediate_____ Advanced_____

Equipment/Models Needed: Mannequin and clamp, classmate, or client.

Supplies Needed: Shampoo supplies, rollers, roller pins, double-prong clips, end wraps, styling lotion, spray bottle, rat-tail and styling combs, brush, hair spray.

Sanitation Supplies and Equipment: Neck strips, protective comb-out cape, sanitized towels.

Teaching Aids Needed: Textbook, Workbook, State Board Review Questions, chalkboard, overhead projector, VCR and videotape(s), computer, printer, setting and combing patterns.

Transparency Master: Figures 10.4 and 10.6.

Theory Objectives

1. Basic materials, shapes, and sizes of rollers.
2. Basic principles used to select roller diameters that are correct for the hair's length and inside and outside movements of hair.
3. Purpose of no-stem, half-stem, and long-stem roller placements.

Practical Objectives

4. Roller curls in four different patterns in the top section of the head.
5. Setting three different patterns in the top, sides, crown, and nape sections of the head.

Word Review:

roller placement
rectangular
natural wave
outside movement
back-combing
partings
cowlick
back-brushing
triangular partings
inside movement

Answers to End-of-Chapter Questions:

1. Distance around the roller. **2.** Half of the distance around the roller (twice its radius). **3.** 1 to 1 1/2 turns. **4.** More than two turns. **5.** The stem placement. **6.** The number of times the hair is wound around the roller. **7.** The same size as the roller's diameter. **8.** Where the roller touches the head. **9.** Yes. **10.** Gives height. **11.** No.

Special Safety Considerations:

Cleansing of hands before and after service; cleansing of bottles etc.; and sanitation of the work area; sanitation of items that can be reused, such as combs and brushes; disposal of used items; return and proper storage of unused supplies.

After use, equipment and supplies, such as mannequins, holders, and clippies, rollers, etc. should be properly stored.

Theory Objective 1: **Explain the basic materials from which rollers are made and describe their shapes and sizes.**

Learning Steps

1. Read chapter in textbook.
2. Complete assignment in workbook.
3. View videotape(s).
4. Proceed to next objective.

Resources

1. *The Professional Cosmetologist*, 4th ed., ch. 10, pp. 176-178.
2. *Theory and Practical Workbook*, ch. 10, p. 67.
3. Videotape library.

Instructor's Resource Notes: ______________________________

____

Theory Objective 2: **Describe the basic principles used to select the correct roller diameter for the hair's length and define inside and outside movements of hair.**

Learning Steps

1. Read chapter in textbook.
2. Complete assignment in workbook.
3. View videotape(s).
4. Proceed to next objective.

Resources

1. *The Professional Cosmetologist*, 4th ed., ch. 10, pp. 178-179.
2. *Theory and Practical Workbook*, ch. 10, p. 67.
3. Videotape library.

Instructor's Resource Notes: ______________________________

____

Theory Objective 3: **Explain the purpose of no-stem, half-stem, and long-stem roller placements.**

Learning Steps

1. Read chapter in textbook.
2. Complete assignment in workbook.
3. View videotape(s).
4. Proceed to next objective.

Resources

1. *The Professional Cosmetologist*, 4th ed., ch. 10, pp. 179-181.
2. *Theory and Practical Workbook*, ch. 10, p. 67.
3. Videotape library.

Instructor's Resource Notes: ______________________________

____

Practical Objective 4: **Set and comb roller curls in four different patterns in the top section of the head.**

Learning Steps

1. Read chapter in textbook.
2. Complete assignment in workbook.
3. View videotape(s).
4. Proceed to next objective.

Resources

1. *The Professional Cosmetologist*, 4th ed., ch. 10, pp. 181-189.
2. *Theory and Practical Workbook*, ch. 10, p. 69.
3. Videotape library.

Instructor's Resource Notes: ______________________________

____

Practical Objective 5: **Set and comb roller curls in three different patterns in the top, sides, crown, and nape sections of the head.**

Learning Steps	*Resources*
1. Read chapter in textbook.	1. *The Professional Cosmetologist,* 4th ed., ch. 10, pp. 189-192.
2. Complete assignment in workbook.	2. *Theory and Practical Workbook,* ch. 10, p. 69.
3. View videotape(s).	3. Videotape library.
4. Proceed to next chapter.	

Instructor's Resource Notes: ______________________________

____

Evaluation of Instruction:

_____ A. Discussed answers to end of chapter questions.
_____ B. Collected completed workbook assignments.
_____ C. Collected student progress charts.
_____ D. State board sheets current.
_____ E. Answered written test(s), and/or computer test questions.
_____ F. Completed Performance/Product Checklist.

Student Assignments: ______________________________

____

11

Lesson Plan

Selecting Hairstyles

Lesson Overview and Motivation: Students will correctly identify the facial shapes of six clients and recommend an appropriate hairstyle for each. For the student who wishes to become a successful hairstylist, executing the desired hairstyle for the different facial shapes is an important aspect of the cosmetology program.

Acceptable Level: Score 85 percent or better on a multiple choice exam.

Location: Theory classroom_____ Lab classroom_____ Clinic_____

Time for Lecture/ Demonstration: 30 min._____ 60 min._____ 90 min._____

Student Level: Beginning_____ Intermediate_____ Advanced_____

Equipment/Models Needed: Chalkboard, chalk.

Teaching Aids Needed: Textbook, Workbook, State Board Review Questions, chalkboard, overhead projector, VCR and videotape(s), computer, printer, patterns of different facial shapes.

Transparency Master: Figure 11.1.

Theory Objectives	*Practical Objectives*
1. Ideal facial and head features. 2. Six facial shapes and ways to create the oval illusion for them. 3. Three common profiles. 4. Six other things to consider in hairstyling. 5. Examples of hair braiding and corn rowing.	None.

Word Review: profile silhouette proportions

Answers to End-of-Chapter Questions: **1.** Compare your answer to the information in the chapter. **2.** Compare your answer to the information in the chapter. **3.** Compare your answer to the information in the chapter. **4.** Compare your answer to the information in the chapter. **5.** Yes. **6.** Yes. **7.** Toward the face. **8.** No, toward the face. **9.** No, inward. **10.** No, outward. **11.** Yes. **12.** Yes (with student's comments).

Theory Objective 1: **Identify the ideal facial and head features.**

Learning Steps

1. Read chapter in textbook.
2. Complete assignment in workbook.
3. View videotape(s).
4. Proceed to next objective.

Resources

1. *The Professional Cosmetologist,* 4th ed., ch. 11, pp. 196-197.
2. *Theory and Practical Workbook,* ch. 11, p. 71.
3. Videotape library.

Instructor's Resource Notes: ____________________

____

Theory Objective 2: **Describe the six facial shapes and identify ways an oval illusion can be created for them.**

Learning Steps

1. Read chapter in textbook.
2. Complete assignment in workbook.
3. View videotape(s).
4. Proceed to next objective.

Resources

1. *The Professional Cosmetologist,* 4th ed., ch. 11, pp. 197-201.
2. *Theory and Practical Workbook,* ch. 11, p. 71.
3. Videotape library.

Instructor's Resource Notes: ____________________

____

Theory Objective 3: **Describe the three common profiles.**

Learning Steps	*Resources*
1. Read chapter in textbook.	1. *The Professional Cosmetologist*, 4th ed., ch. 11, p. 201.
2. Complete assignment in workbook.	2. *Theory and Practical Workbook*, ch. 11, p. 71.
3. View videotape(s).	3. Videotape library.
4. Proceed to next objective.	

Instructor's Resource Notes: ____________________

____

Theory Objective 4: **Identify six other things to consider in hairstyling.**

Learning Steps	*Resources*
1. Read chapter in textbook.	1. *The Professional Cosmetologist*, 4th ed., ch. 11, pp. 201-202.
2. Complete assignment in workbook.	2. *Theory and Practical Workbook*, ch. 11, p. 71.
3. View videotape(s).	3. Videotape library.
4. Proceed to next objective.	

Instructor's Resource Notes: ____________________

____

Theory Objective 5: **Give examples of hair braiding and corn rowing.**

Learning Steps	*Resources*
1. Read chapter in textbook.	1. *The Professional Cosmetologist*, 4th ed., ch. 11, p. 203.
2. Complete assignment in workbook.	2. Videotape library.
3. View videotape(s).	
4. Proceed to next chapter.	

Instructor's Resource Notes: ____________________

____

Evaluation of Instruction:

_____ A. Discussed answers to end of chapter questions.
_____ B. Collected completed workbook assignments.
_____ C. Collected student progress charts.
_____ D. State board sheets current.
_____ E. Answered written test(s), and/or computer test questions.
_____ F. Completed Performance/Product Checklist.

Student Assignments: ____

____

12

Lesson Plan

Hair Shaping

Lesson Overview and Motivation: Students will learn to use the proper shaping techniques and safety precautions in cutting the client's hair, and to use basic procedures with the electric clipper. Since a good hair shaping is the foundation for many other cosmetology services, mastering several basic hair cutting techniques is essential for the basic student.
Natural hair, cut from a classmate or client, could be put away for use later when the hair coloring chapters are studied. If this is done, strands should be at least two-three inches, but not longer than four inches in length.

Acceptable Level: Score 85 percent or better on a multiple choice exam, and complete the performance product checklist for this task.
Complete a hair shaping with a razor in 15 to 25 minutes, or in 25 to 40 minutes with a scissors.

Location: Theory classroom_____ Lab classroom_____ Clinic_____

Time for Lecture/ Demonstration: 30 min._____ 60 min._____ 90 min._____

Student Level: Beginning_____ Intermediate_____ Advanced_____

Equipment/Models Needed: Hydraulic chair, mannequin and clamp, classmate, or client.

Supplies Needed: Double-edge scissors, double-notch scissors, single-notch scissors, single-edge safety razor, electric clipper, styling comb, barber comb, spray applicator bottle for water, sectioning clips, talcum powder, or hair vacuum.

Sanitation Supplies and Equipment: Shampoo cape or chair cloth, neck strips, sanitized towels.

Teaching Aids Needed: Textbook, Workbook, State Board Review Questions, chalkboard, overhead projector, VCR and videotape(s), computer, printer, patterns for school hair cutting techniques. Guest lecturers can also be helpful for advanced classes.

Transparency Master: Figures 12.9, 12.16, and 12.25.

Theory Objectives

1. Hair shaping implements and basic cutting movements.
2. Differences between razor shaping, scissors shaping, and electric clipper shaping.
3. Basic parting sections of the head.
4. Terms used in hair shaping and safety precautions.

Practical Objectives

5. Basic scissors shaping for a female client.
6. Basic scissors shaping for a black female client.
7. Basic scissors shaping for a male client.
8. Basic clipper shaping for a female client.
9. Basic clipper shaping for a male client.
10. Basic razor shaping for a female client.
11. Beard and a mustache trim.

Word Review:

moving point
finger tang
thumb grip
disposable blade
styling comb
effilating
club cut
still point
electric clipper
outliner
side sections
hanging length
low elevation
finger-work
tailored neckline
undercut
clipper-over comb
moving blade
blade receiver
safety guard
handle
double edge scissors
marks on the hair
slither
dry hair cut
natural growth patterns
crepe section
nape section
basic hairshaping
graduation
layer marks (steps)
feathering
bi-level
finger brace
pivot or screw
pivot screw
tang
finger tang
blunt cut
double-notch scissors
wet hair cut
edger
top section
guideline
high elevation
taper
shingling
angle
scissors over comb

Answers to End-of-Chapter Questions:

1. Compare your answer to the information in the chapter. **2.** Sliding the scissors along the hair strand to thin it. **3.** Scissors. **4.** Student's sketches. **5.** Compare your answer to the information in the chapter. **6.** Electric clipper. **7.** Razor (shaper). **8.** The bottom blade . **9.** Barber comb. **10.** Super-curly hair. **11.** Compare your answer to the information in the chapter. **12.** Yes. **13.** Shingle or tailored neckline. **14.** No. **15.** Cloth cape (chair cape). **16.** Consult the client. **17.** False. **18.** Thin subsections. **19.** Yes. **20.** Apply a small amount of talcum powder to the corner of a towel and dust the neck.

Special Safety Considerations:

Students should be warned that small children may move their heads quickly in an unexpected manner. Should the client or student be exposed to blood, Infection Control Procedures described in the Sanitation chapter should be exercised. Stress safety precautions identified in textbook.

Theory Objective 1: **Describe hair-shaping implements and basic cutting movements.**

Learning Steps

1. Read chapter in textbook.
2. Complete assignment in workbook.
3. View videotape(s).
4. Proceed to next objective.

Resources

1. *The Professional Cosmetologist*, 4th ed., ch. 12, pp. 208-213.
2. *Theory and Practical Workbook*, ch. 12, p. 73.
3. Videotape library.

Instructor's Resource Notes: ______________________________

____

Theory Objective 2: **Explain the differences between razor shaping, scissors shaping, and electric clipper shaping.**

Learning Steps

1. Read chapter in textbook.
2. Complete assignment in workbook.
3. View videotape(s).
4. Proceed to next objective.

Resources

1. *The Professional Cosmetologist*, 4th ed., ch. 12, pp. 213-216.
2. *Theory and Practical Workbook*, ch. 12, p. 75.
3. Videotape library.

Instructor's Resource Notes: ______________________________

____

Theory
Objective 3: **Locate the basic parting sections of the head.**

Learning Steps

1. Read chapter in textbook.
2. Complete assignment in workbook.
3. View videotape(s).
4. Proceed to next objective.

Resources

1. *The Professional Cosmetologist,* 4th ed., ch. 12, pp. 216-217.
2. *Theory and Practical Workbook,* ch. 12, p. 76.
3. Videotape library.

Instructor's Resource Notes: ____________________

____

Theory
Objective 4: **Define the terms used in hair shaping and list the necessary safety precautions.**

Learning Steps

1. Read chapter in textbook.
2. Complete assignment in workbook.
3. View videotape(s).
4. Proceed to next objective.

Resources

1. *The Professional Cosmetologist,* 4th ed., ch. 12, pp. 217-229.
2. *Theory and Practical Workbook,* ch. 12, p. 77.
3. Videotape library.

Instructor's Resource Notes: ____________________

____

Practical
Objective 5: **Give a basic scissors shaping for a female client.**

Learning Steps

1. Read chapter in textbook.
2. Complete assignment in workbook.
3. View videotape(s).
4. Proceed to next objective.

Resources

1. *The Professional Cosmetologist,* 4th ed., ch. 12, pp. 229-239.
2. *Theory and Practical Workbook,* ch. 12, p. 79.
3. Videotape library.

Instructor's Resource Notes: ____________________

____

Practical Objective 6: **Give a basic scissors shaping for a black female client.**

Learning Steps	*Resources*
1. Read chapter in textbook.	1. *The Professional Cosmetologist,* 4th ed., ch. 12, pp. 240-243.
2. Complete assignment in workbook.	2. *Theory and Practical Workbook,* ch. 12, p. 79.
3. View videotape(s).	3. Videotape library.
4. Proceed to next objective.	

Instructor's Resource Notes: ______________________________

____

Practical Objective 7: **Give a basic scissors shaping for a male client.**

Learning Steps	*Resources*
1. Read chapter in textbook.	1. *The Professional Cosmetologist,* 4th ed., ch. 12, pp. 243-247.
2. Complete assignment in workbook.	2. Videotape library.
3. View videotape(s).	
4. Proceed to next objective.	

Instructor's Resource Notes: ______________________________

____

Practical Objective 8: **Give a basic clipper shaping for a female client.**

Learning Steps	*Resources*
1. Read chapter in textbook.	1. *The Professional Cosmetologist,* 4th ed., ch. 12, pp. 248-249.
2. Complete assignment in workbook.	2. Videotape library.
3. View videotape(s).	
4. Proceed to next objective.	

Instructor's Resource Notes: ______________________________

____

Practical Objective 9: **Give a basic clipper shaping for a male client.**

Learning Steps

1. Read chapter in textbook.
2. Complete assignment in workbook.
3. View videotape(s).
4. Proceed to next objective.

Resources

1. *The Professional Cosmetologist,* 4th ed., ch. 12, p. 250.
2. Videotape library.

Instructor's Resource Notes: ______________________________

____

Practical Objective 10: **Give a basic razor shaping for a female client.**

Learning Steps

1. Read chapter in textbook.
2. Complete assignment in workbook.
3. View videotape(s).
4. Proceed to next objective.

Resources

1. *The Professional Cosmetologist,* 4th ed., ch. 12, pp. 251-253.
2. Videotape library.

Instructor's Resource Notes: ______________________________

____

Practical Objective 11: **Trim a beard and mustache.**

Learning Steps

1. Read chapter in textbook.
2. Complete assignment in workbook.
3. View videotape(s).
4. Proceed to next chapter.

Resources

1. *The Professional Cosmetologist,* 4th ed., ch. 12, pp. 254-256.
2. Videotape library.

Instructor's Resource Notes: ______________________________

____

Evaluation of Instruction:

_____ A. Discussed answers to end of chapter questions.
_____ B. Collected completed workbook assignments.
_____ C. Collected student progress charts.
_____ D. State board sheets current.
_____ E. Answered written test(s), and/or computer test questions.
_____ F. Completed Performance/Product Checklist.

Student Assignments: ____

____

Lesson Plan 13

Air Waving and Blow Combing

Lesson Overview and Motivation: Using a professional air waver or blow waver, students will learn how to dry the client's hair in a current hairstyle. Since this hairstyling tool has replaced the hair dryer lounge chair, the student should be proficient in the use of the hand dryer for styling the client's hair.

Acceptable Level: Score 85 percent or better on a multiple choice exam, and complete the performance product checklist for this task.
Complete air waving or blow drying within 30 or 40 minutes.

Location: Theory classroom_____ Lab classroom_____ Clinic_____

Time for Lecture/Demonstration: 30 min._____ 60 min._____ 90 min._____

Student Level: Beginning_____ Intermediate_____ Advanced_____

Equipment/Models Needed: Shampoo bowl, shampoo chair, hydraulic chair, mirror, mannequin and clamp, classmate, or client.

Supplies Needed: Shampoo supplies, air waver, blow waver, comb attachment for air waver, nozzle attachment for blow dryer, hard rubber, or heat resistant styling comb, air- (blow drying) waving lotion, vent or round brush, and hair spray.

Sanitation Supplies and Equipment: Cape for client, sanitized towels, neck strips.

Teaching Aids Needed: Textbook, Workbook, State Board Review Questions, chalkboard, overhead projector, VCR and videotape(s), computer, printer.

Transparency Master: Figure 13.7.

Theory Objectives

1. "Quick-service" hairstyling, and implements used.

Practical Objectives

2. Blow wave the hair.
3. Air wave the hair.

Word Review:

air waver	blow comb	blow waver
hand dryer	Underwriter's Laboratories	watt

Answers to End-of-Chapter Questions:

1. Compare your answer to the information in the chapter. **2.** Underwriters Laboratories. **3.** To prevent damage to hair. **4.** Flow of hot air directly on scalp; a burn from allowing hair to be sucked into air inlet vent of blow waver. **5.** Nozzle. **6.** Diffuser. **7.** The hair would become straight. **8.** The edge of your hand.

Special Safety Considerations:

The flow of hot air should always be directed away from the client's scalp. Control of the nozzle of the hand dryer and the brush are of particular importance for mastering this task.

Theory Objective 1: **Explain "quick-service" hairstyling and describe the implements used.**

Learning Steps

1. Read chapter in textbook.
2. Complete assignment in workbook.
3. View videotape(s).
4. Proceed to next objective.

Resources

1. *The Professional Cosmetologist,* 4th ed., ch. 13, pp. 262-264.
2. *Theory and Practical Workbook,* ch. 13, p. 81.
3. Videotape library.

Instructor's Resource Notes:

____

____

Practical Objective 2: **Blow wave the hair.**

Learning Steps

1. Read chapter in textbook.
2. Complete assignment in workbook.
3. View videotape(s).
4. Proceed to next objective.

Resources

1. *The Professional Cosmetologist,* 4th ed., ch. 13, pp. 264-266.
2. *Theory and Practical Workbook,* ch. 13, p. 82.
3. Videotape library.

Instructor's Resource Notes:

____

____

Practical Objective 3: **Air wave the hair.**

Learning Steps

1. Read chapter in textbook.
2. Complete assignment in workbook.
3. View videotape(s).
4. Proceed to next chapter.

Resources

1. *The Professional Cosmetologist*, 4th ed., ch. 13, pp. 267-268.
2. *Theory and Practical Workbook*, ch. 13, p. 82.
3. Videotape library.

Instructor's Resource Notes: ____________________

____

Evaluation of Instruction:

_____ A. Discussed answers to end of chapter questions.
_____ B. Collected completed workbook assignments.
_____ C. Collected student progress charts.
_____ D. State board sheets current.
_____ E. Answered written test(s), and/or computer test questions.
_____ F. Completed Performance/Product Checklist.

Student Assignments: ____________________

____

14

Lesson Plan

Iron Curls

Lesson Overview and Motivation: In this chapter, the student will learn how to curl the client's hair using the curling iron. Study of the previous chapters should make understanding the different hairstyling patterns and desired results easier for the student to comprehend and accomplish. Given adequate practice, the students' psychomotor coordination should be at a level to achieve the skill necessary to master the desired hairstyling results.

Acceptable Level: Score 85 percent or better on a multiple choice exam, and complete the performance product checklist for this task.

Location: Theory classroom_____ Lab classroom_____ Clinic_____

Time for Lecture/ Demonstration: 30 min._____ 60 min._____ 90 min._____

Student Level: Beginning_____ Intermediate_____ Advanced_____

Equipment/Models Needed: Mannequin and clamp, classmate, or client.

Supplies Needed: Student kit, rat-tail comb, rake comb, styling comb, brush, hairpins, bobby pins, single-prong clips, double-prong clips, hair sectioning clips, styling lotion, creme rinse, curling iron(s), hair spray.

Sanitation Supplies and Equipment: Sanitized towels.

Teaching Aids Needed: Textbook, Workbook, State Board Review Questions, chalkboard, overhead projector, VCR and videotape(s), computer, printer.

Transparency Master: Figures 14.7, 14.8, and 14.12.

Theory Objectives

1. Types of electric curling irons and iron sizes.
2. Parts of the curling iron.
3. Types of curls made with the marcel iron.
4. How curls are formed by using the marcel iron.

Practical Objectives

5. Basic hairstyle using the marcel iron.

Word Review:

spring clamp iron
marceling
mini iron
shell clamp
thermostat
croquignole curl
long-stem curls
poker curls
marcel iron
marcel waving
barrel
shell handle
safety rest
half-stem
roller curls
crimping iron
midget iron
rod
swivel base
no-stem curls
candlestick curls
spiral curls

Answers to End-of-Chapter Questions:

1. Thermal or curling irons. **2.** Marcel iron. **3.** The marcel iron is sturdier,opens wider, and heats faster. **4.** The crimping iron is used on longer hair. **5.** Crimping iron. **6.** Mini or midget iron. **7.** Place a comb between the curling iron and the scalp. **8.** Heat resistant. **9.** Steel. **10.** Iron curling. **11.** 70 percent alcohol. **12.** Thermostat. **13.** Pretest the temperature. **14.** Compare your answer to the information in the chapter. **15.** Yes. **16.** Dry hair. **17.** Yes. 18. No. **19.** Thoroughly dry.

Special Safety Considerations:

Since the temperature of a professional curling iron is so much greater than an iron used for home use, it is important to caution the student about this difference. The student's dexterity while using the iron should be demonstrated before they are permitted to work on a classmate or client.

Theory Objective 1: **List the types of curling irons and the different sizes of irons.**

Learning Steps

1. Read chapter in textbook.
2. Complete assignment in workbook.
3. View videotape(s).
4. Proceed to next objective.

Resources

1. *The Professional Cosmetologist*, 4th ed., ch. 14, pp. 272-274.
2. *Theory and Practical Workbook*, ch. 14, p. 85.
3. Videotape library.

Instructor's Resource Notes: ____________________

____

Theory Objective 2: **Identify the parts of a curling iron.**

Learning Steps

1. Read chapter in textbook.
2. Complete assignment in workbook.
3. View videotape(s).
4. Proceed to next objective.

Resources

1. *The Professional Cosmetologist,* 4th ed., ch. 14, pp. 274-275.
2. *Theory and Practical Workbook,* ch. 14, p. 87.
3. Videotape library.

Instructor's Resource Notes: ____________________

____

Theory Objective 3: **Describe basic types of curls made with the marcel iron.**

Learning Steps

1. Read chapter in textbook.
2. Complete assignment in workbook.
3. View videotape(s).
4. Proceed to next objective.

Resources

1. *The Professional Cosmetologist,* 4th ed., ch. 14, pp. 275-276.
2. *Theory and Practical Workbook,* ch. 14, p. 88.
3. Videotape library.

Instructor's Resource Notes: ____________________

____

Theory Objective 4: **Explain how curls are formed using the marcel iron.**

Learning Steps

1. Read chapter in textbook.
2. Complete assignment in workbook.
3. View videotape(s).
4. Proceed to next objective.

Resources

1. *The Professional Cosmetologist,* 4th ed., ch. 14, pp. 277-280.
2. *Theory and Practical Workbook,* ch. 14, p. 89.
3. Videotape library.

Instructor's Resource Notes: ______________________________

____

Theory Objective 5: **Give a basic hairstyle using the marcel iron.**

Learning Steps

1. Read chapter in textbook.
2. Complete assignment in workbook.
3. View videotape(s).
4. Proceed to next chapter.

Resources

1. *The Professional Cosmetologist,* 4th ed., ch. 14, pp. 280-284.
2. *Theory and Practical Workbook,* ch. 14, p. 89.
3. Videotape library.

Instructor's Resource Notes: ______________________________

____

Evaluation of Instruction:

_____ A. Discussed answers to end of chapter questions.
_____ B. Collected completed workbook assignments.
_____ C. Collected student progress charts.
_____ D. State board sheets current.
_____ E. Answered written test(s), and/or computer test questions.
_____ F. Completed Performance/Product Checklist.

Student Assignments: ______________________________

____

15

Lesson Plan

Temporary Hair Coloring

Lesson Overview and Motivation: Students will learn the proper steps in applying temporary hair color(s) to the client's hair. Cosmetology students tend to be more interested in hair coloring than the population at large. This is an opportune time to introduce hair coloring theory, and because of the temporary nature of the product used - experimentation can be most enjoyable by many of the students. Projects using sample hair swatches saved from hair cutting classes can be used effectively now. (See Special Safety Considerations below). You may also want to expand on the pH of temporary hair coloring products.

This would be a good time for a student project applying hair colors to sample hair swatches, which will then be dried, labeled, and taped to a sheet of paper (see swatch chart at the end of this section.) A guest lecturer from a hair color manufacturing company (demonstrator) may also be a presentation to be considered.

Acceptable Level: Score 85 percent or better on a multiple choice exam, and complete the performance product checklist for this task.

Apply a temporary hair color to a client's hair within 3 to 5 minutes.

Location: Theory classroom_____ Lab classroom_____ Clinic_____

Time for Lecture/ Demonstration: 30 min._____ 60 min._____ 90 min._____

Student Level: Beginning_____ Intermediate_____ Advanced_____

Equipment/Models Needed: Mannequin and clamp, classmate, or client, temporary-color chart, shampoo bowl.

Supplies Needed: Shampooing supplies, protective (operator) apron, temporary color rinse.

Sanitation Supplies and Equipment: Sanitized towels, cape, protective gloves (if needed).

Teaching Aids Needed: Textbook, Workbook, State Board Review Questions, chalkboard, overhead projector, VCR and videotape(s), computer, printer, pH meter.

Transparency Master: Figures 15.8, 15.9, 15.10, and 15.11.

Theory Objectives	*Practical Objectives*
1. Temporary hair coloring and early use and development of hair-coloring products.	4. Selecting and applying temporary rinses.
2. Advantages and disadvantages of different types of temporary hair colors.	
3. Primary, secondary, and tertiary colors.	

Word Review:

pigment	melanin	henna
camomile	temporary rinse	cuticle layer
progressive dye	metallic dye	semipermanent hair color
coat	rinse	spray color
creme color	powder color	crayon color
mousse color	achromatic color	chromatic color
red, yellow, blue	primary colors	secondary colors
Food and Drug Administration	complementary colors	tertiary colors

Answers to End-of-Chapter Questions:

1. Cuticle, cortex, and medulla. **2.** Shampoo to shampoo. **3.** No. **4.** Dyes that build up on the hair and make it darker. **5.** Outer. **6.** All colors except black, white, and gray. **7.** Colors that are opposite each other on the color chart; these opposite colors tend to neutralize each other. **8.** Temporary color. **9.** A dye. **10.** The cuticle. **11.** No. **12.** Certified color (FDA approved). **13.** No. **14.** No.

Special Safety Considerations:

Most temporary rinses don't require a preliminary skin test, but students should read label directions for each product used. Caution should be exercised when applying darker colors to natural blondes, or lighter hair colors when the hair is porous because even though these colors are "temporary", they can be difficult to remove from the hair types previously mentioned. In some cases, these temporary colors will not be removed from the hair by shampooing!

Theory Objective 1: **Define temporary hair coloring and describe the early use and development of hair-coloring techniques.**

Learning Steps	*Resources*
1. Read chapter in textbook.	1. *The Professional Cosmetologist*, 4th ed., ch. 15, pp. 290-292.
2. Complete assignment in workbook.	2. *Theory and Practical Workbook*, ch. 15, p. 93.
3. View videotape(s).	3. Videotape library.
4. Proceed to next objective.	

Instructor's Resource Notes: ______________________________

____

Theory Objective 2: **Describe the advantages and disadvantages of different types of temporary hair colors.**

Learning Steps

1. Read chapter in textbook.
2. Complete assignment in workbook.
3. View videotape(s).
4. Proceed to next objective.

Resources

1. *The Professional Cosmetologist,* 4th ed., ch. 15, pp. 292-294.
2. *Theory and Practical Workbook,* ch. 15, p. 95.
3. Videotape library.

Instructor's Resource Notes: ______________________________

____

Theory Objective 3: **Define the primary, secondary, and tertiary colors.**

Learning Steps

1. Read chapter in textbook.
2. Complete assignment in workbook.
3. View videotape(s).
4. Proceed to next objective.

Resources

1. *The Professional Cosmetologist,* 4th ed., ch. 15, pp. 294-296.
2. *Theory and Practical Workbook,* ch. 15, p. 96.
3. Videotape library.

Instructor's Resource Notes: ______________________________

____

Practical Objective 4: **Select and apply temporary rinses.**

Learning Steps

1. Read chapter in textbook.
2. Complete assignment in workbook.
3. View videotape(s).
4. Proceed to next chapter.

Resources

1. *The Professional Cosmetologist,* 4th ed., ch. 15, pp. 296-297.
2. *Theory and Practical Workbook,* ch. 15, p. 97.
3. Videotape library.

Instructor's Resource Notes: ____

____

Evaluation of Instruction:

_____ A. Discussed answers to end of chapter questions.
_____ B. Collected completed workbook assignments.
_____ C. Collected student progress charts.
_____ D. State board sheets current.
_____ E. Answered written test(s), and/or computer test questions.
_____ F. Completed Performance/Product Checklist.

Student Assignments: ____

____

Temporary Color Project

Instructor	Student's Name/Date

Color applied	Color applied	Color applied	Color applied
Original color	Original color	Original color	Original color
Color applied	Color applied	Color applied	Color applied
Original color	Original color	Original color	Original color
Color applied	Color applied	Color applied	Color applied
Original color	Original color	Original color	Original color

16

Lesson Plan

Semipermanent Hair Coloring

Lesson Overview and Motivation: Students will change the client's hair color by following the proper steps. (See Special Safety Considerations below.) You may also want to expand on the pH of semipermanent hair coloring products.
This would be a good time for a student project applying hair colors to sample hair swatches, which will then be dried, labeled, and taped to a sheet of paper. (See swatch chart at the end of this section.) A presentation by a guest lecturer from a hair color manufacturing company (demonstrator) might be considered.
You may also want to introduce the use of a cross-reference color comparison chart, so that if a particular color in one brand is out-of-stock, another color from a different manufacturer may be substituted.

Acceptable Level: Score 85 percent or better on a multiple choice exam, and complete the performance product checklist for this task.
Even application of a semipermanent hair color within 5 to 10 minutes.

Location: Theory classroom_____ Lab classroom_____ Clinic_____

Time for Lecture/ Demonstration: 30 min._____ 60 min._____ 90 min._____

Student Level: Beginning_____ Intermediate_____ Advanced_____

Equipment/Models Needed: Shampoo bowl and chair, semipermanent hair color chart, mannequin and clamp, classmate, or client.

Supplies Needed: Shampooing supplies, talcum powder, timer, color product, color chart, neck strips, protective apron, Q-tips, mixing bottle(s).

Sanitation Supplies and Equipment: Gloves, sanitized towels.

Teaching Aids Needed: Textbook, Workbook, State Board Review Questions, chalkboard, overhead projector, VCR and videotape(s), computer, printer.

Transparency Master: Figure 16.4.

Theory Objectives

1. Semipermanent hair color: Definition, comparison with temporary color, and advantages and disadvantages
2. Identifying the client's natural hair color.

Practical Objectives

3. Selecting and applying semipermanent hair colors.

Word Review:

sulphur	six week rinse	predisposition test
patch test	ammonium thioglycolate	poison control center
blonde	brown	black
levels of color	tone	warm tone
cool tone	drab tone	gloves
manufacturer's directions	dermatitis venenata	positive patch test

Answers to End-of-Chapter Questions:

1. The Federal Food, Drug, and Cosmetic Act. **2.** (Students' answers). **3.** Cuts, abrasions, or disease. **4.** Behind the ear and at the bend of the elbow. **5.** Yes. **6.** Sulfur and ammonium thioglycolate. **7.** Yes. **8.** Yes. **9.** Blonde, brown, and black. **10.** No. **11.** Drab tone. **12.** Warm tone. **13.** Compare your answer to the information in the chapter. **14.** Keep a record. **15.** Yes.

Special Safety Considerations:

Semipermanent colors stain clothing, carpet, upholstery, nails, and the skin. Protective gloves and aprons should be recommended. Some of these colors require a predisposition test for allergies. The cleaning of work areas, bottles and dispensing area should be highlighted. Caution should be exercised when applying darker colors to natural blondes, or lighter hair colors when the hair is porous because even though these colors are "semipermanent", they can be difficult to remove from the hair types previously mentioned.

Theory Objective 1: **Define semipermanent hair color; compare it with temporary color; and list the advantages and disadvantages of semipermanent color.**

Learning Steps

1. Read chapter in textbook.
2. Complete assignment in workbook.
3. View videotape(s).
4. Proceed to next objective.

Resources

1. *The Professional Cosmetologist*, 4th ed., ch. 16, pp. 304-306.
2. *Theory and Practical Workbook,* ch. 16, p. 99.
3. Videotape library.

Instructor's Resource Notes: ____

____

Theory Objective 2: **Identify the client's natural hair color.**

Learning Steps	*Resources*
1. Read chapter in textbook.	1. *The Professional Cosmetologist*, 4th ed., ch. 16, pp. 306-307.
2. Complete assignment in workbook.	2. *Theory and Practical Workbook*, ch. 16, p. 101.
3. View videotape(s).	3. Videotape library.
4. Proceed to next objective.	

Instructor's Resource Notes: ____

____

Practical Objective 3: **Select and apply semipermanent hair colors.**

Learning Steps	*Resources*
1. Read chapter in textbook.	1. *The Professional Cosmetologist*, 4th ed., ch. 16, pp. 307-311.
2. Complete assignment in workbook.	2. *Theory and Practical Workbook*, ch. 16, p. 102.
3. View videotape(s).	3. Videotape library.
4. Proceed to next chapter.	

Instructor's Resource Notes: ____

____

Evaluation of Instruction:

_____ A. Discussed answers to end of chapter questions.
_____ B. Collected completed workbook assignments.
_____ C. Collected student progress charts.
_____ D. State board sheets current.
_____ E. Answered written test(s), and/or computer test questions.
_____ F. Completed Performance/Product Checklist.

Student Assignments: ____

____

Semipermanent Color Project

Instructor **Student's Name/Date**

Color applied	Color applied	Color applied	Color applied
Original color	Original color	Original color	Original color
Color applied	Color applied	Color applied	Color applied
Original color	Original color	Original color	Original color
Color applied	Color applied	Color applied	Color applied
Original color	Original color	Original color	Original color

17

Lesson Plan

Permanent Hair Coloring

Lesson Overview and Motivation: Provided with permanent hair-coloring products and supplies, students will permanently change the client's hair color. (See Special Safety Considerations below.) You may also want to expand on the pH of permanent hair coloring products.

This would be a good time for a student project applying hair colors to sample hair swatches, which will then be dried, labeled, and taped to a sheet of paper (see swatch chart at the end of this section). A guest lecturer from a hair color manufacturing company (demonstrator) may also be a presentation to be considered.

You may also want to introduce how to use a cross-reference color comparison chart, so that if a particular color in one brand is out-of-stock, another color from a different manufacturer may be substituted.

Students also tend to have difficulty "mixing" colors, so practice exercises in this area may be of considerable interest to them.

Acceptable Level: Score 85 percent or better on a multiple choice exam, and complete the performance product checklist for this task.

Following safety precautions and manufacturer's directions, apply permanent hair color to a client in 15 to 20 minutes.

Location: Theory classroom_____ Lab classroom_____ Clinic_____

Time for Lecture/ Demonstration: 30 min._____ 60 min._____ 90 min._____

Student Level: Beginning_____ Intermediate_____ Advanced_____

Equipment/Models Needed: Color chart, comparison chart, timer, mannequin and clamp, classmate, or client.

Supplies Needed: Shampoo supplies, plastic or glass dish, 20-volume peroxide, 28 percent ammonia water, client record card, client release form, shampooing supplies, Q-tips, sanitized tint bottle, talcum powder, tube color, bottle color, or canister color, stain remover.

Sanitation Supplies and Equipment: Sanitized towels, gloves, protective (operator) apron.

Teaching Aids Needed: Textbook, Workbook, State Board Review Questions, chalkboard, overhead projector, VCR and videotape(s), computer, printer, pH meter.

Transparency Master: Figures 17.3, 17.5, 17.6, 17.7, and 17.8.

Theory Objectives

1. Permanent hair-coloring services, terms, and chemicals.
2. Advantages and disadvantages of permanent hair-coloring products and safety measures needed when using them.

Practical Objectives

3. Testing the hair for metallic salts.
4. Applying a virgin tint to lighten or darken hair.
5. Applying a tint retouch.

Word Review:

penetrating tints	bleaching	decolorizing
oxidation tints	single-application	toning
double application	virgin hair	virgin tint
tint retouch	soap cap	oxidation
coal tar	20 volume	hydrogen peroxide
developer	aniline derivative	oxidizer
highlight	H_2O_2	para dyes
3.5-4.0	lighten	darken
tint	developer	para-phenylene-diamine
predisposition test	protective apron	protective gloves
allergy test	patch test	28% ammonia water
virgin tint	lighten	darken
double peroxide	equal peroxide	hydrometer
filler	porosity	plastic
metal	volume reduction	hypersensitive
drabber	bleaching	lightening
pastel toner	line of demarcation	50% gray hair
up to 1/16 inch		

Answers to End-of-Chapter Questions:

1. Hair not previously exposed to chemicals used to permanently curl, straighten, or color the hair. **2.** Shampoo, tint, and peroxide. **3.** H2O2. **4.** Lightening the hair, then applying a pastel tint (a toner) to it. **5.** No—never. **6.** Compare your answer to the information in the chapter. **7.** Yes. **8.** Cuticle and cortex. **9.** Penetrating tint. **10.** Virgin hair. **11.** Tint retouch. **12.** Hydrogen peroxide. **13.** Hydrogen peroxide. **14.** Para-phenylene-diamine. **15.** 3.5 to 4.0. **16.** Tint. **17.** Yes. **18.** Yes. **19.** No. **20.** Yes. **21.** No, use glass or plastic. **22.** Give a strand test. **23.** Add 1 ounce (30 milliliters) hydrogen peroxide (H_2O_2) and 1 ounce (30 milliliters) water (H_2O), then 2 ounces (60 milliliters) tint: 1 oz. (30 ml) H2O2 + 1 oz. (30 ml) H_2O+2 oz. (60 ml) tint. **24.** No. **25.** Yes. **26.** Yes. **27.** Yes. **28.** 1/16 inch (.156 centimeter). **29.** Hydrometer.

Special Safety Considerations:

Since some clients may experience a severe reaction to the color base of the permanent hair color, federal law requires a patch test 24 hours before the application of permanent hair color. These products should *not* be used for coloring eyebrows – to do so may cause blindness.

Like semipermanent hair color, permanent hair color stains just about everything; therefore, working in a neat, orderly fashion is essential. Cleanup and sanitation of shampoo bowls, and bottles used in the service are of equal importance.

The use of the color comparison chart should be introduced at this time. Emphasis should also be placed on the accurate mixing of the different brands of hair colors according to manufacturer's directions.

Color should not be dripped on to the client's eyes, face, or neck.

Students may not realize that because of the oxidation nature of some semipermanent colors, they should only be mixed immediately before application to the client's scalp.

Theory Objective 1: **Define permanent hair-coloring services, terms, and chemicals.**

Learning Steps	Resources
1. Read chapter in textbook.	1. *The Professional Cosmetologist*, 4th ed., ch. 17, pp. 316-319.
2. Complete assignment in workbook.	2. *Theory and Practical Workbook*, ch. 17, p. 105.
3. View videotape(s).	3. Videotape library.
4. Proceed to next objective.	

Instructor's Resource Notes: ______________________________

____

Theory Objective 2: **Describe the advantages and disadvantages of permanent hair color and the safety measures required when using permanent hair-coloring products.**

Learning Steps	Resources
1. Read chapter in textbook.	1. *The Professional Cosmetologist*, 4th ed., ch. 17, pp. 319-322.
2. Complete assignment in workbook.	2. *Theory and Practical Workbook*, ch. 17, p. 107.
3. View videotape(s).	3. Videotape library.
4. Proceed to next objective.	

Instructor's Resource Notes: ______________________________________

____

Practical Objective 3: **Test the hair for metallic salts.**

Learning Steps

1. Read chapter in textbook.
2. Complete assignment in workbook.
3. View videotape(s).
4. Proceed to next objective.

Resources

1. *The Professional Cosmetologist*, 4th ed., ch. 17, pp. 323-324.
2. *Theory and Practical Workbook*, ch. 17, p. 108.
3. Videotape library.

Instructor's Resource Notes: ______________________________________

____

Practical Objective 4: **Apply a virgin tint to lighten or darken hair.**

Learning Steps

1. Read chapter in textbook.
2. Complete assignment in workbook.
3. View videotape(s).
4. Proceed to next objective.

Resources

1. *The Professional Cosmetologist*, 4th ed., ch. 17, pp. 324-339.
2. *Theory and Practical Workbook*, ch. 17, p. 108.
3. Videotape library.

Instructor's Resource Notes: ______________________________________

____

Practical Objective 5: **Apply a tint retouch.**

Learning Steps

1. Read chapter in textbook.
2. Complete assignment in workbook.
3. View videotape(s).
4. Proceed to next chapter.

Resources

1. *The Professional Cosmetologist*, 4th ed., ch. 17, pp. 339-340.
2. *Theory and Practical Workbook*, ch. 17, p. 110.
3. Videotape library.

Instructor's Resource Notes: ______________________________

____

Evaluation of Instruction:

_____ A. Discussed answers to end of chapter questions.
_____ B. Collected completed workbook assignments.
_____ C. Collected student progress charts.
_____ D. State board sheets current.
_____ E. Answered written test(s), and/or computer test questions.
_____ F. Completed Performance/Product Checklist.

Student Assignments: ______________________________

____

Permanent Color Project

Instructor	Student's Name/Date

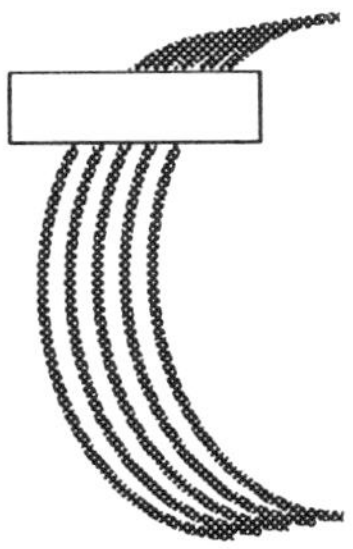

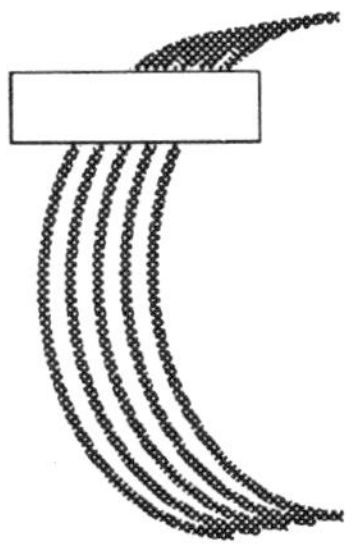

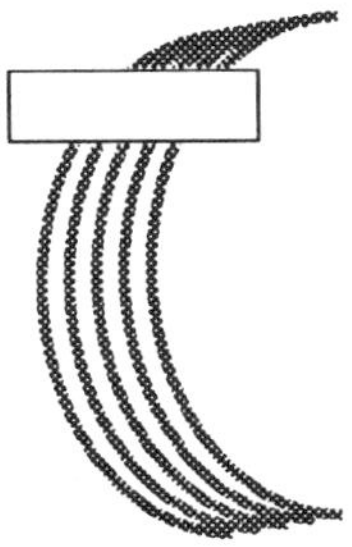

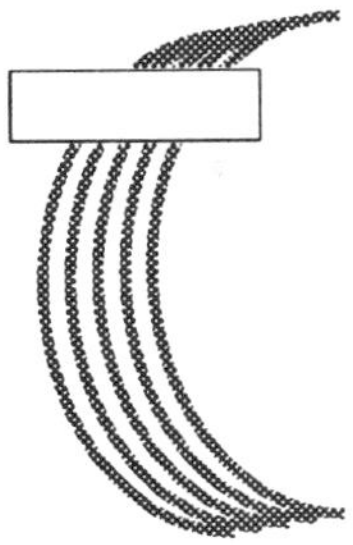

Color applied	Color applied	Color applied	Color applied
Original color	Original color	Original color	Original color
Color applied	Color applied	Color applied	Color applied
Original color	Original color	Original color	Original color
Color applied	Color applied	Color applied	Color applied
Original color	Original color	Original color	Original color

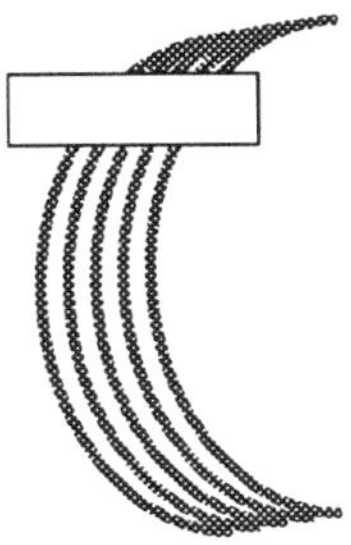

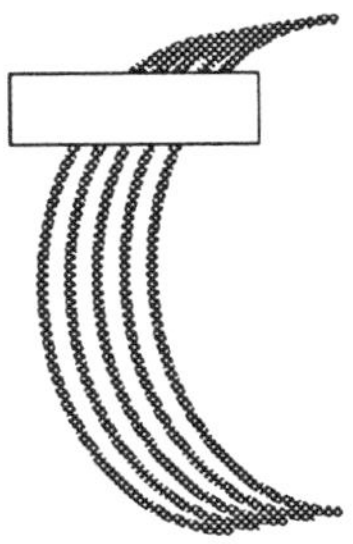

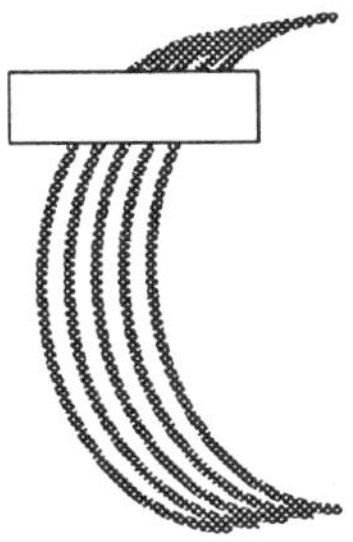

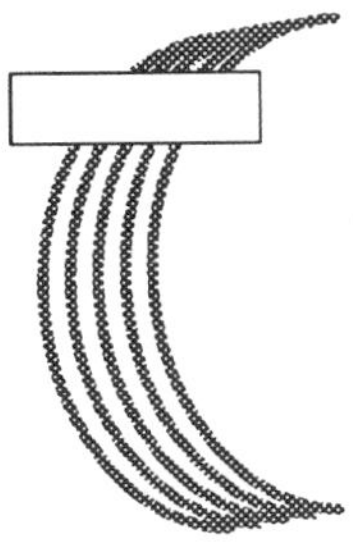

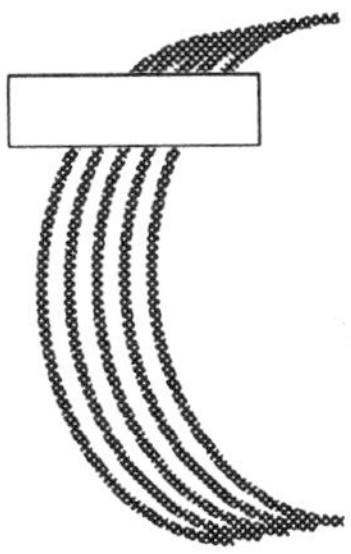

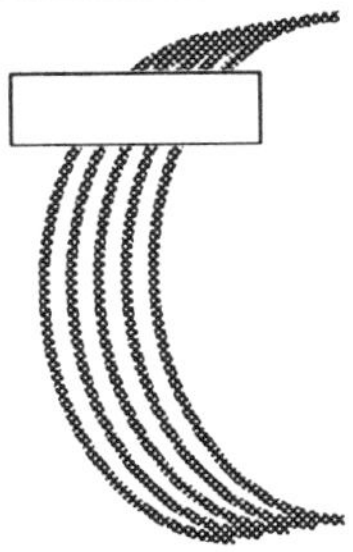

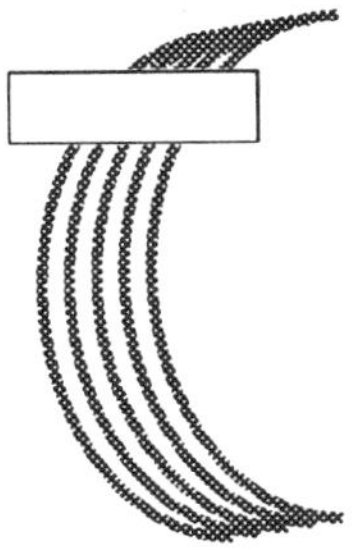

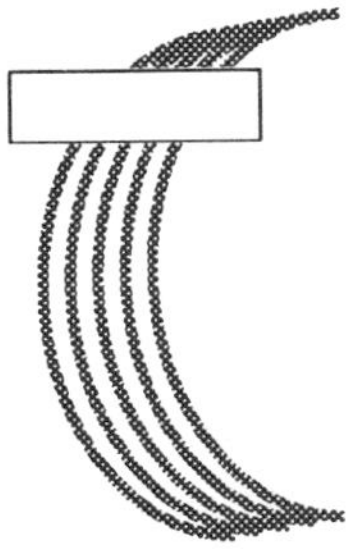

18

Lesson Plan

Lightening and Toning

Lesson Overview and Motivation: Students will learn to follow the proper steps in lightening and toning the client's hair. A guest lecturer from a hair color manufacturing company (demonstrator) may also be a presentation to be considered.
New products are being introduced regularly for lightening and toning the hair, so it is recommended that you survey a at least two supply distributors before presenting this class.

Acceptable Level: Score 85 percent or better on a multiple choice exam, and complete the performance product checklist for this task.
Apply a virgin bleach and a retouch bleach in 30 to 45 minutes (each).

Location: Theory classroom_____ Lab classroom_____ Clinic_____

Time for Lecture/ Demonstration: 30 min._____ 60 min._____ 90 min._____

Student Level: Beginning_____ Intermediate_____ Advanced_____

Equipment/Models Needed: Timer, color chart (toners), color comparison chart.

Supplies Needed: Client release form, client record card, 20-volume peroxide, cream bleach, toner, bleach applicator bottle, shampooing supplies, talcum powder.

Sanitation Supplies and Equipment: Sanitized towels, gloves, operator apron.

Teaching Aids Needed: Textbook, Workbook, State Board Review Questions, chalkboard, overhead projector, VCR and videotape(s), computer, printer, student project for applying colors to sample hair swatches, which will then be dried, labeled, and taped to a sheet of paper. A guest lecturer from a hair color manufacturing company (demonstrator) may also be desired.

Transparency Master: Figure 18.3.

Theory Objectives

1. Hair lightening and toning, their chemical effects on hair and the seven stages of lightening hair.
2. Types of lighteners and lightening and toning services.

Practical Objectives

3. Applying a virgin lightener.
4. Applying a lightener retouch.

Word Review:

Answers to End-of-Chapter Questions: **1.** Student's dictionary. **2.** Hydrogen peroxide. **3.** Powder lightener. **4.** Yellow, gold, orange, red, and brown. **5.** Double-application service. **6.** 8 to 9.5. **7.** Yes. **8.** Cortex. **9.** Yes. **10.** Compare your answer to the information in the chapter. **11.** Cream, powder, and oil. **12.** Compare your answer to the information in the chapter. **13.** No. **14.** No. **15.** Yes. **16.** 1/2 inch (1.25 centimeter). **17.** 1/8 inch (.31 centimeter). **18.** Yes. **19.** Yes. **20.** Applying a lightener on previously lightened hair when giving a lightening retouch. **21.** Yes.

Special Safety Considerations: The model's scalp should be carefully examined before proceeding with lightening services. Since the product used will be applied to the scalp, it should not be too strong for the model with a sensitive scalp. Brushing, or scalp manipulations, before this service should be avoided. Particularly during the application, the student should work quickly and accurately.

Students may not realize that because of the oxidation nature of permanent colors, they should only be mixed immediately before application to the client's scalp.

Lightener should not be dripped on to the client's eyes, face, or neck.

Theory Objective 1: **Define hair lightening and toning; describe their chemical effects on hair; and identify the seven stages of lightening the hair.**

Learning Steps

1. Read chapter in textbook.
2. Complete assignment in workbook.
3. View videotape(s).
4. Proceed to next objective.

Resources

1. *The Professional Cosmetologist*, 4th ed., ch. 18, pp. 346-347.
2. *Theory and Practical Workbook*, ch. 18, p. 113.
3. Videotape library.

Instructor's Resource Notes: ______________________________

____

Theory Objective 2: **Identify types of lighteners and services used for lightening and toning and identify the toning colors.**

Learning Steps

1. Read chapter in textbook.
2. Complete assignment in workbook.
3. View videotape(s).
4. Proceed to next objective.

Resources

1. *The Professional Cosmetologist*, 4th ed., ch. 18, pp. 347-349.
2. *Theory and Practical Workbook*, ch. 18, p. 114.
3. Videotape library.

Instructor's Resource Notes: ______________________________

____

Practical Objective 3: **Apply a virgin lightener.**

Learning Steps

1. Read chapter in textbook.
2. Complete assignment in workbook.
3. View videotape(s).
4. Proceed to next objective.

Resources

1. *The Professional Cosmetologist*, 4th ed., ch. 18, pp. 349-352.
2. *Theory and Practical Workbook*, ch. 18, p. 115.
3. Videotape library.

Instructor's Resource Notes: ______________________________

____

Practical Objective 4: **Apply a lightener retouch.**

Learning Steps

1. Read chapter in textbook.
2. Complete assignment in workbook.
3. View videotape(s).
4. Proceed to next chapter.

Resources

1. *The Professional Cosmetologist*, 4th ed., ch. 18, p. 353.
2. *Theory and Practical Workbook*, ch. 18, p. 116.
3. Videotape library.

Instructor's Resource Notes: ______________________________

____

Evaluation of Instruction:

_____ A. Discussed answers to end of chapter questions.
_____ B. Collected completed workbook assignments.
_____ C. Collected student progress charts.
_____ D. State board sheets current.
_____ E. Answered written test(s), and/or computer test questions.
_____ F. Completed Performance/Product Checklist.

Student Assignments: ____

____

19

Lesson Plan

Creative Lightening and Toning Techniques

Lesson Overview and Motivation: Students will learn the proper steps to streak, frame, frost, and paint the hair, and to tint it back to its original color. Since there are many techniques for creative lightening and toning, you may want to have a meeting with other staff members to determine exactly which methods you want to teach your students for use in the clinical experience center.

Acceptable Level: Score 85 percent or better on a multiple choice exam, and complete the performance product checklist for this task.
Follow the proper steps to achieve special lightening effects.

Location: Theory classroom_____ Lab classroom_____ Clinic_____

Time for Lecture/ Demonstration: 30 min._____ 60 min._____ 90 min._____

Student Level: Beginning_____ Intermediate_____ Advanced_____

Equipment/Models Needed: Color chart, dispensary scissors, crochet hook, toner color chart, hair-setting tape, filler color chart.

Supplies Needed: Client release form, client color form, aluminum foil, powder bleach, 20-volume hydrogen peroxide, shampoo supplies, hair clips, permanent hair colors, applicator bottle, talcum powder, plastic under-cap, frosting cap, plastic over-cap, orangewood stick, cellophane, oil bleach, color fillers, dye solvent.

Sanitation Supplies and Equipment: Protective gloves, protective apron, sanitized towels, cholesterol creme, cotton.

Teaching Aids Needed: Textbook, Workbook, State Board Review Questions, chalkboard, overhead projector, VCR and videotape(s), computer, printer, student project for applying colors to sample hair swatches, which will then be dried, labeled, and taped to a sheet of paper. A guest lecturer from a hair color manufacturing company (demonstrator) may also be desired.

Transparency Master: Figures 19.14 and 19.15.

Theory Objectives

None

Practical Objectives

1. Foil frosting the hair.
2. Framing the hair.
3. Frosting the hair.
4. Painting (freehand lighten) the hair.
5. Tinting the hair back to original color.

Word Review:

hair frosting	hair painting	powder bleach
reverse frosting	undercap	over-cap
weave the hair	equal peroxide	double peroxide
orangewood stick	tint-back	dye solvent
spot lightening	color filler	

Answers to End-of-Chapter Questions:

1. (a) Using foil and lightener to lighten large sections of hair around the face;
(b) lightening or darkening small strands of hair around the face;
(c) applying a solvent or lightener to lighten certain dark spots on the hair.
2. Compare your answer to the information in the chapter. **3.** Before the tint application. **4.** No. **5.** No. **6.** Yes. **7.** Yes. **8.** A reverse frosting. **9.** False. **10.** Yes. **11.** Thin strips. **12.** A tint-back. **13.** A filler. **14.** Spot lightening. **15.** Dye solvent.

Special Safety Considerations:

Caution the students to work carefully because when they are working with foil, caps, and cellophane, the lightener may seep down onto the scalp. This not only discolors the hair, but may irritate the scalp causing a chemical burn.

Practical Objective 1: **Foil frost the hair.**

Learning Steps

1. Read chapter in textbook.
2. Complete assignment in workbook.
3. View videotape(s).
4. Proceed to next objective.

Resources

1. *The Professional Cosmetologist*, 4th ed., ch. 19, pp. 358-359.
2. *Theory and Practical Workbook*, ch. 19, p. 119.
3. Videotape library.

Instructor's Resource Notes: ______________________________

____

Practical Objective 2: **Frame the hair.**

Learning Steps

1. Read chapter in textbook.
2. Complete assignment in workbook.
3. View videotape(s).
4. Proceed to next objective.

Resources

1. *The Professional Cosmetologist,* 4th ed., ch. 19, pp. 360-361.
2. *Theory and Practical Workbook,* ch. 19, p. 120.
3. Videotape library.

Instructor's Resource Notes: ______________________________

____

Practical Objective 3: **Frost the hair.**

Learning Steps

1. Read chapter in textbook.
2. Complete assignment in workbook.
3. View videotape(s).
4. Proceed to next objective.

Resources

1. *The Professional Cosmetologist,* 4th ed., ch. 19, pp. 361-363.
2. *Theory and Practical Workbook,* ch. 19, p. 120.
3. Videotape library.

Instructor's Resource Notes: ______________________________

____

Practical Objective 4: **Paint (freehand lighten) the hair.**

Learning Steps

1. Read chapter in textbook.
2. Complete assignment in workbook.
3. View videotape(s).
4. Proceed to next objective.

Resources

1. *The Professional Cosmetologist,* 4th ed., ch. 19, pp. 363-365.
2. *Theory and Practical Workbook,* ch. 19, p. 120.
3. Videotape library.

Instructor's Resource Notes: ______________________________

____

Practical Objective 5: **Tint hair back to its original color, lighter or darker.**

Learning Steps

1. Read chapter in textbook.
2. Complete assignment in workbook.
3. View videotape(s).
4. Proceed to next chapter.

Resources

1. *The Professional Cosmetologist,* 4th ed., ch. 19, pp. 365-369.
2. *Theory and Practical Workbook,* ch. 19, p. 122.
3. Videotape library.

Instructor's Resource Notes: ______________________________

____

Evaluation of Instruction:

______ A. Discussed answers to end of chapter questions.
______ B. Collected completed workbook assignments.
______ C. Collected student progress charts.
______ D. State board sheets current.
______ E. Answered written test(s), and/or computer test questions.
______ F. Completed Performance/Product Checklist.

Student Assignments: ______________________________

____

20

Lesson Plan

Permanent Wave

Lesson Overview and Motivation: Students will learn the proper procedure to permanently curl the client's hair. Permanent waving is so popular - students are typically eager to learn about this service. It tends to be less confusing for the student if the number of brands of permanent waves can be limited to no more than six. Since procedures for the different permanent waves may vary substantially, it is recommended that you carefully weigh the benefits of using a permanent wave that employ unusual steps that are not typical of all the other permanent waves used in your school.
You may also want to evaluate the pH of the different chemicals used for curling the hair.
Careful analysis of the condition of the hair and scalp are prerequisite to determining whether to proceed with this service, and which product to use.

Acceptable Level: Score 85 percent or better on a multiple choice exam, and complete the performance product checklist for this task.
Using water, wrap the client's hair on permanent wave rods in 45 minutes.

Location: Theory classroom_____ Lab classroom_____ Clinic_____

Time for Lecture/ Demonstration: 30 min._____ 60 min._____ 90 min._____

Student Level: Beginning_____ Intermediate_____ Advanced_____

Equipment/Models Needed: Cold-waving rods, hair-cutting implements, timer, processing overcap, applicator bottle, neutralizing bib.

Supplies Needed: Client release form, client permanent record form, shampoo supplies, protein conditioner, styling comb or rat-tail comb, cold (acid)-waving lotion and neutralizer, tube or cholesterol, mixing brush, end wraps, clips, rubber bands, a comb with coarse (widely-spaced) teeth. Long hair may require extra rods, rubber binders, or special rods.

Sanitation Supplies and Equipment: Shampoo cape, sanitized towels, operator apron, protective garment for client (if available), gloves, protective cream, cotton coil, neutralizing bib.

Teaching Aids Needed: Textbook, Theory and Practical Workbook, State Board Review Questions, chalkboard, overhead projector, VCR and videotape(s), computer, printer, pH meter.

Transparency Master: Figures 20.8, 20.9, 20.18, 20.27, and 20.31.

Theory Objectives

1. Three historical permanent-waving methods and the advantages of permanent cold-waving services.
2. Difference between acid waves and neutral waves.
3. Effects of cold waving, basic cold-waving chemicals, comparison of pH, cost, and procedures of the acid wave and the regular thio cold wave.
4. Other service included in cold waving.

Practical Objectives

5. Analyzing the hair and selecting proper cold-wave lotion and rods.
6. Sectioning (blocking) and wrapping the hair on permanent wave rods.
7. Processing and neutralizing the cold wave.
8. Giving a perm on long hair with a ponytail wrap
9. Relaxing an overly curly perm or naturally wavy hair.

Word Review:

permanent waving
chemical pads
end wraps
superheat permanent wave
machineless permanent
chemical burn
wrapping
self-timing
neutralizing
body heat
ammonium thioglycolate
rod size
leaving client unattended
single-end straight
hair breakage
rod length
plastic cap
hair breakage
neutralizing bib
spiral wrap
softens and swells hair
cold wave
cotton coil
neutralizer
acid wave
neutral wave
dryer heat
wrapping
cystine
hydrogen peroxide
scalp analysis
number of rods
hair analysis
elastic straps
double-end straight
body heat
S pattern
skin irritation
triangle net
pony tail wrap
spiral wrap
hardens and shrinks hair
cold wave rod
machine permanent
permanent wave
tension
chemical heat
processing
disulfide bonds
sodium bromate
times around the rod
solution strength
test curl
book-end fold
rod diameter
even, moderate tension
over-cap
neutralizing methods
stack wrap
subsections

Answers to End-of-Chapter Questions:

1. Physical, by winding; chemical, by waving lotion. **2.** It softens and swells the hair shaft. **3.** It shrinks and hardens the hair shaft. **4.** The diameter (size) of the rods and the number used. **5.** To prevent a chemical burn on the skin. **6.** Both. **7.** No. **8.** True. **9.** Yes. **10.** Yes. **11.** Ammonium thioglycolate. **12.** 8.5 to 9.5. **13.** Yes. **14.** Bromate. **15.** Yes. **16.** The size of the rods used. **17.** 2 1/2 turns. **18.** Blot with damp towels, and allow hair to air dry naturally.

Special Safety Considerations:

Cleansing of hands before and after service; chemicals coming in contact with clients' skin (neck and hairline), eyes, or ears; cleansing of bottles etc.; and sanitation of the work area; sanitation of items that can be reused, such as rods, combs and brushes; disposal of used items, such as end wraps; return and proper storage of unused supplies; disposable gloves.

Emphasize safety precautions described in textbook. Special attention should be directed to the removal of saturated cotton around hairline and neck towels because this may cause a chemical burn to develop.

Advise students to work quickly and accurately. Avoid dripping waving solution or neutralizer into the client's eyes or ears.

Caution the students about applying the "neutralizer" - when they actually intended to use the "waving solution" to begin the processing of a permanent wave.

Theory Objective 1: **Describe three historical permanent-waving methods and list the advantages of the permanent cold-waving services.**

Learning Steps

1. Read chapter in textbook.
2. Complete assignment in workbook.
3. View videotape(s).
4. Proceed to next objective.

Resources

1. *The Professional Cosmetologist,* 4th ed., ch. 20, pp. 374-376.
2. *Theory and Practical Workbook,* ch. 20, p. 125.
3. Videotape library.

Instructor's Resource Notes: ____________________

____

Theory Objective 2: **Explain the difference between acid waves and neutral waves.**

Learning Steps

1. Read chapter in textbook.
2. Complete assignment in workbook.
3. View videotape(s).
4. Proceed to next objective.

Resources

1. *The Professional Cosmetologist,* 4th ed., ch. 20, pp. 376-377.
2. *Theory and Practical Workbook,* ch. 20, p. 126.
3. Videotape library.

Instructor's Resource Notes: ____________________

____

Theory
Objective 3: **Describe the effects of cold waving, identify the basic cold-waving chemicals, and compare the pH, cost, and methods of giving the acid wave and the regular thio wave.**

Learning Steps

1. Read chapter in textbook.
2. Complete assignment in workbook.
3. View videotape(s).
4. Proceed to next objective.

Resources

1. *The Professional Cosmetologist,* 4th ed., ch. 20, pp. 377-378.
2. *Theory and Practical Workbook,* ch. 20, p. 127.
3. Videotape library.

Instructor's Resource Notes: ____

____

Theory
Objective 4: **List other services included with cold waving.**

Learning Steps

1. Read chapter in textbook.
2. Complete assignment in workbook.
3. View videotape(s).
4. Proceed to next objective.

Resources

1. *The Professional Cosmetologist,* 4th ed., ch. 20, pp. 378-379.
2. *Theory and Practical Workbook,* ch. 20, p. 127.
3. Videotape library.

Instructor's Resource Notes: ____

____

Practical
Objective 5: **Analyze the hair and select the proper cold-wave lotion and rods.**

Learning Steps

1. Read chapter in textbook.
2. Complete assignment in workbook.
3. View videotape(s).
4. Proceed to next objective.

Resources

1. *The Professional Cosmetologist,* 4th ed., ch. 20, pp. 379-384.
2. *Theory and Practical Workbook,* ch. 20, p. 129.
3. Videotape library.

Instructor's Resource Notes: ____

____

Practical Objective 6: **Section (block) and wrap the hair on permanent wave rods.**

Learning Steps	*Resources*
1. Read chapter in textbook.	1. *The Professional Cosmetologist,* 4th ed., ch. 20, pp. 384-391.
2. Complete assignment in workbook.	2. *Theory and Practical Workbook,* ch. 20, p. 130.
3. View videotape(s).	3. Videotape library.
4. Proceed to next objective.	

Instructor's Resource Notes: ______________________________

____

Practical Objective 7: **Process and neutralize the cold wave.**

Learning Steps	*Resources*
1. Read chapter in textbook.	1. *The Professional Cosmetologist,* 4th ed., ch. 20, pp. 391-396.
2. Complete assignment in workbook.	2. *Theory and Practical Workbook,* ch. 20, p. 131.
3. View videotape(s).	3. Videotape library.
4. Proceed to next objective.	

Instructor's Resource Notes: ______________________________

____

Practical Objective 8: **Give a perm on long hair using a ponytail wrap.**

Learning Steps	*Resources*
1. Read chapter in textbook.	1. *The Professional Cosmetologist,* 4th ed., ch. 20, pp. 397-401.
2. Complete assignment in workbook.	2. *Theory and Practical Workbook,* ch. 20, p. 135.
3. View videotape(s).	3. Videotape library.
4. Proceed to next objective.	

Instructor's Resource Notes: ______________________________

____

Practical Objective 9: **Relax an overly curly perm or naturally wavy hair.**

Learning Steps	*Resources*
1. Read chapter in textbook.	1. *The Professional Cosmetologist*, 4th ed., ch. 20, pp. 402-404.
2. Complete assignment in workbook.	2. *Theory and Practical Workbook*, ch. 20, p. 135.
3. View videotape(s).	3. Videotape library.
4. Proceed to next chapter.	

Instructor's Resource Notes: ______________________________

____

Evaluation of Instruction:

_____ A. Discussed answers to end of chapter questions.
_____ B. Collected completed workbook assignments.
_____ C. Collected student progress charts.
_____ D. State board sheets current.
_____ E. Answered written test(s), and/or computer test questions.
_____ F. Completed Performance/Product Checklist.

Student Assignments: ______________________________

____

21

Lesson Plan
Chemical Hair Relaxing

Lesson Overview and Motivation: Students will learn how to relax the client's hair for a hair style with less natural curl. The relaxing of super-curly hair is a popular service offered by the beauty salon, so student typically very interested in learning about this service. The chemical aspects of the service should be explained in detail.
Careful analysis of the condition of the hair and scalp are prerequisite to determining whether to proceed with this service, and which product to use. This service requires that the student work quickly and accurately - otherwise, the client's skin may sustain a chemical burn.

Acceptable Level: Score 85 percent or better on a multiple choice exam, and complete the performance product checklist for this task.
Apply a no-base relaxer in 15 minutes; apply a base relaxer (with base) in 30 minutes.

Location: Theory classroom_____ Lab classroom_____ Clinic_____

Time for Lecture/ Demonstration: 30 min._____ 60 min._____ 90 min._____

Student Level: Beginning_____ Intermediate_____ Advanced_____

Equipment/Models Needed: Timer, label/manufacturer's directions.

Supplies Needed: Client chemical services form, shampoo cape, rake and rat-tail combs, base chemical relaxing kit, chemical relaxing creme, neutralizing (stabilizing) shampoo, hair conditioner, scalp conditioner, styling lotion.

Sanitation Supplies and Equipment: Sanitized towels, protective gloves, protective base creme.

Teaching Aids Needed: Textbook, Workbook, State Board Review Questions, chalkboard, overhead projector, VCR and videotape(s), computer, printer, pH meter. Guest lecturers can also be helpful for advanced classes.

Transparency Master: Figures 21.7 and 21.8.

Theory Objectives

1. Chemical relaxing and straightening.
2. Differences between a base and a no-base relaxer.
3. Safety precautions used in chemical relaxing and straightening.

Practical Objectives

4. Applying a base chemical relaxer to virgin hair.
5. Giving a chemical blowout relaxer.

Word Review:

ammonium thioglycolate
perms
fixative
caustic soda
regular strength
dilute the relaxer
2–3 shampoos
sodium hydroxide
neutralizing shampoo
stabilizer
1/4 inch sections
super strength
silky/shiny appearance
relaxer retouch
petrolatum
straightener
straightening service
mild strength
virgin relaxer
tepid

Answers to End-of-Chapter Questions:

1. Sodium hydroxide. **2.** Neutralizing shampoo, stabilizer, or fixative. **3.** No. It would most likely break. **4.** No. **5.** The base relaxer uses a protective scalp cream, the no-base relaxer does not. **6.** No. **7.** Yes. **8.** Chemical relaxing. **9.** 11.5 to 14; 8.5 to 9.5. **10.** To neutralize the hair in the straighter position. **11.** Yes. **12.** Yes. **13.** No; several. **14.** Yes. **15.** False; flush with cool water. **16.** Yes. **17.** No; in the bottom. **18.** No; 1/4-inch (.625-centimeter) subsections. **19.** No. **20.** Pressure (friction). **21.** False. **22.** False.

Special Safety Considerations:

Cleansing of hands before and after service; chemicals coming in contact with clients' skin (neck and hairline), eyes, or ears; cleansing of bottles etc.; and sanitation of the work area; sanitation of items that can be reused, such as combs and brushes; disposal of used items; return and proper storage of unused supplies; disposable gloves.

Due to the caustic nature of the chemicals used for this service, students should be careful not to allow chemicals to come in contact with the client's ears, neckline, or hairline. Neck towels should be changed frequently as chemicals drip on to them.

Theory Objective 1: **Describe chemical relaxing and straightening.**

Learning Steps	Resources
1. Read chapter in textbook.	1. *The Professional Cosmetologist*, 4th ed., ch. 21, pp. 411-414.
2. Complete assignment in workbook.	2. *Theory and Practical Workbook*, ch. 21, p. 139.
3. View videotape(s).	3. Videotape library.
4. Proceed to next objective.	

Instructor's Resource Notes: ______________________________

____

Theory Objective 2: **Explain the difference between a base and no-base relaxer.**

Learning Steps	Resources
1. Read chapter in textbook.	1. *The Professional Cosmetologist*, 4th ed., ch. 21, p. 414.
2. Complete assignment in workbook.	2. *Theory and Practical Workbook*, ch. 21, p. 140.
3. View videotape(s).	3. Videotape library.
4. Proceed to next objective.	

Instructor's Resource Notes: ______________________________

____

Theory Objective 3: **Identify safety precautions used in chemical relaxing and straightening.**

Learning Steps	Resources
1. Read chapter in textbook.	1. *The Professional Cosmetologist*, 4th ed., ch. 21, pp. 414-416.
2. Complete assignment in workbook.	2. *Theory and Practical Workbook*, ch. 21, p. 141.
3. View videotape(s).	3. Videotape library.
4. Proceed to next objective.	

Instructor's Resource Notes: ______________________________

____

Practical Objective 4: **Apply a base chemical relaxer to virgin hair; apply a retouch relaxer.**

Learning Steps

1. Read chapter in textbook.
2. Complete assignment in workbook.
3. View videotape(s).
4. Proceed to next objective.

Resources

1. *The Professional Cosmetologist*, 4th ed., ch. 21, pp. 416-424.
2. *Theory and Practical Workbook*, ch. 21, p. 142.
3. Videotape library.

Instructor's Resource Notes: ______________________________

____

Practical Objective 5: **Give a chemical blowout relaxer.**

Learning Steps

1. Read chapter in textbook.
2. Complete assignment in workbook.
3. View videotape(s).
4. Proceed to next chapter.

Resources

1. *The Professional Cosmetologist*, 4th ed., ch. 21, pp. 425-427.
2. Videotape library.

Instructor's Resource Notes: ______________________________

____

Evaluation of Instruction:

_____ A. Discussed answers to end of chapter questions.
_____ B. Collected completed workbook assignments.
_____ C. Collected student progress charts.
_____ D. State board sheets current.
_____ E. Answered written test(s), and/or computer test questions.
_____ F. Completed Performance/Product Checklist.

Student Assignments: ______________________________

____

22

Lesson Plan

Thermal Pressing

Lesson Overview and Motivation: Students will learn how to straighten the hair with the pressing comb, curl the hair with the curling iron, and comb the curls into a hairstyle. This is a temporary hairstyling method. Once the hair is exposed to humidity or moisture - it reverts back to its original degree of curliness.
Careful analysis of the condition of the hair and scalp are prerequisite to determining whether to proceed with this service.
Because of the extreme heat of the pressing comb, practice on a mannequin is recommended prior to working on a classmate or client.

Acceptable Level: Score 85 percent or better on a multiple choice exam, and complete the performance product checklist for this task.
Silk the hair in 30 to 45 minutes, then curl and style the hair in 45 to 60 minutes.

Location: Theory classroom_____ Lab classroom_____ Clinic_____

Time for Lecture/ Demonstration: 30 min._____ 60 min._____ 90 min._____

Student Level: Beginning_____ Intermediate_____ Advanced_____

Equipment/Models Needed: Electric heater for irons.

Supplies Needed: Shampoo supplies, chair cloth, hard rubber combs (rake, rat-tail, styling), pressing combs (regular and midget), pressing creme or oil, curling wax (optional), hair spray, white tissue, sectioning clips, brush, curling irons, electric curling iron.

Sanitation Supplies and Equipment: Neck strips, sanitized towels.

Teaching Aids Needed: Textbook, Workbook, State Board Review Questions, chalkboard, overhead projector, VCR and videotape(s), computer, printer.

Theory Objectives	***Practical Objectives***
1. Equipment and supplies used for pressing and curling super-curly hair. 2. Use of the pressing comb. 3. Techniques used to produce thermal curls.	4. Pressing the hair. 5. Curling the hair with marcel-style irons.

Word Review:

pressing comb	electric stove	heat resistant comb
heat resistant cape	pressing oils	pressing brilliantine
lusterizing spray	lanolin sheep wool	thermostat
silking	revert	hard press
hair textures	soft press	roller technique
candlestick curl	spiral technique	poker curl
croquignole technique	scorched hair	temperature setting
physical burn	pressing cape	natural growth direction

Answers to End-of-Chapter Questions:

1. Straighten it. **2.** About two weeks. **3.** Pressing comb. **4.** Yes. **5.** In an electric heater. **6.** Straightening. **7.** Moisture. **8.** Double press. **9.** It will need to be curled. **10.** Yes. **11.** "000" steel wool, very fine sandpaper, emery board file. **12.** Yes. **13.** Pretest for temperature. **14.** Compare your answer to the information in the chapter. **15.** Yes. **16.** Lower. **17.** Yes. **18.** No. **19.** Thoroughly dried.

Special Safety Considerations:

These irons are extremely hot, and the new student will need to develop dexterity before attempting to press the client's hair.

Theory Objective 1: **Describe the equipment and supplies used for pressing and curling super-curly hair.**

Learning Steps	***Resources***
1. Read chapter in textbook. 2. Complete assignment in workbook. 3. View videotape(s). 4. Proceed to next objective.	1. *The Professional Cosmetologist*, 4th ed., ch. 22, pp. 432-433. 2. *Theory and Practical Workbook*, ch. 22, p. 147. 3. Videotape library.

Instructor's Resource Notes: ____

____

Theory Objective 2: **Explain the use of the pressing iron.**

Learning Steps

1. Read chapter in textbook.
2. Complete assignment in workbook.
3. View videotape(s).
4. Proceed to next objective.

Resources

1. *The Professional Cosmetologist,* 4th ed., ch. 22, pp. 433-434.
2. *Theory and Practical Workbook,* ch. 22, p. 148.
3. Videotape library.

Instructor's Resource Notes: ______________________________

____

Theory Objective 3: **Describe the techniques used to produce thermal curls.**

Learning Steps

1. Read chapter in textbook.
2. Complete assignment in workbook.
3. View videotape(s).
4. Proceed to next objective.

Resources

1. *The Professional Cosmetologist,* 4th ed., ch. 22, pp. 434-435.
2. *Theory and Practical Workbook,* ch. 22, p. 149.
3. Videotape library.

Instructor's Resource Notes: ______________________________

____

Practical Objective 4: **Press the hair.**

Learning Steps

1. Read chapter in textbook.
2. Complete assignment in workbook.
3. View videotape(s).
4. Proceed to next objective.

Resources

1. *The Professional Cosmetologist,* 4th ed., ch. 22, pp. 435-439.
2. *Theory and Practical Workbook,* ch. 22, p. 149.
3. Videotape library.

Instructor's Resource Notes: ______________________________

____

Practical Objective 5: **Curl the hair with marcel-type irons.**

Learning Steps	*Resources*
1. Read chapter in textbook.	1. *The Professional Cosmetologist,* 4th ed., ch. 22, pp. 439-444.
2. Complete assignment in workbook.	2. *Theory and Practical Workbook,* ch. 22, p. 151.
3. View videotape(s).	3. Videotape library.
4. Proceed to next chapter.	

Instructor's Resource Notes: ______________________________

____

Evaluation of Instruction:

_____ A. Discussed answers to end of chapter questions.
_____ B. Collected completed workbook assignments.
_____ C. Collected student progress charts.
_____ D. State board sheets current.
_____ E. Answered written test(s), and/or computer test questions.
_____ F. Completed Performance/Product Checklist.

Student Assignments: ______________________________

____

23

Lesson Plan

Recurling the Hair

Lesson Overview and Motivation: Students will learn how to relax and reform (recurl) super-curly hair into a different curl formation. Because this is an expensive school or salon service, students are eager to learn how to perform this service. Since recurling (soft curl) is actually a combination of chemical relaxing and permanent waving, more skill and concentration are required of the student to achieve the desired result, and maintain the proper condition of the client's scalp and hair.

Careful analysis of the condition of the hair and scalp are prerequisite to determining whether to proceed with this service, and which product to use. This service requires that the student work quickly and accurately - otherwise, the client's skin may sustain a chemical burn.

Acceptable Level: Score 85 percent or better on a multiple choice exam, and complete the performance product checklist for this task.

Relax the hair in 30 to 45 minutes and then wrap the hair on permanent-wave rods in 45 to 75 minutes.

Location: Theory classroom_____ Lab classroom_____ Clinic_____

Time for Lecture/ Demonstration: 30 min._____ 60 min._____ 90 min._____

Student Level: Beginning_____ Intermediate_____ Advanced_____

Equipment/Models Needed: Shampoo bowl, dryer with chair, timer.

Supplies Needed: Shampoo cape, neutralizing bib, rat-tail comb, end wraps, large-tooth comb, cold-wave rods, plastic cap, tint brush, hair relaxer, waving solution, neutralizer, protein conditioner, instant moisturizer, curl activator, conditioning shampoo, polymer pretreatment, clips, protective base.

Sanitation Supplies and Equipment: Sanitized towels, cotton coil, protective gloves.

Teaching Aids Needed: Textbook, Workbook, State Board Review Questions, chalkboard, overhead projector, VCR and videotape(s), computer, printer. Guest lecturers can also be helpful for advanced classes.

Transparency Master: Figures 23.3, 23.7, and 23.13.

Theory Objectives	*Practical Objectives*
1. Basic curl re-formation service and its advantages.	5. Analyzing the hair and applying the chemical curl relaxer.
2. Chemical processes of the curl re-formation service.	6. Sectioning and subsectioning the client's hair and wrapping it on cold-wave rods.
3. Evaluating the condition of the hair and scalp.	7. Processing and neutralizing the curl re-formation.
4. Important safety and after-care considerations for the curl re-formation service.	

Word Review:

curl rearranger	thinly parted subsections	recurl
rubber gloves	wrapping (rodding)	manufacturer's directions
apron	curl booster	acid
curl booster	alkaline	pH
small rod sizes	test curl	resistant area
accelerated chemical processing	even tension	

Answers to End-of-Chapter Questions:

1. Curl rearranger or recurl. **2.** Double-application service. **3.** No. **4.** False; ammonium thioglycolate. **5.** No; sodium bromate. **6.** Yes. **7.** Yes. **8.** Yes. **9.** No; very thin subsections. **10.** False; firm, even tension. **11.** Yes. **12.** Yes. **13.** No; 9.6. **14.** To straighten the hair. **15.** Yes. **16.** No; a shorter time. **17.** False; hair must be cut first. **18.** No. **19.** No; cool water. **20.** No; do not brush the hair.

Special Safety Considerations:

Because of the duration of this service and the strength of the chemicals used, the sensitivity of the scalp must be considered at all times. Whether shampooing, rinsing chemicals, or neutralizers from the hair, it is important to use tepid water to start, and ask clients if they are comfortable.

Theory Objective 1: **Define the basic curl re-formation service and its advantages.**

Learning Steps	*Resources*
1. Read chapter in textbook.	1. *The Professional Cosmetologist,* 4th ed., ch. 23, pp. 448-450.
2. Complete assignment in workbook.	2. *Theory and Practical Workbook,* ch. 23, p. 153.
3. View videotape(s).	3. Videotape library.
4. Proceed to next objective.	

Instructor's Resource Notes: ______________________________

____

Theory Objective 2: **Describe the chemical processes of the curl re-formation service.**

Learning Steps

1. Read chapter in textbook.
2. Complete assignment in workbook.
3. View videotape(s).
4. Proceed to next objective.

Resources

1. *The Professional Cosmetologist*, 4th ed., ch. 23, pp. 450-451.
2. *Theory and Practical Workbook*, ch. 23, p. 155.
3. Videotape library.

Instructor's Resource Notes: ______________________________

____

Theory Objective 3: **Evaluate the condition of the hair and scalp.**

Learning Steps

1. Read chapter in textbook.
2. Complete assignment in workbook.
3. View videotape(s).
4. Proceed to next objective.

Resources

1. *The Professional Cosmetologist*, 4th ed., ch. 23, pp. 451-452.
2. *Theory and Practical Workbook*, ch. 23, p. 156.
3. Videotape library.

Instructor's Resource Notes: ______________________________

____

Theory Objective 4: **Identify important safety and after-care considerations for the curl re-formation service.**

Learning Steps

1. Read chapter in textbook.
2. Complete assignment in workbook.
3. View videotape(s).
4. Proceed to next objective.

Resources

1. *The Professional Cosmetologist*, 4th ed., ch. 23, pp. 452-454.
2. *Theory and Practical Workbook*, ch. 23, p. 157.
3. Videotape library.

Instructor's Resource Notes: ______________________

____

Theory Objective 5: **Analyze the hair and apply the chemical curl relaxer.**

Learning Steps

1. Read chapter in textbook.
2. Complete assignment in workbook.
3. View videotape(s).
4. Proceed to next objective.

Resources

1. *The Professional Cosmetologist*, 4th ed., ch. 23, pp. 454-457.
2. *Theory and Practical Workbook*, ch. 23, p. 158.
3. Videotape library.

Instructor's Resource Notes: ______________________

____

Theory Objective 6: **Section and subsection the client's hair and wrap it on cold-wave rods.**

Learning Steps

1. Read chapter in textbook.
2. Complete assignment in workbook.
3. View videotape(s).
4. Proceed to next objective.

Resources

1. *The Professional Cosmetologist*, 4th ed., ch. 23, pp. 457-459.
2. *Theory and Practical Workbook*, ch. 23, p. 159.
3. Videotape library.

Instructor's Resource Notes: ______________________

____

Theory Objective 7: **Process and neutralize the curl re-formation.**

Learning Steps

1. Read chapter in textbook.
2. Complete assignment in workbook.
3. View videotape(s).
4. Proceed to next chapter.

Resources

1. *The Professional Cosmetologist*, 4th ed., ch. 23, pp. 459-462.
2. *Theory and Practical Workbook*, ch. 23, p. 160.
3. Videotape library.

Instructor's Resource Notes: ______________________________

____

Evaluation of Instruction:

_____ A. Discussed answers to end of chapter questions.
_____ B. Collected completed workbook assignments.
_____ C. Collected student progress charts.
_____ D. State board sheets current.
_____ E. Answered written test(s), and/or computer test questions.
_____ F. Completed Performance/Product Checklist.

Student Assignments: ______________________________

____

24

Lesson Plan

Describing the Skin

Lesson Overview and Motivation: Students will learn to recognize common skin disorders that may be treated in the salon, and diseases that should be referred to a medical doctor/dermatologist. Emphasis should be placed on the preservation of the skin by avoiding harmful ultraviolet light from the sun, and on the value of using Retin-A for restoring the elasticity of the skin, and reducing or eliminating liver spots.
Recognizing various lesions of the skin is also interesting to the students.

Acceptable Level: Score 85 percent or better on a multiple choice exam.

Location: Theory classroom_____ Lab classroom_____ Clinic_____

Time for Lecture/ Demonstration: 30 min._____ 60 min._____ 90 min._____

Student Level: Beginning_____ Intermediate_____ Advanced_____

Teaching Aids Needed: Textbook, Workbook, State Board Review Questions, chalkboard, overhead projector, VCR and videotape(s), computer, printer

Transparency Master: Figures 24.1, 24.2, 24.3, and 24.8.

Theory Objectives

1. Structure and functions of the skin.
2. Layers of the epidermis and their functions.
3. Appendages of the skin classified by name and function.
4. Diseases of the sweat glands.
5. Skin pigmentation and its abnormalities.
6. Skin keratinization.
7. Primary and secondary lesions.

Practical Objectives

None.

Word Review:

histology
esthetician
heat regulation
shock
basal layer
prickle layer
glands
melanin cells
PABA
photodermatitis
Chloasma
hypopigmentation
nevus flammeus
callus
secondary lesion
vesicle
premature aging and wrinkling

dermatology
practitioner
sensation
absorption
lucid layer
keratinized cells
secretions
tyrosine
skin cancer
melanoderma
ephelides
albinism
Retina A
lesion
furuncle
pustules
scars

dermatologist
protection
secretion
horny layer
granular layer
appendage
sebaceous glands
SPF
freckles
liver spots
lentigines
vitiligo
primary lesion
carbuncles
cyst
fissures

Answers to End-of-Chapter Questions:

1. Outermost (top) layer of skin; layer below the epidermis; fatty subcutaneous tissue; same as dermis; protein of the skin; any abnormal skin condition. **2.** Prickly heat or heat rash. **3.** Fissure. **4.** The cause of a disease or disorder. **5.** Below the epidermis and dermis (corium). **6.** Dermatology. **7.** Any abnormal skin condition. **8.** Yes. **9.** Yes. **10.** No. **11.** Monthly. **12.** Yes. **13.** Dermis. **14.** No. **15.** Secretions. **16.** They empty in both locations. **17.** Hyperhidrosis. **18.** Sun protection factor. **19.** False. **20.** False; good protection. **21.** Melanin. **22.** Yes. **23.** Nevus or nevi. **24.** Collagen.

Theory Objective 1: **Explain the structure and function of the skin.**

Learning Steps

1. Read chapter in textbook.
2. Complete assignment in workbook.
3. View videotape(s).
4. Proceed to next objective.

Resources

1. *The Professional Cosmetologist,* 4th ed., ch. 24, pp. 466-469.
2. *Theory and Practical Workbook,* ch. 24, p. 163.
3. Videotape library.

Instructor's Resource Notes: ____

____

Theory Objective 2: **Describe the layers of the epidermis and explain their functions.**

Learning Steps	*Resources*
1. Read chapter in textbook.	1. *The Professional Cosmetologist,* 4th ed., ch. 24, pp. 469-471.
2. Complete assignment in workbook.	2. *Theory and Practical Workbook,* ch. 24, p. 164.
3. View videotape(s).	3. Videotape library.
4. Proceed to next objective.	

Instructor's Resource Notes: ______________________________

____

Theory Objective 3: **Classify the appendages of the skin by name and function.**

Learning Steps	*Resources*
1. Read chapter in textbook.	1. *The Professional Cosmetologist,* 4th ed., ch. 24, pp. 471-473.
2. Complete assignment in workbook.	2. *Theory and Practical Workbook,* ch. 24, p. 166.
3. View videotape(s).	3. Videotape library.
4. Proceed to next objective.	

Instructor's Resource Notes: ______________________________

____

Theory Objective 4: **Describe the diseases of the sweat gland.**

Learning Steps	*Resources*
1. Read chapter in textbook.	1. *The Professional Cosmetologist,* 4th ed., ch. 24, pp. 473-474.
2. Complete assignment in workbook.	2. *Theory and Practical Workbook,* ch. 24, p. 167.
3. View videotape(s).	3. Videotape library.
4. Proceed to next objective.	

Instructor's Resource Notes: ______________________________

____

Theory Objective 5: **Explain skin pigmentation and its abnormalities.**

Learning Steps

1. Read chapter in textbook.
2. Complete assignment in workbook.
3. View videotape(s).
4. Proceed to next objective.

Resources

1. *The Professional Cosmetologist*, 4th ed., ch. 24, pp. 474-479.
2. *Theory and Practical Workbook*, ch. 24, p. 168.
3. Videotape library.

Instructor's Resource Notes: ______________________________

____

Theory Objective 6: **Explain skin keratinization.**

Learning Steps

1. Read chapter in textbook.
2. Complete assignment in workbook.
3. View videotape(s).
4. Proceed to next objective.

Resources

1. *The Professional Cosmetologist*, 4th ed., ch. 24, pp. 479-480.
2. *Theory and Practical Workbook*, ch. 24, p. 169.
3. Videotape library.

Instructor's Resource Notes: ______________________________

____

Theory Objective 7: **List the more common primary and secondary lesions.**

Learning Steps

1. Read chapter in textbook.
2. Complete assignment in workbook.
3. View videotape(s).
4. Proceed to next chapter.

Resources

1. *The Professional Cosmetologist*, 4th ed., ch. 24, pp. 480-484.
2. *Theory and Practical Workbook*, ch. 24, p. 170.
3. Videotape library.

Instructor's Resource Notes: ______________________________

____

Evaluation of Instruction:

_____ A. Discussed answers to end of chapter questions.
_____ B. Collected completed workbook assignments.
_____ C. Collected student progress charts.
_____ D. State board sheets current.
_____ E. Answered written test(s), and/or computer test questions.
_____ F. Completed Performance/Product Checklist.

Student Assignments: ____

____

25

Lesson Plan

Facial Treatments

Lesson Overview and Motivation:	Students will learn how to give a facial massage after a careful analysis of the client's skin condition. In this chapter the students will learn how to improve the elasticity of facial muscles, and apply lotions for simple skin conditions. Because this service is so relaxing and sometimes beneficial for the client, it is a service of high demand in certain geographic locations.
Acceptable Level:	Score 85 percent or better on a multiple choice exam, and complete the performance product checklist for this task. Give a facial treatment within 45 minutes.
Location:	Theory classroom_____ Lab classroom_____ Clinic_____
Time for Lecture/ Demonstration:	30 min._____ 60 min._____ 90 min._____
Student Level:	Beginning_____ Intermediate_____ Advanced_____
Equipment/Models Needed:	Facial chair for client, chair, facial steamer, comedone extractor, Wood's light, infrared or red dermal lamp, high-frequency electrode (optional).
Supplies Needed:	Cold creme, cleansing creme, cleansing lotion, emollient creme, astringent lotion, skin freshener, cotton, cotton pledgets or tissue, spatula(s), abrasive facial cleanser, medicated soap, antiseptic lotion.
Sanitation Supplies and Equipment:	Sanitized towels for head band, spatulas, tissue.
Teaching Aids Needed:	Textbook, Workbook, State Board Review Questions, chalkboard, overhead projector, VCR and videotape(s), computer, printer, chart of facial procedures.
Transparency Master:	Figure two page spread of facial manipulations.

Theory Objectives

1. Five basic massage movements.
2. Considerations when giving a facial.
3. Nature and benefits of light therapy.

Practical Objectives

4. Facial treatment for normal skin, dry skin, and oily skin: proper steps and safety precautions.

Word Review:

effleurage	petrissage	tapotement
friction	vibration	frontalis
emollient cream	gel	facial sponge
sanitation procedures	visible light	ultraviolet light
sunlight	actinic rays	ultraviolet rays
hot oil mask	witch hazel	Wood's light
facial pack	clay pack	milia
acne	comedone	high-frequency treatment

Answers to End-of-Chapter Questions:

1. After every client. **2.** Sanitized spatula. **3.** Upward. **4.** Yes. **5.** No; the forehead. **6.** Yes. **7.** Yes. **8.** No; the back of the neck and shoulder area. **9.** No. **10.** Yes. **11.** Yes.

Special Safety Considerations:

To prevent the spread of disease through the orifaces of the eyes and nose, washing hands before and after this service is important. A careful analysis of the model's/client's skin is essential. The proper disposal of used supplies, such as cotton balls, pledgets, tissue, etc., and replacement/storage of containers should be advised. Work areas should be thoroughly sanitized after use.

Theory Objective 1: **Describe the five basic massage movements.**

Learning Steps

1. Read chapter in textbook.
2. Complete assignment in workbook.
3. View videotape(s).
4. Proceed to next objective.

Resources

1. *The Professional Cosmetologist*, 4th ed., ch. 25, pp. 492-493.
2. *Theory and Practical Workbook*, ch. 25, p. 173.
3. Videotape library.

Instructor's Resource Notes: ______________________________

____

Theory Objective 2: **Explain the basic considerations when giving a facial.**

Learning Steps

1. Read chapter in textbook.
2. Complete assignment in workbook.
3. View videotape(s).
4. Proceed to next objective.

Resources

1. *The Professional Cosmetologist,* 4th ed., ch. 25, pp. 493-494.
2. *Theory and Practical Workbook,* ch. 25, p. 174.
3. Videotape library.

Instructor's Resource Notes: ______________________________

____

Theory Objective 3: **Describe the nature and benefits of light therapy.**

Learning Steps

1. Read chapter in textbook.
2. Complete assignment in workbook.
3. View videotape(s).
4. Proceed to next objective.

Resources

1. *The Professional Cosmetologist,* 4th ed., ch. 25, pp. 494-497.
2. *Theory and Practical Workbook,* ch. 25, p. 175.
3. Videotape library.

Instructor's Resource Notes: ______________________________

____

Practical Objective 4: **Use the proper steps and safety precautions to give a facial treatment for normal skin, dry skin, and oily skin.**

Learning Steps

1. Read chapter in textbook.
2. Complete assignment in workbook.
3. View videotape(s).
4. Proceed to next chapter.

Resources

1. *The Professional Cosmetologist,* 4th ed., ch. 25, pp. 497-509.
2. *Theory and Practical Workbook,* ch. 25, p. .
3. Videotape library.

Instructor's Resource Notes: ______________________________

____

Evaluation of Instruction:

_____ A. Discussed answers to end of chapter questions.
_____ B. Collected completed workbook assignments.
_____ C. Collected student progress charts.
_____ D. State board sheets current.
_____ E. Answered written test(s), and/or computer test questions.
_____ F. Completed Performance/Product Checklist.

Student Assignments: ____

____

26

Lesson Plan

Applying Makeup

Lesson Overview and Motivation: Students will learn how to apply makeup to enhance the client's facial features. One of the truly artistic components of the cosmetology course, makeup is very important in providing a "complete look" for the client in conjunction with the client's hairstyle. Students tend to be very interested in this chapter because techniques learned may be applied to themselves as well as their clients.

Acceptable Level: Score 85 percent or better on a multiple choice exam, and complete the performance product checklist for this task.
Apply makeup on a client in 40 to 60 minutes.

Location: Theory classroom_____ Lab classroom_____ Clinic_____

Time for Lecture/ Demonstration: 30 min._____ 60 min._____ 90 min._____

Student Level: Beginning_____ Intermediate_____ Advanced_____

Equipment/Models Needed: Client release form, tissue, small terry cloth, lip brush, makeup chair.

Supplies Needed: Cleansing cream, sanitized towels, skin freshener, astringent, moisturizer, corrective stick, liquid base, blusher, powder, powder or cream eyeshadow, eyeliner, eyebrow pencil, mascara, lipstick, cotton pledgets, water, contour makeup, rouge.

Sanitation Supplies and Equipment: Cape, laundered towel, sanitized spatula, makeup cape.

Teaching Aids Needed: Textbook, Workbook, State Board Review Questions, chalkboard, overhead projector, VCR and videotape(s), computer, printer.

Transparency Master: Figure 26.10.

Theory Objectives	***Practical Objectives***
1. Basic cosmetics used on the face. 2. Selecting an appropriate color of foundation (base). 3. Using cosmetics and techniques to correct specific problems. 4. Techniques for applying false (strip) eyelashes and semipermanent lashes (eye tabbing) for tinting lashes and brows. 5. Makeup techniques for black women.	6. Applying makeup for a black client.

Word Review:

epidermal layer	pH	astringent
emollient cream	mascara	eyebrow pencil
cleanser	bar soap	liquid soap
toners	moisturizer	foundation
blusher	lipstick	powder
eye shadow	eyeliners	natural pH
oval shape	round shape	oblong shape
square shape	shadowing effect	protruding
receding	sagging double chin	tweezers
lash and brow tint	eye shields	artificial eyelashes
tabbing	false strip eyelashes	

Answers to End-of-Chapter Questions:

1. It closes them. **2.** Yes. **3.** To outline the eyes. **4.** Cleanser. **5.** An astringent. **6.** An emollient cream. **7.** Eye shadow. **8.** 4.5 to 5.5. **9.** Oval. **10.** A quick movement. **11.** The same direction as hair growth. **12.** No. **13.** Yes. **14.** No.

Special Safety Considerations:

Special practices should be adopted to prevent the spread of bacteria and viruses that may cause disease via eye makeup and lip makeup applied to the skin. Since the students will be working around the orifaces of the eyes, nose, and mouth, only the client's own makeup or that of a freshly opened package should be used.

Theory Objective 1: **Describe the basic cosmetics used on the face.**

Learning Steps	***Resources***
1. Read chapter in textbook. 2. Complete assignment in workbook. 3. View videotape(s). 4. Proceed to next objective.	1. *The Professional Cosmetologist,* 4th ed., ch. 26, pp. 514-516. 2. *Theory and Practical Workbook,* ch. 26, p. 181. 3. Videotape library.

Instructor's Resource Notes: ______________________________

____

Theory Objective 2: **Explain how to select an appropriate color of foundation (base).**

Learning Steps

1. Read chapter in textbook.
2. Complete assignment in workbook.
3. View videotape(s).
4. Proceed to next objective.

Resources

1. *The Professional Cosmetologist*, 4th ed., ch. 26, pp. 516-517.
2. *Theory and Practical Workbook*, ch. 26, p. 182.
3. Videotape library.

Instructor's Resource Notes: ______________________________

____

Theory Objective 3: **Describe the cosmetics and techniques used to enhance facial features and correct specific problems.**

Learning Steps

1. Read chapter in textbook.
2. Complete assignment in workbook.
3. View videotape(s).
4. Proceed to next objective.

Resources

1. *The Professional Cosmetologist*, 4th ed., ch. 26, pp. 517-521.
2. *Theory and Practical Workbook*, ch. 26, p. 183.
3. Videotape library.

Instructor's Resource Notes: ______________________________

____

Theory Objective 4: **Describe the techniques used to apply false (strip) eyelashes and semipermanent lashes (eye tabbing) and to tint lashes and brows.**

Learning Steps

1. Read chapter in textbook.
2. Complete assignment in workbook.
3. View videotape(s).
4. Proceed to next objective.

Resources

1. *The Professional Cosmetologist*, 4th ed., ch. 26, pp. 521-523.
2. *Theory and Practical Workbook*, ch. 26, p. 184.
3. Videotape library.

Instructor's Resource Notes: ______________________________

____

Theory Objective 5: **Describe the basic cosmetics used for black clients.**

Learning Steps

1. Read chapter in textbook.
2. Complete assignment in workbook.
3. View videotape(s).
4. Proceed to next objective.

Resources

1. *The Professional Cosmetologist*, 4th ed., ch. 26, pp. 523-525.
2. *Theory and Practical Workbook*, ch. 26, p. 184.
3. Videotape library.

Instructor's Resource Notes: ______________________________

____

Practical Objective 6: **Apply makeup for a black client.**

Learning Steps

1. Read chapter in textbook.
2. Complete assignment in workbook.
3. View videotape(s).
4. Proceed to next chapter.

Resources

1. *The Professional Cosmetologist*, 4th ed., ch. 26, pp. 525-527.
2. *Theory and Practical Workbook*, ch. 26, p. 184.
3. Videotape library.

Instructor's Resource Notes: ______________________________

____

Evaluation of Instruction:

_____ A. Discussed answers to end of chapter questions.
_____ B. Collected completed workbook assignments.
_____ C. Collected student progress charts.
_____ D. State board sheets current.
_____ E. Answered written test(s), and/or computer test questions.
_____ F. Completed Performance/Product Checklist.

Student Assignments: ______________________________

____

27

Lesson Plan

Nail Anatomy, Disorders, and Diseases

Lesson Overview and Motivation: Students will learn to recognize, describe, and label nail shapes, disorders, diseases, and the main bones of the arm and hand. Recognition of nail disorders and diseases is of particular importance as a preliminary step to the actual manicuring procedures described in the following chapter.

Acceptable Level: Score 85 percent or better on a multiple choice exam.

Location: Theory classroom_____ Lab classroom_____ Clinic_____

Time for Lecture/ Demonstration: 30 min._____ 60 min._____ 90 min._____

Student Level: Beginning_____ Intermediate_____ Advanced_____

Teaching Aids Needed: Textbook, Workbook, State Board Review Questions, chalkboard, overhead projector, VCR and videotape(s), computer, printer.

Transparency Master: Figures 27.2, 27.17, and 27.18.

Theory Objectives

1. Four basic nail shapes, anatomy of the fingernail, its surrounding structures, and nail growth.
2. Nail irregularities.
3. Nail diseases.
4. The main bones of the arm and hand.
5. Disorders and diseases of the feet.

Practical Objectives

None.

Word Review:

appendage
cuticle
nail groove
matrix
onychosis
leukonychia
blue nails
corrugations (furrows)
paronychia (felon)
phalanges
ingrown nails
podiatry
onychocryptosis (ingrown nail)
nail plate
eponychium
nail root
lunula
onychatrophia
onychauxis onyx
eggshell nails
bruised nails
onycholysis (separated nail)
radius
metacarpals
athlete's foot
podiatrist
free edge
nail wall
nail mantle
rate of growth
hangnail
pumice powder
Pterygium
onychomycosis (tinea)
onychogryposis (claw nails)
ulna carpals
callouses
plantar warts

Answers to End-of-Chapter Questions:

1. Free edge. **2.** Hyponychium. **3.** Nail groove. **4.** Matrix. **5.** Yes. **6.** No. **7.** Onychosis. **8.** No. **9.** Onychatrophia. **10.** Yes. **11.** Onychauxis. **12.** No. **13.** Yes. **14.** Carpals. **15.** Callus. **16.** Plantar warts.

Theory Objective 1: **Describe four basic nail shapes, the anatomy of the fingernail, its surrounding structures, and nail growth.**

Learning Steps

1. Read chapter in textbook.
2. Complete assignment in workbook.
3. View videotape(s).
4. Proceed to next objective.

Resources

1. *The Professional Cosmetologist,* 4th ed., ch. 27, pp. 532-534.
2. *Theory and Practical Workbook,* ch. 27, p. 187.
3. Videotape library.

Instructor's Resource Notes: ______________________________

____

Theory Objective 2: **Describe nail irregularities.**

Learning Steps

1. Read chapter in textbook.
2. Complete assignment in workbook.
3. View videotape(s).
4. Proceed to next objective.

Resources

1. *The Professional Cosmetologist,* 4th ed., ch. 27, pp. 534-537.
2. *Theory and Practical Workbook,* ch. 27, p. 189.
3. Videotape library.

Instructor's Resource Notes: ______________________________

____

Theory Objective 3: **Identify nail diseases.**

Learning Steps	*Resources*
1. Read chapter in textbook.	1. *The Professional Cosmetologist*, 4th ed., ch. 27, pp. 537-539.
2. Complete assignment in workbook.	2. *Theory and Practical Workbook*, ch. 27, p. 191.
3. View videotape(s).	3. Videotape library.
4. Proceed to next objective.	

Instructor's Resource Notes: ______________________________

____

Theory Objective 4: **Identify and label the main bones of the arms, hands, feet, and legs.**

Learning Steps	*Resources*
1. Read chapter in textbook.	1. *The Professional Cosmetologist*, 4th ed., ch. 27, p. 539.
2. Complete assignment in workbook.	2. *Theory and Practical Workbook*, ch. 27, p. 192.
3. View videotape(s).	3. Videotape library.
4. Proceed to next objective.	

Instructor's Resource Notes: ______________________________

____

Theory Objective 5: **Describe the disorders and diseases of the feet.**

Learning Steps	*Resources*
1. Read chapter in textbook.	1. *The Professional Cosmetologist*, 4th ed., ch. 27, pp. 539-541.
2. Complete assignment in workbook.	2. *Theory and Practical Workbook*, ch. 27, p. 193.
3. View videotape(s).	3. Videotape library.
4. Proceed to next chapter.	

Instructor's Resource Notes: ______________________________

____

Evaluation of Instruction:

_____ A. Discussed answers to end of chapter questions.
_____ B. Collected completed workbook assignments.
_____ C. Collected student progress charts.
_____ D. State board sheets current.
_____ E. Answered written test(s), and/or computer test questions.
_____ F. Completed Performance/Product Checklist.

Student Assignments: ______________________________

____

28

Lesson Plan

Manicuring and Pedicuring

Lesson Overview and Motivation: Students will learn how to shape and apply polish to the nails, and be able to give special nail services. Because this procedure is applicable to both men and women, students tend to learn the basic procedures quickly. The application of artificial nail and acrylic nails require extensive practice. For the application of new nail products, it may be helpful to invite a guest lecturer to demonstrate for the class.

Due to the adhesive quality of many of the manicuring products used in this service, cleaning/sanitizing of implements, drawers, and table-tops is essential for maintaining a clean and orderly environment for this service. Controlling the spread of bacteria, and exposure to blood products are also considerations when teaching this service.

Acceptable Level: Score 85 percent or better on a multiple choice exam, and complete the performance product checklist for this task.

Give a plain manicure in 25 to 40 minutes, and an oil manicure in 45 to 50 minutes.

Location: Theory classroom_____ Lab classroom_____ Clinic_____

Time for Lecture/ Demonstration: 30 min._____ 60 min._____ 90 min._____

Student Level: Beginning_____ Intermediate_____ Advanced_____

Equipment/Models Needed: Manicure table, cosmetologist's chair, client's chair, hot-oil heater, closed cotton container, manicure tray, small glass implement container, two foot-bath containers.

Supplies Needed: Finger bowl, two new emery boards, metal pusher, manicure scissors, buffer, orangewood stick, cuticle nippers and scissors, nail brush, spatula, a fresh paper cup for hot-oil heater, cotton, cuticle softener, cuticle remover (solvent), base coat, sealer (top coat), hand lotion or creme, absorbent tissue, enamel thinner, enamel remover, nail builder, nail enamel, aerosol enamel dry (or powder or paste) nail polish, manicure oil, pumice powder, fast-drying glue, linen or silk wrapping fiber, nail forms or tips, brush, round nail file/buffer, acrylic nail kit, toenail clipper, nail massage cream, moisturizing cream, moisturizing lotion, protective gloves (for control of infection should bleeding of finger(s) occur).

Sanitation Supplies and Equipment: Sanitized towels, disposable plastic bag, 70 percent alcohol, soap, anti-fungus nail solution, antiseptic/disinfectant for feet.

Teaching Aids Needed: Textbook, Workbook, State Board Review Questions, chalkboard, overhead projector, VCR and videotape(s), computer, printer. Artificial, rubber-like hands and counter-top clamps are helpful for providing initial practice for students.

Transparency Master: Figures 28.18 and 28.24.

Theory Objectives

1. Different nail services and when they are given.

Practical Objectives

2. Giving a plain or oil manicure (including hand and arm massage).
3. Giving a nail wrap.
4. Applying different types of artificial nails.
5. Giving a sculptured nail repair and fills.
6. Giving a pedicure.

Word Review:

oil manicure	regular manicure	sculptured nails
nail tips	nail caps	nail shells
flammable materials	Acetone	acrylic sculptured nails

Answers to End-of-Chapter Questions:

1. Manicuring. **2.** Pedicuring. **3.** False. **4.** Yes. **5.** No; strengthen it. **6.** No. **7.** Yes. **8.** Yes. **9.** Yes. **10.** Yes. **11.** Yes. **12.** No. **13.** Yes. **14.** No; remove all polish from cuticle. **15.** Yes. **16.** No. **17.** Yes. **18.** Yes. **19.** Yes. **20.** False. **21.** No; cotton. **22.** Yes.

Special Safety Considerations:

Since nail polish removers , enamel drying spray chemicals, and adhesives are flammable, advise students to avoid excess heat, or open flame when using these products. Wash hands before and after service.

Cleaning of table tops is essential to remove nail adhesives, and artificial nail sealers, etc. Disposal of used supplies, such as cotton balls and emery boards, and proper storage of nail supplies are important.

Theory Objective 1: **Identify different nail services and explain when they are given.**

Learning Steps

1. Read chapter in textbook.
2. Complete assignment in workbook.
3. View videotape(s).
4. Proceed to next objective.

Resources

1. *The Professional Cosmetologist*, 4th ed., ch. 28, pp. 548-549.
2. *Theory and Practical Workbook*, ch. 28, p. 195.
3. Videotape library.

Instructor's Resource Notes: ______________________________

____

Practical Objective 2: **Give a plain or oil manicure (including hand and arm massage).**

Learning Steps

1. Read chapter in textbook.
2. Complete assignment in workbook.
3. View videotape(s).
4. Proceed to next objective.

Resources

1. *The Professional Cosmetologist*, 4th ed., ch. 28, pp. 549-560.
2. *Theory and Practical Workbook*, ch. 28, p. 197.
3. Videotape library.

Instructor's Resource Notes: ______________________________

____

Practical Objective 3: **Give a nail wrap.**

Learning Steps

1. Read chapter in textbook.
2. Complete assignment in workbook.
3. View videotape(s).
4. Proceed to next objective.

Resources

1. *The Professional Cosmetologist*, 4th ed., ch. 28, pp. 560-562.
2. *Theory and Practical Workbook*, ch. 28, p. 198.
3. Videotape library.

Instructor's Resource Notes: ______________________________

____

Practical Objective 4: **Apply different types of artificial nails.**

Learning Steps

1. Read chapter in textbook.
2. Complete assignment in workbook.
3. View videotape(s).
4. Proceed to next objective.

Resources

1. *The Professional Cosmetologist*, 4th ed., ch. 28, pp. 563-564.
2. *Theory and Practical Workbook*, ch. 28, p. 199.
3. Videotape library.

Instructor's Resource Notes: ______________________________

____

Practical Objective 5: **Give a sculptured nail repair with fills.**

Learning Steps

1. Read chapter in textbook.
2. Complete assignment in workbook.
3. View videotape(s).
4. Proceed to next objective.

Resources

1. *The Professional Cosmetologist*, 4th ed., ch. 28, pp. 564-566.
2. *Theory and Practical Workbook*, ch. 28, p. 199.
3. Videotape library.

Instructor's Resource Notes: ______________________________

____

Practical Objective 6: **Give a pedicure.**

Learning Steps

1. Read chapter in textbook.
2. Complete assignment in workbook.
3. View videotape(s).
4. Proceed to next chapter.

Resources

1. *The Professional Cosmetologist*, 4th ed., ch. 28, pp. 566-569.
2. *Theory and Practical Workbook*, ch. 28, p. 200.
3. Videotape library.

Instructor's Resource Notes: ______________________________

____

Evaluation of Instruction:

_____ A. Discussed answers to end of chapter questions.
_____ B. Collected completed workbook assignments.
_____ C. Collected student progress charts.
_____ D. State board sheets current.
_____ E. Answered written test(s), and/or computer test questions.
_____ F. Completed Performance/Product Checklist.

Student Assignments: ____

____

29

Lesson Plan
Wigs and Hairpieces

Lesson Overview and Motivation: Using professional wiggery supplies and implements, students will learn how to fit, shape, clean, set, and style a wig and hairpiece.

Acceptable Level: Score 85 percent or better on a multiple choice exam, and complete the performance product checklist for this task.
Clean a wig within 20 minutes, set it within 25 minutes, and comb it out within 20 minutes. Clean a hairpiece within 15 minutes, set it in 10 to 20 minutes, and comb it into the client's hair in 15 to 30 minutes.

Location: Theory classroom_____ Lab classroom_____ Clinic_____

Time for Lecture/ Demonstration: 30 min._____ 60 min._____ 90 min._____

Student Level: Beginning_____ Intermediate_____ Advanced_____

Equipment/Models Needed: Client release form, canvas block and clamp, glass bowl, pencil, tape measure.

Supplies Needed: Wig dry cleaner or shampoo, T-pins, styling comb, wig brush, rollers, clips, styling lotion, conditioner.

Sanitation Supplies and Equipment: Plastic cover, 2 towels, protective gloves.

Teaching Aids Needed: Textbook, Workbook, State Board Review Questions, chalkboard, overhead projector, VCR and videotape(s), computer, printer.

Theory Objectives	Practical Objectives
1. Types of wigs and hairpieces and their construction, coloring, and styling. 2. Measuring and altering wigs.	None.

Word Review:

cascade	chignon	fall
hand-tied	JL color ring	postiche
switches	synthetic fibers	toupee
weft	wig	wiggery
wiglet	yak hair	canvas block
wig block	wig clamp	T-pins
plastic bag		

Answers to End-of-Chapter Questions:

1. A special dry cleaning fluid for wigs. **2.** Material to which hair is sewn in a wig or hairpiece. **3.** A toupee covers only part of the scalp, and a wig usually covers the entire scalp. **4.** Yes.

Special Safety Considerations:

If a dry cleaning type of cleanser is used, follow label directions for fire hazard. It is necessary that the student be able to determine whether the wig or hairpiece they are servicing is human or artificial hair.

Theory Objective 1:

Describe the various types of wigs and hairpieces, and explain how they are made, colored, and styled.

Learning Steps

1. Read chapter in textbook.
2. Complete assignment in workbook.
3. View videotape(s).
4. Proceed to next objective.

Resources

1. *The Professional Cosmetologist*, 4th ed., ch. 29, pp. 574-577.
2. *Theory and Practical Workbook*, ch. 29, p. 203.
3. Videotape library.

Instructor's Resource Notes:

____

____

Theory Objective 2:

Explain how wigs are measured and altered.

Learning Steps

1. Read chapter in textbook.
2. Complete assignment in workbook.
3. View videotape(s).
4. Proceed to next chapter.

Resources

1. *The Professional Cosmetologist*, 4th ed., ch. 29, pp. 577-580.
2. *Theory and Practical Workbook*, ch. 29, p. 204.
3. Videotape library.

Instructor's Resource Notes: ____

____

Evaluation of Instruction:

_____ A. Discussed answers to end of chapter questions.
_____ B. Collected completed workbook assignments.
_____ C. Collected student progress charts.
_____ D. State board sheets current.
_____ E. Answered written test(s), and/or computer test questions.

Student Assignments: ____

____

30

Lesson Plan

Shaving

Lesson Overview and Motivation: Because so many beauty and barber regulatory agencies have been combined, the introduction of shaving has been included. Except for the basic shaving procedure, the primary concern in this chapter is control of disease should the client be cut with the razor - resulting in the student being exposed to blood, which could spread the HIV virus.

Acceptable Level: Score 85 percent or better on a multiple choice exam.

Location: Theory classroom_____ Lab classroom_____ Clinic_____

Time for Lecture/ Demonstration: 30 min._____ 60 min._____ 90 min._____

Student Level: Beginning_____ Intermediate_____ Advanced_____

Equipment/Models Needed: Latherizing machine, razor (straight, or disposable), strop, stone, barber chair, shampoo bowl.

Supplies Needed: Neck and face towels.

Sanitation Supplies and Equipment: Antiseptic, cotton swabs.

Teaching Aids Needed: Textbook, Workbook, State Board Review Questions, chalkboard, overhead projector, VCR and videotape(s), computer, printer.

Theory Objectives

1. Shaving supplies, implements, and equipment.
2. Shaving safety precautions.

Practical Objectives

3. Shaving the client.

Word Review:

electric latherizer	barber chair	lather
straight razor	razor's balance	point of the razor
hone	strop	

Answers to End-of-Chapter Questions:

1. Latherizer. **2.** Softens the hair; provides a protective surface. **3.** Razor balance. **4.** Hone and strop. **5.** Coarse. **6.** Irritated or diseased skin. **7.** No. **8.** Adam's apple. **9.** Put on rubber gloves; observe other precautions detailed in the discussion of sanitation in Chapter 3. **10.** Antiseptic and styptic powder.

Special Safety Considerations:

Whenever there is the possibility of exposure to blood, it is important that the student know Infection Control procedures described in the Sanitation chapter of the textbook. The student needs to be particularly careful when using the razor because any incorrect movement may result in the cutting of the client's skin.

Theory Objective 1: **Describe the supplies, implements, and equipment used in shaving.**

Learning Steps	*Resources*
1. Read chapter in textbook.	1. *The Professional Cosmetologist*, 4th ed., ch. 30, pp. 584-586.
2. Complete assignment in workbook.	2. *Theory and Practical Workbook*, ch. 30, p. 207.
3. View videotape(s).	3. Videotape library.
4. Proceed to next objective.	

Instructor's Resource Notes: ______________________________

____

Theory Objective 2: **Identify shaving safety precautions.**

Learning Steps	*Resources*
1. Read chapter in textbook.	1. *The Professional Cosmetologist*, 4th ed., ch. 30, pp. 586-587.
2. Complete assignment in workbook.	2. *Theory and Practical Workbook*, ch. 30, p. 208.
3. View videotape(s).	3. Videotape library.
4. Proceed to next objective.	

Instructor's Resource Notes: ______________________________

____

Practical Objective 3: **Shave the client.**

Learning Steps

1. Read chapter in textbook.
2. Complete assignment in workbook.
3. View videotape(s).
4. Proceed to next chapter.

Resources

1. *The Professional Cosmetologist,* 4th ed., ch. 30, pp. 587-590.
2. *Theory and Practical Workbook,* ch. 30, p. 210.
3. Videotape library.

Instructor's Resource Notes: ______________________________

____

Evaluation of Instruction:

_____ A. Discussed answers to end of chapter questions.
_____ B. Collected completed workbook assignments.
_____ C. Collected student progress charts.
_____ D. State board sheets current.
_____ E. Answered written test(s), and/or computer test questions.

Student Assignments: ______________________________

____

31

Lesson Plan

Planning a Salon

Lesson Overview and Motivation: Students will be able to describe the basic principles needed to plan a salon as a successful business. Since we are teaching the student how to perform skills for making a living, it also seems logical to provide information that will enhance their chances for success. The information in this chapter will not only assist the student that intends to open their own salon, but give an appreciation of what is involved in opening a business to the student planning to work for someone else.

Acceptable Level: Score 85 percent or better on a multiple choice exam.

Location: Theory classroom_____ Lab classroom_____ Clinic_____

Time for Lecture/ Demonstration: 30 min._____ 60 min._____ 90 min._____

Student Level: Beginning_____ Intermediate_____ Advanced_____

Teaching Aids Needed: Textbook, Workbook, State Board Review Questions, chalkboard, overhead projector, VCR and videotape(s), computer, printer.

Transparency Master: Figure 31.3.

Theory Objectives

1 Basic forms of business ownership.
2. Selecting a good salon site and building.
3. Negotiating a salon lease.
4. Salon insurance needs.
5. Importance of the salon reception area.
6. Retailing in the salon.

Practical Objectives

None.

Word Review:

sole proprietorship	partnership	corporation
profits	liabilities	shareholders
population density	socioeconomic factors	accessibility
surrounding businesses	gross income	fixed costs
percentage rents	variable costs	lease
lessor	lessee	long-term lease
form lease	lease amendments	tax escalator clause
liability insurance	malpractice insurance	long-term lease
competitive price	retailing	private label

Answers to End-of-Chapter Questions:

1. A partnership. **2.** No. **3.** Yes. **4.** Yes. **5.** False. **6.** Ordinances. **7.** The income level of families in a certain area. **8.** No. **9.** No; remain the same or increase. **10.** Lessee. **11.** Lessor. **12.** Lease. **13.** Yes. **14.** No. **15.** False. **16.** Liability insurance. **17.** Malpractice insurance. **18.** Receptionist.

Theory Objective 1: **Identify the basic forms of business ownership.**

Learning Steps

1. Read chapter in textbook.
2. Complete assignment in workbook.
3. View videotape(s).
4. Proceed to next objective.

Resources

1. *The Professional Cosmetologist,* 4th ed., ch. 31, pp. 594-595.
2. *Theory and Practical Workbook,* ch. 31, p. 211.
3. Videotape library.

Instructor's Resource Notes: ______________________________

____

Theory Objective 2: **Explain how to select a good salon site and building.**

Learning Steps

1. Read chapter in textbook.
2. Complete assignment in workbook.
3. View videotape(s).
4. Proceed to next objective.

Resources

1. *The Professional Cosmetologist,* 4th ed., ch. 31, pp. 596-598.
2. *Theory and Practical Workbook,* ch. 31, p. 213.
3. Videotape library.

Instructor's Resource Notes: ______________________________

____

Theory Objective 3: **List points to consider in negotiating a salon lease.**

Learning Steps

1. Read chapter in textbook.
2. Complete assignment in workbook.
3. View videotape(s).
4. Proceed to next objective.

Resources

1. *The Professional Cosmetologist*, 4th ed., ch. 31, pp. 598-600.
2. *Theory and Practical Workbook*, ch. 31, p. 215.
3. Videotape library.

Instructor's Resource Notes: ______________________________

____

Theory Objective 4: **Identify salon insurance needs.**

Learning Steps

1. Read chapter in textbook.
2. Complete assignment in workbook.
3. View videotape(s).
4. Proceed to next objective.

Resources

1. *The Professional Cosmetologist*, 4th ed., ch. 31, p. 600.
2. *Theory and Practical Workbook*, ch. 31, p. 217.
3. Videotape library.

Instructor's Resource Notes: ______________________________

____

Theory Objective 5: **Describe the importance of the salon reception area.**

Learning Steps

1. Read chapter in textbook.
2. Complete assignment in workbook.
3. View videotape(s).
4. Proceed to next objective.

Resources

1. *The Professional Cosmetologist*, 4th ed., ch. 31, pp. 600-601.
2. *Theory and Practical Workbook*, ch. 31, p. 217.
3. Videotape library.

Instructor's Resource Notes: ______________________________

____

Theory Objective 6: **Explain the importance of retailing in the salon.**

Learning Steps	*Resources*
1. Read chapter in textbook.	1. *The Professional Cosmetologist,* 4th ed., ch. 31, pp. 601-602.
2. Complete assignment in workbook.	2. *Theory and Practical Workbook,* ch. 31, p. 217.
3. View videotape(s).	3. Videotape library.
4. Proceed to next chapter.	

Instructor's Resource Notes: ______________________________

____

Evaluation of Instruction:

_____ A. Discussed answers to end of chapter questions.
_____ B. Collected completed workbook assignments.
_____ C. Collected student progress charts.
_____ D. State board sheets current.
_____ E. Answered written test(s), and/or computer test questions.

Student Assignments: ______________________________

____

32

Lesson Plan
Salon Operations

Lesson Overview and Motivation: Students will be able to describe the basic principles involved in the operation of a salon. This chapter should provide you with an opportunity to involve the student in the operation of the school to the extent that the student can learn about ordering products, inventory control, and operating the appointment desk.
Topics, such as, booth rental should also be discussed while teaching this subject.
These are some of the tasks that they will be performing when working in a beauty salon.

Acceptable Level: Score 85 percent or better on a multiple choice exam.

Location: Theory classroom_____ Lab classroom_____ Clinic_____

Time for Lecture/ Demonstration: 30 min._____ 60 min._____ 90 min._____

Student Level: Beginning_____ Intermediate_____ Advanced_____

Teaching Aids Needed: Textbook, Theory and Practical Workbook, State Board Review Questions, chalkboard, overhead projector, VCR. This is an opportune time to address issues and practices such as inventory control, and working at the appointment/reception/retail desk. A guest lecturer may also be helpful to emphasize certain business practices.

Transparency Master: Table 32.1 and 32.2.

Theory Objectives	*Practical Objectives*
1. Purchasing salon equipment and supplies.	None.
2. Developing salon operating policies and interviewing prospective employees.	
3. Salon operating costs.	
4. Client supply charge system.	
5. Basic accounting principles and taxation.	
6. Advantages of accepting credit cards.	
7. Booth rental system.	

Word Review:

request for bids	installment plan	service charges
balloon clause	consumable supplies	product duplication
invoice	statement	operating policies
job interview	applicant	seminars
fixed costs	variable costs	commission
client supply charge system	service charge	assets
liabilities	proprietorship	income statement
net income	gross income	Tax acts
payroll deductions	FUTA	SUTA
FICA	tips	Workman's Compensation
Basic accounting equation	credit card	credit check
Booth rental system		

Answers to End-of-Chapter Questions:

1. Operating (consumable) supplies. **2.** 8 percent. **3.** Salesperson. **4.** Yes. **5.** False; on the invoice. **6.** No; 90 days. **7.** Yes. **8.** No; 15 minutes early. **9.** No. **10.** False; on or before the appointment. **11.** No. **12.** No. **13.** Remain the same. **14.** Economics. **15.** Yes. **16.** Yes. **17.** True. **18.** FUTA, SUTA and FICA. **19.** An equal percentage. **20.** True. **21.** (a) Renter does not have to follow salon policies; (b) salon equipment gets additional use. See the material in the chapter for other disadvantages.

Theory Objective 1: **Explain the factors to be considered in purchasing salon equipment and supplies.**

Learning Steps	*Resources*
1. Read chapter in textbook.	1. *The Professional Cosmetologist*, 4th ed., ch. 32, pp. 606-610.
2. Complete assignment in workbook.	2. *Theory and Practical Workbook*, ch. 32, p. 221.
3. View videotape(s).	3. Videotape library.
4. Proceed to next objective.	

Instructor's Resource Notes: ______________________________

____

Theory Objective 2: **Identify the considerations involved in developing salon operating policies, and describe the techniques used in interviewing prospective employees.**

Learning Steps

1. Read chapter in textbook.
2. Complete assignment in workbook.
3. View videotape(s).
4. Proceed to next objective.

Resources

1. *The Professional Cosmetologist,* 4th ed., ch. 32, pp. 610-612.
2. *Theory and Practical Workbook,* ch. 32, p. 224.
3. Videotape library.

Instructor's Resource Notes: ______________________________

____

Theory Objective 3: **Describe how the salon's operating costs are computed.**

Learning Steps

1. Read chapter in textbook.
2. Complete assignment in workbook.
3. View videotape(s).
4. Proceed to next objective.

Resources

1. *The Professional Cosmetologist,* 4th ed., ch. 32, pp. 612-614.
2. *Theory and Practical Workbook,* ch. 32, p. 225.
3. Videotape library.

Instructor's Resource Notes: ______________________________

____

Theory Objective 4: **Explain the client supply charge system.**

Learning Steps

1. Read chapter in textbook.
2. Complete assignment in workbook.
3. View videotape(s).
4. Proceed to next objective.

Resources

1. *The Professional Cosmetologist,* 4th ed., ch. 32, pp. 614-615.
2. *Theory and Practical Workbook,* ch. 32, p. 226.
3. Videotape library.

Instructor's Resource Notes: ____

____

Theory Objective 5: **Explain basic accounting and taxation principles.**

Learning Steps

1. Read chapter in textbook.
2. Complete assignment in workbook.
3. View videotape(s).
4. Proceed to next objective.

Resources

1. *The Professional Cosmetologist,* 4th ed., ch. 32, pp. 616-620.
2. *Theory and Practical Workbook,* ch. 32, p. 226.
3. Videotape library.

Instructor's Resource Notes: ____

____

Theory Objective 6: **List the advantages of accepting credit cards.**

Learning Steps

1. Read chapter in textbook.
2. Complete assignment in workbook.
3. View videotape(s).
4. Proceed to next objective.

Resources

1. *The Professional Cosmetologist,* 4th ed., ch. 32, pp. 620-621.
2. *Theory and Practical Workbook,* ch. 32, p. 229.
3. Videotape library.

Instructor's Resource Notes: ____

____

Theory Objective 7: **Explain the booth rental system.**

Learning Steps

1. Read chapter in textbook.
2. Complete assignment in workbook.
3. View videotape(s).
4. Proceed to next chapter.

Resources

1. *The Professional Cosmetologist,* 4th ed., ch. 32, pp. 621-622.
2. *Theory and Practical Workbook,* ch. 32, p. 230.
3. Videotape library.

Instructor's Resource Notes: ____

____

Evaluation of Instruction:

_____ A. Discussed answers to end of chapter questions.
_____ B. Collected completed workbook assignments.
_____ C. Collected student progress charts.
_____ D. State board sheets current.
_____ E. Answered written test(s), and/or computer test questions.

Student Assignments: ____

____

33

Lesson Plan

The Psychology of Interpersonal Skills and Retailing

Lesson Overview and Motivation: Since most stylists are required to "sell" products to their clients in addition to hairstyling services, this chapter provides some proven methods for teaching students how to interact with their clients and sell them products that they would normally purchase anyway.

Acceptable Level: Score 85 percent or better on a multiple choice exam.

Location: Theory classroom_____ Lab classroom_____ Clinic_____

Time for Lecture/ Demonstration: 30 min._____ 60 min._____ 90 min._____

Student Level: Beginning_____ Intermediate_____ Advanced_____

Theory Objectives

1. Developing successful salon communications.
2. Using psychology to develop communication strategies and salon sales.
3. Four income-producing strategies.

Practical Objectives

4. Recognizing and using effective client-handling techniques.

Word Review:

rapport
salesperson
non-verbal communication
discovery process
extra services
referrals
client handling
verbal communication
the "look"
consulting
bonding
"Big Four" income strategies
fear of rejection
extra-verbal communication
bonding
full book
client retention
client handling

Answers to End-of-Chapter Questions: **1.** Rapport (a set of common thoughts and a comfortable style of communicating). **2.** Client-handling skills. **3.** Salesperson. **4.** Rejection. **5.** By realizing that the client is not rejecting you as a person. **6.** Clients are afraid to ask or don't know that the products and services are available in your salon. **7.** How you communicate. **8.** The "look" they want to achieve. **9.** Verbally, extra-verbally through the tone and quality of your voice, and nonverbally through your body movements. **10.** Interpersonal communications. **11.** 60 percent. **12.** Becoming sincerely interested in and wanting to help the client. **13.** The positive emotional connection between you and the client. **14.** Employ the strategy of discovery. **15.** Consultation. **16.** Ask the client. **17.** Make a follow-up phone call. **18.** Full book. **19.** Extra services. **20.** Products sold in the salon are generally of higher quality. **21.** Referral. **22.** Advertising and promotions by the salon. **23.** 4 to 6 percent. **24.** Client retention. **25.** Client-handling techniques.

Theory Objective 1: **Understand the process for developing successful salon communications.**

Learning Steps

1. Read chapter in textbook.
2. Complete assignment in workbook.
3. View videotape(s).
4. Proceed to next objective.

Resources

1. *The Professional Cosmetologist,* 4th ed., ch. 33, pp. 628-631.
2. *Theory and Practical Workbook,* ch. 33, p. 233.
3. Videotape library.

Instructor's Resource Notes: ______________________________

____

Theory Objective 2: **Use psychology to develop communication strategies and improve salon sales.**

Learning Steps

1. Read chapter in textbook.
2. Complete assignment in workbook.
3. View videotape(s).
4. Proceed to next objective.

Resources

1. *The Professional Cosmetologist,* 4th ed., ch. 33, pp. 631-633.
2. *Theory and Practical Workbook,* ch. 33, p. 235.
3. Videotape library.

Instructor's Resource Notes: ____________________

____

Theory Objective 3: **Identify four income-producing strategies.**

Learning Steps	*Resources*
1. Read chapter in textbook.	1. *The Professional Cosmetologist,* 4th ed., ch. 33, pp. 633-636.
2. Complete assignment in workbook.	2. *Theory and Practical Workbook,* ch. 33, p. 236.
3. View videotape(s).	3. Videotape library.
4. Proceed to next objective.	

Instructor's Resource Notes: ____________________

____

Practical Objective 4: **Recognize and use effective client-handling techniques.**

Learning Steps	*Resources*
1. Read chapter in textbook.	1. *The Professional Cosmetologist,* 4th ed., ch. 33, pp. 636-639.
2. Complete assignment in workbook.	2. Videotape library.
3. View videotape(s).	
4. Proceed to next chapter.	

Instructor's Resource Notes: ____________________

____

Evaluation of Instruction:

_____ A. Discussed answers to end of chapter questions.
_____ B. Collected completed workbook assignments.
_____ C. Collected student progress charts.
_____ D. State board sheets current.
_____ E. Answered written test(s), and/or computer test questions.

Student Assignments: ____________________

____

Lesson Plan 34

Principles of Electricity

Lesson Overview and Motivation: Students will be able to define and describe professional electrical terms in cosmetology. Because the science of electricity is relatively complex, where you place the emphasis with respect to what the student needs to know is somewhat arbitrary. You may choose to cover the basics of electricity and include the use of the high-frequency facial unit, or offer a more comprehensive course.

Acceptable Level: Score 85 percent or better on a multiple choice exam.

Location: Theory classroom_____ Lab classroom_____ Clinic_____

Time for Lecture/ Demonstration: 30 min._____ 60 min._____ 90 min._____

Student Level: Beginning_____ Intermediate_____ Advanced_____

Equipment/Models Needed: High-frequency unit, 1 glass-rake electrode (indirect treatment), or 1 glass-rod electrode attachment (indirect treatment), timer.

Supplies Needed: Protective cape.

Sanitation Supplies and Equipment: Sanitized towels or neck strips.

Teaching Aids Needed: High-frequency machine and glass electrodes.

Theory Objectives

1. Basic electrical concepts.
2. Producing and controlling electricity.
3. Types of electrotherapy.
4. Electrolysis and thermolysis (diathermy).
5. Benefits of a high-frequency scalp treatment.

Practical Objectives

6. High-frequency scalp treatment.

Word Review:

voltage	current	resistance
wattage	ohm	ampere (amp)
110 volt	220 volt	electron
insulator	alternating current	60 Hz
dry cell	wet cell	generator
rectifier	thermocouple	photocell
fuse	circuit breaker	electrotherapy
faradic therapy	galvanic therapy	sinusoidal therapy
"wall plate"	phoresis	anaphoresis
cataphoresis	electrodes	cathode
anode	acidic reaction	direct method
indirect method	induced current	Tesla current
nitrous oxide	alkaline electrotherapy	thermolysis
ozone	electrolysis	blend (or dual) method
diathermy	sodium hydroxide	high-frequency therapy
low-frequency galvanic current	"inactive" and "active" electrodes	electro-suction-cup treatment

Answers to End-of-Chapter Questions:

1. Volt. **2.** Yes. **3.** Alternating current. **4.** Yes. **5.** Nucleus. **6.** Electron. **7.** Resistance. **8.** Transformer. **9.** Fuse; circuit breaker. **10.** Direct current. **11.** Yes. **12.** Anode. **13.** Cathode. **14.** Phoresis. **15.** Yes. **16.** Yes. **17.** Yes. **18.** No, "0.". **19.** Yes. **20.** Yes. **21.** Yes. **22.** Compare your answer to the information in the chapter. **23.** No, Tesla current. **24.** Yes. **25.** No, electrolysis. **26.** Yes. **27.** Yes. **28.** Yes. **29.** True. **30.** False.

Special Safety Considerations:

Be sure to keep electrodes sanitized. Demonstration and student practice will allow the individual student to become comfortable using the high frequency unit. Advise student to establish contact with the finger on the client's scalp before applying the high frequency electrode to the client's scalp.

Theory Objective 1: **Explain basic electrical concepts.**

Learning Steps	*Resources*
1. Read chapter in textbook.	1. *The Professional Cosmetologist*, 4th ed., ch. 34, pp. 644-649.
2. Complete assignment in workbook.	2. *Theory and Practical Workbook*, ch. 34, p. 239.
3. View videotape(s).	3. Videotape library.
4. Proceed to next objective.	

Instructor's Resource Notes: ______________________________

____

Theory Objective 2: **Explain how electricity is produced and controlled.**

Learning Steps	Resources
1. Read chapter in textbook.	1. *The Professional Cosmetologist*, 4th ed., ch. 34, pp. 649-652.
2. Complete assignment in workbook.	2. *Theory and Practical Workbook*, ch. 34, p. 241.
3. View videotape(s).	3. Videotape library.
4. Proceed to next objective.	

Instructor's Resource Notes: ____

____

Theory Objective 3: **Describe the types of electrotherapy and the precautions needed when using it.**

Learning Steps	Resources
1. Read chapter in textbook.	1. *The Professional Cosmetologist*, 4th ed., ch. 34, pp. 653-660.
2. Complete assignment in workbook.	2. *Theory and Practical Workbook*, ch. 34, p. 242.
3. View videotape(s).	3. Videotape library.
4. Proceed to next objective.	

Instructor's Resource Notes: ____

____

Theory Objective 4: **Describe the processes of electrolysis and thermolysis (diathermy).**

Learning Steps	Resources
1. Read chapter in textbook.	1. *The Professional Cosmetologist*, 4th ed., ch. 34, pp. 660-662.
2. Complete assignment in workbook.	2. *Theory and Practical Workbook*, ch. 34, p. 247.
3. View videotape(s).	3. Videotape library.
4. Proceed to next objective.	

Instructor's Resource Notes: ____

____

Theory Objective 5: **Describe the benefits of a high-frequency scalp treatment.**

Learning Steps	*Resources*
1. Read chapter in textbook.	1. *The Professional Cosmetologist*, 4th ed., ch. 34, pp. 662-663.
2. Complete assignment in workbook.	2. *Theory and Practical Workbook*, ch. 34, p. 248.
3. View videotape(s).	3. Videotape library.
4. Proceed to next objective.	

Instructor's Resource Notes: ______________________________

____

Practical Objective 6: **Give a high-frequency scalp treatment.**

Learning Steps	*Resources*
1. Read chapter in textbook.	1. *The Professional Cosmetologist*, 4th ed., ch. 34, pp. 663-665.
2. Complete assignment in workbook.	2. Videotape library.
3. View videotape(s).	
4. Proceed to next chapter.	

Instructor's Resource Notes: ______________________________

____

Evaluation of Instruction:

_____ A. Discussed answers to end of chapter questions.
_____ B. Collected completed workbook assignments.
_____ C. Collected student progress charts.
_____ D. State board sheets current.
_____ E. Answered written test(s), and/or computer test questions.

Student Assignments: ______________________________

____

35

Lesson Plan

Chemistry of Cosmetology

Lesson Overview and Motivation: Students will be able to describe, define, and identify the basic principles of chemistry related to the practice of cosmetology. Since chemistry related to a particular service has be included in the chapter for that service, this chapter is a general overview of some general chemistry concepts. At the end of this section you will note a listing of potentially hazardous chemicals used in the salon. It is located here to provide rationale for adequate ventilation laws promulgated by state boards and agencies of cosmetology.

Acceptable Level: Score 85 percent or better on a multiple choice exam.

Location: Theory classroom_____ Lab classroom_____ Clinic_____

Time for Lecture/ Demonstration: 30 min._____ 60 min._____ 90 min._____

Student Level: Beginning_____ Intermediate_____ Advanced_____

Teaching Aids Needed: Textbook, Theory and Practical Workbook, State Board Review Questions, chalkboard, overhead projector, VCR. Listing of chemicals used in the salon

Transparency Master: Figures 35.4 and 35.5.

Theory Objectives

1. Matter, substance, and organic and inorganic chemistry, and the ways matter can be changed.
2. Elements, compounds, atoms, ions, and molecules.
3. Physical and chemical properties.
4. Kinds of mixtures: solutions, colloids, and suspensions.
5. Acids, bases, salts and pH.

Practical Objectives

None.

Word Review:

matter
inorganic chemistry
physical changes
element
electron
chemical properties
mixture
suspension
saturated solution
liquid emulsion
hydroxyl ions
forms of matter
substances
chemical changes
proton
ion
synthesis
solution
solute
colloidal particle
emulsifying agent
litmus papers
organic chemistry
antioxidants
compound
neutron
physical properties
decomposition
colloid
solvent
dispersing medium
hydrogen ions
neutralization

Answers to End-of-Chapter Questions:

1. Matter. **2.** Inorganic. **3.** Organic. **4.** Chemistry. **5.** Yes. **6.** A compound. **7.** Chemistry. **8.** Yes. **9.** No; indefinite shape. **10.** True. **11.** Yes. **12.** A compound. **13.** Atom. **14.** Protons, electrons, and neutrons. **15.** True. **16.** True. **17.** Water, acetone, alcohol, glycerine. **18.** Yes. **19.** Yes.

Special Safety Considerations:

Most of the related chemistry is included in the respective chapter where the information would normally be useful. This is a separate chapter to cover some other chemistry topics.

Following the objective is a listing of some of the effects of various chemicals used in beauty products. This should be helpful in emphasizing the need for proper ventilation in the beauty salons and beauty schools.

Theory Objective 1:

Define matter, substance, and organic and inorganic chemistry, and explain how matter can be changed.

Learning Steps	Resources
1. Read chapter in textbook.	1. *The Professional Cosmetologist*, 4th ed., ch. 35, pp. 672-675.
2. Complete assignment in workbook.	2. *Theory and Practical Workbook*, ch. 35, p. 249.
3. View videotape(s).	3. Videotape library.
4. Proceed to next objective.	

Instructor's Resource Notes:

___

___

Theory Objective 2: **Explain what elements, compounds, atoms, ions, and molecules are.**

Learning Steps	*Resources*
1. Read chapter in textbook.	1. *The Professional Cosmetologist,* 4th ed., ch. 35, pp. 675-678.
2. Complete assignment in workbook.	2. *Theory and Practical Workbook,* ch. 35, p. 250.
3. View videotape(s).	3. Videotape library.
4. Proceed to next objective.	

Instructor's Resource Notes: ______________________________

____

Theory Objective 3: **Define physical and chemical properties.**

Learning Steps	*Resources*
1. Read chapter in textbook.	1. *The Professional Cosmetologist,* 4th ed., ch. 35, pp. 678-679.
2. Complete assignment in workbook.	2. *Theory and Practical Workbook,* ch. 35, p. 252.
3. View videotape(s).	3. Videotape library.
4. Proceed to next objective.	

Instructor's Resource Notes: ______________________________

____

Theory Objective 4: **Identify and describe the kinds of mixtures: solutions, colloids, and suspensions.**

Learning Steps	*Resources*
1. Read chapter in textbook.	1. *The Professional Cosmetologist,* 4th ed., ch. 35, pp. 679-681.
2. Complete assignment in workbook.	2. *Theory and Practical Workbook,* ch. 35, p. 252.
3. View videotape(s).	3. Videotape library.
4. Proceed to next objective.	

Instructor's Resource Notes: ______________________________

____

Theory Objective 5: **Describe acids, bases, salts and pH.**

Learning Steps	*Resources*
1. Read chapter in textbook.	1. *The Professional Cosmetologist*, 4th ed., ch. 35, pp. 681-682.
2. Complete assignment in workbook.	2. *Theory and Practical Workbook*, ch. 35, p. 254.
3. View videotape(s).	3. Videotape library.
4. Proceed to next chapter.	

Instructor's Resource Notes: ______________________________

____

Evaluation of Instruction:

_____ A. Discussed answers to end of chapter questions.
_____ B. Collected completed workbook assignments.
_____ C. Collected student progress charts.
_____ D. State board sheets current.
_____ E. Answered written test(s), and/or computer test questions.

Student Assignments: ______________________________

____

Source materials	Chemical name	Concentration	Comments
Oxidizing materials (trace)	ACETIC ACID	10 ppm*	Mild eye and skin irritant
Nail glue remover Polish remover Nail sterilizer Brush cleaner	ACETONE	1000 ppm	Fire danger; skin & throat irritant; headache.
Bleach powders	ALKYLATED SILICATES	—**	Caustic to skin layer; may lead to eczema.
Alkaline wave lotions Bleach oils Oxidation hair dyes Permanent wave solutions Permanent hair color	AMMONIA	50 ppm	Strong eye & respiratory irritant; swelling of eyelids; corneal burns to the eye if contact is made.
Oxidation hair color	AMINOPHENOL	—	Allergy, skin & eye irritant, toxic if ingested.
Hair spray (trace) Waving lotions Thioglycolate waving lotions Oxidation dyes	AMMONIUM HYDROXIDE	—	Eye irritant; toxic via oral and inhalation routes.
Bleaching agents Pre-lightners	AMMONIUM PERSULFATE	—	Tissue irritant & allergen; fire hazard.
Permanent waving solution	AMM0NIUM THIOGLYCOLATE	—	Toxic via oral and inhalation routes; can cause dermatitis.
Nail enamel dryer Aerosol propellants	BUTANE	—	This is an asphyxiant; breathing causes drowsiness.
Permanent wave solution	BENZYL ALCOHOL	—	Moderately toxic via ingestion & inhalation; skin & eye irritant.
Direct non oxidation dyes	BUTOXYETHANOL	50 ppm	Skin, eye, and respiratory irritant and narcosis.
Nail lacquer	*n*-BUTYL ACETATE	150 ppm	Skin & eye irritant; allergen; can cause respiratory irritation.
Nail lacquer	*n*-BUTYL PHTHALATE	—	Low oral/inhalation toxicity; can cause eye damage.
Hair relaxers	CALCIUM OXIDE	5 mg/m3	Caustic, capable of burning eyes and skin.

* Parts per million.
** Not given.

Source materials	Chemical name	Concentration	Comments
Hair relaxer	CAMPHOR	2 mg/m3	High to moderate ingestion hazard. Local exposure causes irritation.
Hair relaxer	CETYL ALCOHOL	—	Low oral toxicity, irritant via inhalation, skin or eye contact.
Shampoo (trace) Perm neutralizer Thioglycolate permanent waves Products remove coatings from hair	ETHALINE DIAMINE TETRACETIC ACID	—	Eye irritation; salt has moderate to high toxicity.
Waving lotions Oxidation dyes	ETHANOLAMINE	3 ppm	Causes severe eye tissue damage; low inhalation tolerance.
Nail lacquer solvent	ETHYL ACETATE	400 ppm	Irritant to mucous lining in eyes, respiratory tract and gums; dermatitis.
Hair spray Setting lotions Mousse Conditioner Nail sterilizer	ETHYL ALCOHOL	1000 ppm	Flammability.
Shampoo	FORMALDEHYDE	3 ppm	Vapor can cause skin/eye/respiratory tract irritant; allergic response even in low dosage.
Oxidation hair dye developer Neutralizers for permanent waves Hair lighteners Peroxide base neutralizers Permanent wave activator solutions Oxidizers Enzyme developers	HYDROGEN PEROXIDE	—	Highly toxic at high concentrations (35%) can blister skin; fire & explosive risk.
Aerosol propellants	ISOBUTANE	—	Dangerous fire risk when exposed to heat, flame, or oxidizers.
Permanent dyes Hair spray Nail enamel dryer Oil hair dressing Hair sling mousse Setting gels/lotions Bleach oils Semipermanent & oxidation hair dyes Peroxide based neutralizers	ISOPROPYL ALCOHOL	—	Mild narcosis, corneal burns and eye damage; de-fats & dries skin. Prolonged exp. may cause dermatitis, liver, and brain damage.

Source materials	Chemical name	Concentration	Comments
Mousse Oxidation hair colors Permanent hair colors	GLYCEROL	—	Respiratory irritant.
Hair spray propellants	LPG (liquefied petroleum gas)	1000 ppm	Asphyxiant; fire risk from heat, flame, and oxidizers.
Nail bonding agents (acrylic)	METHACRYLIC ACID	500 ppm	Skin irritant; moderate fire risk when exposed to heat, flame, & oxidizers.
Nail enamel dryer Oil hair dressing aerosols Hair spray	METHYLENE CHLORIDE (dichloromethane)	—	Fatigue, headache, dizziness; prolonged-dermatitis, liver, and brain damage; suspected carcinogen.
Hairdressings	MINERAL SPIRITS	—	Irritates skin, eyes, and mucous membranes; serious hazard and risk.
Hairdressing	NONIONIC DETERGENTS	—	Fire danger; Irritates skin, eyes, and mucous membranes; serious hazard and risk.
Peroxide based neutralizers	PHENACETIN	—	Experimental carcinogen and mutagen.
Oxidation hair dyes Permanent hair dye Semi-permanent hair dyes	PARA-PHENYLENEDIAMINE	.1 mg/m3	Skin irritant; suspected carcinogen; known to cause vertigo, anemia, gastritis, exfol.dermatitis; suspect in one death.
Oxidizers Neutralizers	PHOSPHORIC ACID	1 mg/m3	Skin, eye, and respiratory tract irritant.
Bleach powders Lightener powders	POTASSIUM PERSULFATE	—	Moderate tissue irritant and allergen. fire risk; decomposes if not stored properly.
Aerosol propellants MANP-50 propellant Nail enamel dryer	PROPANE	1000 ppm	Asphyxiant, fire risk-heat, sparks, flame, oxidizers.
Oxidation hair dye base Semi-permanent hair dye base Hair relaxer Thioglycolate permanent wave lotion	PROPYLENE GLYCOL	—	Skin and eye irritant.

Source materials	Chemical name	Concentration	Comments
Oxidation hair dyes	RESORCINOL	—	Can cause serious eye and skin injury to some. Dermatitis, edema, corrosion of skin; lymph gland swelling.
Frosts Activator powders	SILICAS	—	If inhaled for prolonged period of time, can lead to scarring of lung tissue.
Oxidation shampoos	SODIUM BISULFITE	—	Strong solutions can irritate skin and other tissue; allergen.
Sodium bromate neutralizers Hot tub/spa anti-algaecides	SODIUM BROMATE	—	Reacts violently with metals. High oral toxicity.
Hair relaxer Thioglycolate permanent waves	SODIUM PEROXIDE	—	Prolonged exposure can cause burns and ulcerations of skin and other tissue; severe eye damage.
Bleach powders Lightener powders	SODIUM PERSULFATE	—	Strong tissue irritant; toxic by ingestion; decomposes if not properly stored.
Persulfate and peroxide oxidizers	STRONTIUM PEROXIDE	—	Powder which is an irritant to eyes, skin and mucous membranes; because of reactivity - caution must be used.
Oxidizers (trace)	TETRASODIUM PYROPHOSPHATE	—	Toxic by ingestion.
Waving lotions Oxidation dyes	THIOGLYCOLIC ACID	—	Corrosive & irritant to skin, eyes, and mucous membranes.
Hair relaxers Dyes Nail powder	TITANIUM DIOXIDE	15 mg/m^3	Skin irritant; experimental tumorogenic agent.
Nail lacquer	TRICRESYL PHOSPHATE	—	Eye irritant; toxic when ingested.
Nail lacquer solvent	TOLUENE	200 ppm	Main ingredient of gasoline; skin & eye irritation. Vapors: narcotic action causing headache & nausea; experimental mutagen.

GLOSSARY

Allergen:................................ A material which can trigger an allergic reaction.
Asphyxiant: .... A material which can cause suffocation.
Carcinogen; .... A cancer causing agent.
Conjunctivitis: .... Irritation of the conjunctiva lining of the eye, leading to swelling and redness.
Dermatitis:............................. General inflammation of the skin.
Dyspnea:................................ Difficult or painful breathing.
Eczema; .... A disease of the skin characterized by itching, redness or scaling.
Edema:.................................. A swelling of tissue due to the collection of fluids.
Exfoliative Dermatitis: .... Shedding of skin tissue due to irritation.
Isomers: .... Molecules of a compound in which the atoms have a slightly different configuration.
Mutagen:................................ A material which can cause inheritable genetic changes in offspring.
NeoplasticAgent:................... A material capable of causing an abnormal growth of tissue.
Teratogen:............................. An agent which can cause non-inheritable mutations in offspring.
Tumerogenic: .... Capable of inducing growth of a tumor.
Vertigo:................................. Dizziness characterized by a sensation of whirling movement.

36

Lesson Plan

Anatomy and Physiology of Cosmetology

Lesson Overview and Motivation: Students will be able to define anatomy and physiology, and important bone structures, muscles, and nerves.

Acceptable Level: Score 85 percent or better on a multiple choice exam.

Location: Theory classroom_____ Lab classroom_____ Clinic_____

Time for Lecture/ Demonstration: 30 min._____ 60 min._____ 90 min._____

Student Level: Beginning_____ Intermediate_____ Advanced_____

Equipment/Models Needed: Anatomy map, and/or skeleton.

Teaching Aids Needed: Textbook, Theory and Practical Workbook, State Board Review Questions, chalkboard, overhead projector, VCR and videotape(s), computer, printer.

Theory Objectives	*Practical Objectives*
1. Physiology and anatomy, physiological cells and tissues, and systems of the body affected by school and salon services. 2. Osteology and the structure and function of bones, cartilage, ligaments, and joints, and synovial fluid. 3. Major bones of the head, neck, trunk, arm, and hand. 4. Myology, the functions and types of muscles, and muscle contraction, origin, and insertion. 5. Muscles of the head, face, trunk, and arm. 6. Neurological terms and the divisions of the nervous system and brain. 7. Types and functions of nerves in the head, face, neck, arm, hand, and finger; reflex arc.	None.

Word Review:

osteology	cancellous tissue	red marrow
compact bone	periosteum	ligament
cartilage	synovial fluid	cranium
frontal bone	occipital bone	parietal bone
temporal bone	zygomaticus	maxillae
mandible	cervical vertibrae	hyoid bone
sternum	clavicles	scapulae
carpals	metacarpals	phlanges
buccinator	corrugator	frontalis
epicranius	masseter	mentalis
nasalis	orbicularis oculi	platysma
risorius	temporalis	orbicularis oris
depressor labii inferioris	levitor palpabrae superioris	trifacial (trigeminal) nerve
supratrochlear nerve	auriculotemporal nerve	nasal nerve

Answers to End-of-Chapter Questions:

1. Physiology is the study of body function. **2.** Anatomy. **3.** Cell membrane. **4.** Cytoplasm is the jelly-like substance inside the cell. **5.** Metabolism. **6.** Tissue is a group of similar cells that perform a specialized function. For example, muscle tissue is made up of the same type of cells. **7.** Connective tissue binds, supports, protects and nourishes the body. **8.** The tissue that covers the surfaces (outside coverings) of the body. **9.** Organ. **10.** System. **11.** Osteology. **12.** Yes. **13.** Yes. **14.** Yes. **15.** Myology. **16.** No; the arm. **17.** The head.

Theory Objective 1: **Define the terms physiology and anatomy, describe physiological cells and tissues, and list the systems of the body that may be affected by school and salon services.**

Learning Steps

1. Read chapter in textbook.
2. Complete assignment in workbook.
3. View videotape(s).
4. Proceed to next objective.

Resources

1. *The Professional Cosmetologist,* 4th ed., ch. 36, pp. 688-689.
2. *Theory and Practical Workbook,* ch. 36, p. 257.
3. Videotape library.

Instructor's Resource Notes: ______________________________

____

Theory Objective 2: **Define osteology, and explain the structure and function of bones, cartilage, ligaments, joints, and synovial fluid.**

Learning Steps

1. Read chapter in textbook.
2. Complete assignment in workbook.
3. View videotape(s).
4. Proceed to next objective.

Resources

1. *The Professional Cosmetologist,* 4th ed., ch. 36, pp. 689-691.
2. *Theory and Practical Workbook,* ch. 36, p. 257.
3. Videotape library.

Instructor's Resource Notes: ______________________________

____

Theory Objective 3: **Describe the major bones of the head, neck, trunk, arm, and hand.**

Learning Steps

1. Read chapter in textbook.
2. Complete assignment in workbook.
3. View videotape(s).
4. Proceed to next objective.

Resources

1. *The Professional Cosmetologist,* 4th ed., ch. 36, pp. 691-693.
2. *Theory and Practical Workbook,* ch. 36, p. 258.
3. Videotape library.

Instructor's Resource Notes: ______________________________

____

Theory Objective 4: **Define myology; describe the functions of the muscles and identify three types of muscles; and explain muscle contraction, origin, and insertion.**

Learning Steps

1. Read chapter in textbook.
2. Complete assignment in workbook.
3. View videotape(s).
4. Proceed to next objective.

Resources

1. *The Professional Cosmetologist,* 4th ed., ch. 36, pp. 693-694.
2. *Theory and Practical Workbook,* ch. 36, p. 260.
3. Videotape library.

Instructor's Resource Notes: ____________________

____

Theory Objective 5: **Describe the muscles of the head, face, trunk, and arm.**

Learning Steps

1. Read chapter in textbook.
2. Complete assignment in workbook.
3. View videotape(s).
4. Proceed to next objective.

Resources

1. *The Professional Cosmetologist,* 4th ed., ch. 36, pp. 694-697.
2. *Theory and Practical Workbook,* ch. 36, p. 261.
3. Videotape library.

Instructor's Resource Notes: ____________________

____

Theory Objective 6: **Define neurological terms and explain the divisions of the nervous system and the brain.**

Learning Steps

1. Read chapter in textbook.
2. Complete assignment in workbook.
3. View videotape(s).
4. Proceed to next objective.

Resources

1. *The Professional Cosmetologist,* 4th ed., ch. 36, pp. 697-698.
2. *Theory and Practical Workbook,* ch. 36, p. 262.
3. Videotape library.

Instructor's Resource Notes: ____________________

____

Theory Objective 7: **Explain the types and functions of nerves found in the head, face, neck, arm, hand, and fingers, and describe the arc reflex.**

Learning Steps	***Resources***
1. Read chapter in textbook.	1. *The Professional Cosmetologist*, 4th ed., ch. 36, pp. 698-700.
2. Complete assignment in workbook.	2. Videotape library.
3. View videotape(s).	
4. Proceed to next chapter.	

Instructor's Resource Notes: ______________________________

____

Evaluation of Instruction:

_____ A. Discussed answers to end of chapter questions.
_____ B. Collected completed workbook assignments.
_____ C. Collected student progress charts.
_____ D. State board sheets current.
_____ E. Answered written test(s), and/or computer test questions.
_____ F. Completed Performance/Product Checklist.

Student Assignments: ______________________________

____

37

Lesson Plan

Anatomy and Physiology: Vascular and Endocrine Systems

Lesson Overview and Motivation: Students will define, describe, and classify the parts of the vascular and endocrine systems of the human body.

Acceptable Level: Score 85 percent or better on a multiple choice exam.

Location: Theory classroom_____ Lab classroom_____ Clinic_____

Time for Lecture/ Demonstration: 30 min._____ 60 min._____ 90 min._____

Student Level: Beginning_____ Intermediate_____ Advanced_____

Teaching Aids Needed: Textbook, Theory and Practical Workbook, State Board Review Questions, chalkboard, overhead projector, VCR and videotape(s), computer, printer.

Theory Objectives	Practical Objectives
1. Angiology and the three subdivisions of the vascular system, parts and functions of the heart and blood vessels, and the function of pulmonary circulation. 2. Arteries and veins of the head, face, neck, arm, and hand; the composition of blood; and the lymphatic system. 3. Endocrine system and its five major glands.	None.

Word Review:

blood vessels	arteries	veins
capillaries	carotid artery	internal carotid
jugular vein	plasma	brachial artery
radial arteries	ulna arteries	lymph
hemoglobin	red blood cells	white blood cells
platelets	external carotid	

Answers to End-of-Chapter Questions:

Objective 1.

1. Blood. **2.** The circulatory system. **3.** Pericardium. **4.** To bring food and oxygen to the body and remove waste products and carbon dioxide from the blood cells. **5.** The chest cavity. **6.** Yes. **7.** Yes. **8.** Yes. **9.** Yes. **10.** Small—can only be seen with the aid of a microscope. **11.** The lungs.

Objective 2.

1. The aorta. **2.** Carotid. **3.** Brachial. **4.** 8-10 pints. **5.** Yes. **6.** Yes. **7.** Leukocytes. **8.** Platelets.

Objective 3.

1. Yes. **2.** Yes. **3.** The base of the brain. **4.** Yes. **5.** Yes. **6.** The thyroid gland. **7.** The pancreas

Theory Objective 1: **Define angiology, and identify the three subdivisions of the vascular system, the parts and functions of the heart and blood vessels, and the function of pulmonary circulation.**

Learning Steps

1. Read chapter in textbook.
2. Complete assignment in workbook.
3. View videotape(s).
4. Proceed to next objective.

Resources

1. *The Professional Cosmetologist,* 4th ed., ch. 37, pp. 710-713.
2. *Theory and Practical Workbook,* ch. 37, p. 263.
3. Videotape library.

Instructor's Resource Notes: ______________________________

____

Theory Objective 2: **Identify the arteries and veins of the head, face, neck, arm, and hand.**

Learning Steps

1. Read chapter in textbook.
2. Complete assignment in workbook.
3. View videotape(s).
4. Proceed to next objective.

Resources

1. *The Professional Cosmetologist,* 4th ed., ch. 37, pp. 713-715.
2. *Theory and Practical Workbook,* ch. 37, p. 263.
3. Videotape library.

Instructor's Resource Notes: ____

____

Theory Objective 3: **Describe the endocrine system and its five major glands.**

Learning Steps

1. Read chapter in textbook.
2. Complete assignment in workbook.
3. View videotape(s).
4. Congratulations you have completed the basic competencies for this course.

Resources

1. *The Professional Cosmetologist*, 4th ed., ch. 37, pp. 715-717.
2. Videotape library.

Instructor's Resource Notes: ____

____

Evaluation of Instruction:

_____ A. Discussed answers to end of chapter questions.
_____ B. Collected completed workbook assignments.
_____ C. Collected student progress charts.
_____ D. State board sheets current.
_____ E. Answered written test(s), and/or computer test questions.

Student Assignments: ____

____

STUDENT PROGRESS CHARTS

You can use the progress charts on the following pages to keep track of the theory and practical exercises completed during the first 6-10 weeks of basic cosmetology training. For instance, at the end of a school month, the instructor can glance at this progress chart and determine - almost immediately - exactly **what was taught, what work students have completed**, and **when it was done**.

In the following example of the first section of a chart, please note under the "Sanitation" heading, the abbreviations. These are examples of daily duties that students should perform to assist in maintaining a sanitary and safe work environment in their school. These are the same duties students will be performing in a beauty salon. You will note that abbreviations, such as "SB," are used to indicate "Shampoo Bowl", "PW" for the cleaning of permanent wave trays and rods, etc. You may wish to assign a different system of abbreviations. It is suggested that **all** of the Sanitation boxes be assigned when your students begin using this chart. Then, **each day**, as the students complete the assignment, they should ask you to **initial** and **date** the Sanitation Procedure box for the procedure done. For example, each day that a student sanitized the shampoo bowl, you would signoff on one "SB" box. So, if he or she completed one sanitation procedure per day, this chart could be used for 18 school days. Since sanitation is part of every school day, this section will be located at the top of all the progress charts.

If you decide to copy these charts, rather than use those in the Theory and Practical Workbook, color coding each chart works very nicely. For example, Chart 1 could be copied on regular, white paper, Chart 2 on yellow colored paper, and Chart 3 on orange colored paper, etc.

CHART NO. 2	**Cosmetology Program**					
Instructor(s)	**Date**			**Student's Name**		
SANITATION: **Examples:** **SB - Sh. bowls** **SP - Put away supplies** **PW - PW rods** **RC - Recept. area**	SB					

Continued on next page...

The second section of the progress chart **defines the name of the chapter** your class is currently studying. In the first part of the following example, the subject is Condition, Chapter 5. Usually, you would give the students a theory assignment that would include the reading of certain pages from the textbook. This may also follow the assignment of workbook pages to be completed, videotapes to be viewed, tests to be taken, and the recording of test results, etc. The blanks provided will give the students a place to write down these assignments and related information.

The third section of the Sanitation chapter **provides spaces (boxes) to record practical exercises** related to the chapter you are teachinging. In this example, the exercise is conditioning the hair using different types of conditioners. On another chart, this practical exercise may be wrapping a certain number of mannequins with permanent wave rods, or applying a certain number of hair colors. **Remember** to initial and date each box for the exercise completed.

TASK (CHAPTER) NAMES					
CONDITION 5	Read: The Professional Cosmetologist (TPC) Pages_______________ Workbook: Study Guide for TPC Pages_______________ Instr. Init./Date______________ Other (AV, Tests, Assignments)__________________________ Written Test Score _______ Practical Test Results__________				
Select/Give Conditioner w/ hair analysis Examples: P - Protein M - Moisturizing I - Instant	M				
Instructor's Directions or Comments:					

<table>
<tr><td>CHART NO. 1</td><td colspan="6" rowspan="2">Cosmetology Program

Date ______________________ Student's Name</td></tr>
<tr><td>Instructor(s)</td></tr>
<tr><td rowspan="3">SANITATION:
Examples:
SB - Sh. bowls
SP - Put away supplies
PW - PW rods
RC - Recept. area</td><td>SB</td><td></td><td></td><td></td><td></td><td></td></tr>
<tr><td></td><td></td><td></td><td></td><td></td><td></td></tr>
<tr><td></td><td></td><td></td><td></td><td></td><td></td></tr>
<tr><td>TASK (CHAPTER) NAMES</td><td colspan="6"></td></tr>
<tr><td>CAREERS
1</td><td colspan="6">Read: The Professional Cosmetologist (TPC), John W. Dalton
Pages__________
Workbook: Study Guide for TPC
Pages__________ Instr. Init./Date__________
Other (AV, Tests, Assignments)__________
Written Test Score ______ Practical Test Results______</td></tr>
<tr><td>ETHICS
2</td><td colspan="6">Read: The Professional Cosmetologist (TPC)
Pages__________
Workbook: Study Guide for TPC
Pages__________ Instr. Init./Date__________
Other (AV, Tests, Assignments)__________
Written Test Score ______ Practical Test Results______</td></tr>
<tr><td>SANITATION
3</td><td colspan="6">Read: The Professional Cosmetologist (TPC)
Pages__________
Workbook: Study Guide for TPC
Pages__________ Instr. Init./Date__________
Other (AV, Tests, Assignments)__________
Written Test Score ______ Practical Test Results______</td></tr>
<tr><td rowspan="3">Sanitation Practical</td><td>Work Area</td><td>Work Area</td><td>Work Area</td><td>Work Area</td><td colspan="2">Work Area</td></tr>
<tr><td>Work Area</td><td>Work Area</td><td>Work Area</td><td>Work Area</td><td colspan="2">Work Area</td></tr>
<tr><td>Work Area</td><td>Work Area</td><td>Work Area</td><td>Work Area</td><td colspan="2">Work Area</td></tr>
<tr><td colspan="7">Instructor's Directions or Comments:</td></tr>
</table>

CHART NO. 2	Cosmetology Program					
Instructor(s)	Date			Student's Name		
SANITATION: Examples: SB - Sh. bowls SP - Put away supplies PW - PW rods RC - Recept. area	SB					
TASK (CHAPTER) NAMES						

SHAMPOO 4	Read: The Professional Cosmetologist (TPC), John W. Dalton Pages ______ Workbook: Study Guide for TPC Pages ______ Instr. Init./Date ______ Other (AV, Tests, Assignments) ______ Written Test Score ______ Practical Test Results ______

Shampoo practical Examples: DM - Dandruff medicated G - General O/D - Oily or dry SP - Conditioning	G						

CONDITION 5	Read: The Professional Cosmetologist (TPC) Pages ______ Workbook: Study Guide for TPC Pages ______ Instr. Init./Date ______ Other (AV, Tests, Assignments) ______ Written Test Score ______ Practical Test Results ______

Select/Give Conditioner w/ hair analysis Examples: P - Protein M - Moisturizing I - Instant	M				

Instructor's Directions or Comments:

CHART NO. 3	Cosmetology Program					
Instructor(s)	Date			Student's Name		
SANITATION: Sanitation Examples: SB - Sh. bowls SP - Put away supplies PW - PW rods RC - Recept. area	SB					

TASK (CHAPTER) NAMES

SCALP CARE 6

Read: The Professional Cosmetologist (TPC), John W. Dalton

Pages________________

Workbook: Study Guide for TPC

Pages________________ Instr. Init./Date________________

Other (AV, Tests, Assignments)________________________________

Written Test Score ________ Practical Test Results____________

Scalp Care Practical Examples: DM - Dandruff medicated G - General O/D - Oily or dry Spec - Conditioning	G						

FINGER WAVE 7

Read: The Professional Cosmetologist (TPC)

Pages________________

Workbook: Study Guide for TPC

Pages________________ Instr. Init./Date________________

Other (AV, Tests, Assignments)________________________________

Written Test Score ________ Practical Test Results____________

Finger Wave Practical Examples: B - Back S - Sides Wh - Whole head T - Top section					

Instructor's Directions or Comments:

<table>
<tr><td>CHART NO. 4</td><td colspan="7">Cosmetology Program</td></tr>
<tr><td>Instructor(s)</td><td colspan="7">Date ______________________ Student's Name</td></tr>
<tr><td rowspan="3">SANITATION
Examples:
SB - Sh. bowls
SP - Put away supplies
PW - PW rods
RC - Recept. area</td><td>SB</td><td></td><td></td><td></td><td></td><td></td><td></td></tr>
<tr><td></td><td></td><td></td><td></td><td></td><td></td><td></td></tr>
<tr><td></td><td></td><td></td><td></td><td></td><td></td><td></td></tr>
<tr><td>TASK (CHAPTER) NAMES</td><td colspan="7"></td></tr>
<tr><td>SCULPTURE CURLS
9</td><td colspan="7">Read: The Professional Cosmetologist (TPC), John W. Dalton
Pages__________________
Workbook: Study Guide for TPC
Pages__________________ Instr. Init./Date________________
Other (AV, Tests, Assignments)____________________________________
Written Test Score ________ Practical Test Results___________</td></tr>
<tr><td rowspan="2">Sculpture curl Practical
Examples:
TP - Top set
TS - Top & sides
Wh - Whole head
St - Stem...No, half, and long</td><td>TP</td><td></td><td></td><td></td><td></td><td></td><td></td></tr>
<tr><td></td><td></td><td></td><td></td><td></td><td></td><td></td></tr>
<tr><td>SETTING THE HAIR WITH ROLLERS
10</td><td colspan="7">Read: The Professional Cosmetologist (TPC)
Pages__________________
Workbook: Study Guide for TPC
Pages__________________ Instr. Init./Date________________
Other (AV, Tests, Assignments)____________________________________
Written Test Score ________ Practical Test Results___________</td></tr>
<tr><td rowspan="4">Roller set/comb Practical
Examples:
TP - Top set
TS - Top & sides
Wh - Whole head
Sp - Special Pattern set</td><td></td><td></td><td></td><td></td><td></td><td colspan="2"></td></tr>
<tr><td></td><td></td><td></td><td></td><td></td><td colspan="2"></td></tr>
<tr><td></td><td></td><td></td><td></td><td></td><td colspan="2"></td></tr>
<tr><td></td><td></td><td></td><td></td><td></td><td colspan="2"></td></tr>
<tr><td colspan="8">Instructor's Directions or Comments:</td></tr>
</table>

<table>
<tr><td>CHART NO. 5</td><td colspan="7">Cosmetology Program</td></tr>
<tr><td>Instructor(s)</td><td colspan="7">Date ______ Student's Name</td></tr>
<tr><td rowspan="3">SANITATION
Examples:
SB - Sh. bowls
SP - Put away supplies
PW - PW rods
RC - Recept. area</td><td>SB</td><td></td><td></td><td></td><td></td><td></td><td></td></tr>
<tr><td></td><td></td><td></td><td></td><td></td><td></td><td></td></tr>
<tr><td></td><td></td><td></td><td></td><td></td><td></td><td></td></tr>
<tr><td>TASK (CHAPTER) NAMES</td><td colspan="7"></td></tr>
<tr><td>HAIR DESIGN 11</td><td colspan="7">Read: The Professional Cosmetologist (TPC), John W. Dalton
Pages________________
Workbook: Study Guide for TPC
Pages________________ Instr. Init./Date_______________
Other (AV, Tests, Assignments)__________________________________
Written Test Score ________ Practical Test Results__________</td></tr>
<tr><td rowspan="2">Hair Design Practical
Examples:
F - Facial shapes
FH - Odd shaped foreheads
G - Eyeglasses</td><td>F</td><td></td><td></td><td></td><td></td><td></td><td></td></tr>
<tr><td></td><td></td><td></td><td></td><td></td><td></td><td></td></tr>
<tr><td>HAIR SHAPING 12</td><td colspan="7">Read: The Professional Cosmetologist (TPC)
Pages________________
Workbook: Study Guide for TPC
Pages________________ Instr. Init./Date_______________
Other (AV, Tests, Assignments)__________________________________
Written Test Score ________ Practical Test Results__________</td></tr>
<tr><td rowspan="4">Hair Shaping Practical
Examples:
R - Razor
S - Scissors
AE - Around ears
B - Basic cut
N - Neckline
B - Basic Sch. Cut</td><td>R</td><td></td><td></td><td></td><td></td><td colspan="2"></td></tr>
<tr><td></td><td></td><td></td><td></td><td></td><td colspan="2"></td></tr>
<tr><td></td><td></td><td></td><td></td><td></td><td colspan="2"></td></tr>
<tr><td></td><td></td><td></td><td></td><td></td><td colspan="2"></td></tr>
<tr><td colspan="8">Instructor's Directions or Comments:</td></tr>
</table>

CHART NO. 6	Cosmetology Program					
Instructor(s)	Date	_____ Student's Name				
SANITATION Examples: SB - Sh. bowls SP - Put away supplies PW - PW rods RC - Recept. area	SB					
TASK (CHAPTER) NAMES						
AIR WAVE & BLOW-DRY 13	Read: The Professional Cosmetologist (TPC), John W. Dalton Pages_____ Workbook: Study Guide for TPC Pages_____ Instr. Init./Date_____ Other (AV, Tests, Assignments)_____ Written Test Score _____ Practical Test Results_____					
Air Wave Practical Examples: W - Waves U - Under TF - Toward face AF - Away fr face	W					
IRON CURLS 14	Read: The Professional Cosmetologist (TPC) Pages_____ Workbook: Study Guide for TPC Pages_____ Instr. Init./Date_____ Other (AV, Tests, Assignments)_____ Written Test Score _____ Practical Test Results_____					
Iron Curls Practical Examples: M - Marcel iron EM - Electric iron CI - Clamp iron W - Waves C - Curls specify type	W					

Instructor's Directions or Comments:

CHART NO. 7	Cosmetology Program					
Instructor(s)	Date			Student's Name		
SANITATION Examples: SB - Sh. bowls SP - Put away supplies PW - PW rods RC - Recept. area	SB					
TASK (CHAPTER) NAMES						

TEMPORARY COLOR 15	**Read: The Professional Cosmetologist (TPC), John W. Dalton** **Pages**__________ **Workbook: Study Guide for TPC** **Pages**__________ **Instr. Init./Date**__________ **Other (AV, Tests, Assignments)**__________ **Written Test Score** _____ **Practical Test Results**_______
SEMI-PERMANENT COLOR 16	**Read: The Professional Cosmetologist (TPC)** **Pages**__________ **Workbook: Study Guide for TPC** **Pages**__________ **Instr. Init./Date**__________ **Other (AV, Tests, Assignments)**__________ **Written Test Score** _____ **Practical Test Results**_______

Temporary Color Practical Examples: C - Color swatches CM - Classmate M - Mannequin A - Applications	A						

Semipermanent Color Practical Examples: C - Color swatches CM - Classmate M - Mannequin CC - Color client A - Applications	CM				

Instructor 's Directions or Comments:

CHART NO. 8	Cosmetology Program					
Instructor(s)	Date		Student's Name			
SANITATION Examples: SB - Sh. bowls SP - Put away supplies PW - PW rods RC - Recept. area	SB					
TASK (CHAPTER) NAMES						

PERMANENT COLOR 17

Read: The Professional Cosmetologist (TPC), John W. Dalton

Pages________________

Workbook: Study Guide for TPC

Pages________________ Instr. Init./Date______________

Other (AV, Tests, Assignments)________________________________

Written Test Score _______ Practical Test Results__________

Permanent Color Practical Examples: V - Virgin lightener R - Retouch SC - Soap cap CM - Classmate CC - Color client A - Applications	V						

LIGHTEN - TONE HAIR 18

Read: The Professional Cosmetologist (TPC)

Pages________________

Workbook: Study Guide for TPC

Pages________________ Instr. Init./Date______________

Other (AV, Tests, Assignments)________________________________

Written Test Score _______ Practical Test Results__________

Lighten & Tone Practical Examples: V - Virgin lightener R - Retouch T - Toner F - Frost A - Applications	R				

Instructor's Directions or Comments:

<table>
<tr><td>CHART NO. 9</td><td colspan="7">Cosmetology Program</td></tr>
<tr><td>Instructor(s)</td><td colspan="3">Date</td><td colspan="4">Student's Name</td></tr>
<tr><td>SANITATION
Examples:
SB - Sh. bowls
SP - Put away supplies
PW - PW rods
RC - Recept. area</td><td>SB</td><td></td><td></td><td></td><td></td><td></td><td></td></tr>
<tr><td>TASK (CHAPTER) NAMES</td><td></td><td></td><td></td><td></td><td></td><td></td><td></td></tr>
<tr><td>Multicolor Techniques 19</td><td colspan="7">Read: The Professional Cosmetologist (TPC), John W. Dalton
Pages________________
Workbook: Study Guide for TPC
Pages________________ Instr. Init./Date______________
Other (AV, Tests, Assignments)________________________________
Written Test Score _______ Practical Test Results__________</td></tr>
<tr><td>Multi-Color Practical
Examples:
SP - Special effects
W - Weave color
F - Foil
P - Paint
A - Applications</td><td>SP</td><td></td><td></td><td></td><td></td><td></td><td></td></tr>
<tr><td>Permanent Waving 20</td><td colspan="7">Read: The Professional Cosmetologist (TPC)
Pages________________
Workbook: Study Guide for TPC
Pages________________ Instr. Init./Date______________
Other (AV, Tests, Assignments)________________________________
Written Test Score _______ Practical Test Results__________</td></tr>
<tr><td>Permanent Wave Practical
Examples:
B - Basic wrap
PT - Pony tail wrap
SP - Spiral wrap
O - Other
SA - Select & Apply
RPW - Relax/PW</td><td>R</td><td></td><td></td><td></td><td></td><td></td><td></td></tr>
<tr><td colspan="8">Instructor's Directions or Comments:</td></tr>
</table>

CHART NO. 10	Cosmetology Program					
Instructor(s)	Date			Student's Name		
SANITATION **Examples:** **SB - Sh. bowls** **SP - Put away supplies** **PW - PW rods** **RC - Recept. area**	SB					
TASK (CHAPTER) NAMES						

HAIR RELAXING 21

Read: The Professional Cosmetologist (TPC), John W. Dalton

Pages________________

Workbook: Study Guide for TPC

Pages________________ Instr. Init./Date________________

Other (AV, Tests, Assignments)________________________________

Written Test Score ________ Practical Test Results____________

Hair Relaxer Practical Examples: A - Applications T - Timing S - Selection of product R - Retouch V - Virgin	R						

THERMAL PRESS AND CURL 22

Read: The Professional Cosmetologist (TPC)

Pages________________

Workbook: Study Guide for TPC

Pages________________ Instr. Init./Date________________

Other (AV, Tests, Assignments)________________________________

Written Test Score ________ Practical Test Results____________

Thermal Press & Curl Practical Examples: B - Basic press DP - Double press SP - Spec. case CH - Curled & combed hairstyle	B				

Instructor's Directions or Comments:

CHART NO. 11	Cosmetology Program					
Instructor(s)	Date			Student's Name		
SANITATION Examples: SB - Sh. bowls SP - Put away supplies PW - PW rods RC - Recept. area	SB					
TASK (CHAPTER) NAMES						

RECURLING (SOFT CURL) 23	Read: The Professional Cosmetologist (TPC), John W. Dalton Pages________ Workbook: Study Guide for TPC Pages________ Instr. Init./Date________ Other (AV, Tests, Assignments)________ Written Test Score ____ Practical Test Results______

Recurl Practical Examples: A - Applications T - Timing S - Selection of product R - Retouch V - Virgin	R						

DESCRIBING THE SKIN 24	Read: The Professional Cosmetologist (TPC) Pages________ Workbook: Study Guide for TPC Pages________ Instr. Init./Date________ Other (AV, Tests, Assignments)________ Written Test Score ____ Practical Test Results______
FACIALS 25	Read: The Professional Cosmetologist (TPC) Pages________ Workbook: Study Guide for TPC Pages________ Instr. Init./Date________ Other (AV, Tests, Assignments)________ Written Test Score ____ Practical Test Results______

Instructor's Directions or Comments:

<table>
<tr><td>CHART NO. 12</td><td colspan="6">Cosmetology Program</td></tr>
<tr><td>Instructor(s)</td><td colspan="2">Date</td><td colspan="4">Student's Name</td></tr>
<tr><td rowspan="3">SANITATION
Examples:
SB - Sh. bowls
SP - Put away supplies
PW - PW rods
RC - Recept. area</td><td>SB</td><td></td><td></td><td></td><td></td><td></td></tr>
<tr><td></td><td></td><td></td><td></td><td></td><td></td></tr>
<tr><td></td><td></td><td></td><td></td><td></td><td></td></tr>
<tr><td>TASK (CHAPTER) NAMES</td><td></td><td></td><td></td><td></td><td></td><td></td></tr>
<tr><td rowspan="3">Facial Practical
Examples:
B - Basic
O - For Oily Skin
D - Dry Skin
HF - High freq.</td><td>B</td><td></td><td></td><td></td><td></td><td></td></tr>
<tr><td></td><td></td><td></td><td></td><td></td><td></td></tr>
<tr><td></td><td></td><td></td><td></td><td></td><td></td></tr>
<tr><td>MAKE UP
26</td><td colspan="6">Read: The Professional Cosmetologist (TPC), John W. Dalton
Pages________________
Workbook: Study Guide for TPC
Pages________________ Instr. Init./Date________________
Other (AV, Tests, Assignments)________________________________
Written Test Score ________ Practical Test Results__________</td></tr>
<tr><td rowspan="3">Make up Practical
Examples:
B - Basic
MO - Make over</td><td>B</td><td></td><td></td><td></td><td></td><td></td></tr>
<tr><td></td><td></td><td></td><td></td><td></td><td></td></tr>
<tr><td></td><td></td><td></td><td></td><td></td><td></td></tr>
<tr><td>NAIL DISEASES AND DISORDERS
27</td><td colspan="6">Read: The Professional Cosmetologist (TPC)
Pages________________
Workbook: Study Guide for TPC
Pages________________ Instr. Init./Date________________
Other (AV, Tests, Assignments)________________________________
Written Test Score ________ Practical Test Results__________</td></tr>
<tr><td colspan="7">Instructor's Directions or Comments:</td></tr>
</table>

<table>
<tr><td>CHART NO. 13</td><td colspan="6">Cosmetology Program</td></tr>
<tr><td>Instructor(s)</td><td colspan="6">Date Student's Name</td></tr>
<tr><td rowspan="3">SANITATION
Examples:
SB - Sh. bowls
SP - Put away supplies
PW - PW rods
RC - Recept. area</td><td>SB</td><td></td><td></td><td></td><td></td><td></td></tr>
<tr><td></td><td></td><td></td><td></td><td></td><td></td></tr>
<tr><td rowspan="2"></td><td rowspan="2"></td><td rowspan="2"></td><td rowspan="2"></td><td rowspan="2"></td><td rowspan="2"></td></tr>
<tr><td>TASK (CHAPTER) NAMES</td></tr>
<tr><td>Manicure - Pedicure the Nails 28</td><td colspan="6">Read: The Professional Cosmetologist (TPC), John W. Dalton
Pages________
Workbook: Study Guide for TPC
Pages________ Instr. Init./Date________
Other (AV, Tests, Assignments)________
Written Test Score ________ Practical Test Results________</td></tr>
<tr><td rowspan="3">Manicure - Pedicure Practical
Examples:
BM - Basic mani.
BP - Basic ped.
HO - Hot oil
SN - Sculp. nails
W - Nail wrap</td><td></td><td></td><td></td><td></td><td></td><td></td></tr>
<tr><td></td><td></td><td></td><td></td><td></td><td></td></tr>
<tr><td></td><td></td><td></td><td></td><td></td><td></td></tr>
<tr><td>Wigs and Hairpieces 29</td><td colspan="6">Read: The Professional Cosmetologist (TPC)
Pages________
Workbook: Study Guide for TPC
Pages________ Instr. Init./Date________
Other (AV, Tests, Assignments)________
Written Test Score ________ Practical Test Results________</td></tr>
<tr><td rowspan="2">Wigs and Hairpiece Practical
Examples:
HH - Human hair
SYNH - Synthetic Hair
CS - Clean & style
C - Color wig or HP</td><td></td><td></td><td></td><td></td><td colspan="2"></td></tr>
<tr><td></td><td></td><td></td><td></td><td colspan="2"></td></tr>
<tr><td colspan="7">Instructor's Directions or Comments:</td></tr>
</table>

CHART NO. 14	Cosmetology Program					
Instructor(s)	Date			Student's Name		
SANITATION Examples: SB - Sh. bowls SP - Put away supplies PW - PW rods RC - Recept. area	SB					
TASK (CHAPTER) NAMES						
SHAVING (May be optional) 30	Read: The Professional Cosmetologist (TPC), John W. Dalton Pages________ Workbook: Study Guide for TPC Pages________ Instr. Init./Date________ Other (AV, Tests, Assignments)________ Written Test Score ____					
PLAN A SALON 31	Read: The Professional Cosmetologist (TPC) Pages________ Workbook: Study Guide for TPC Pages________ Instr. Init./Date________ Other (AV, Tests, Assignments)________ Written Test Score ____					
SALON OPERATIONS 32	Read: The Professional Cosmetologist (TPC) Pages________ Workbook: Study Guide for TPC Pages________ Instr. Init./Date________ Other (AV, Tests, Assignments)________ Written Test Score ____					

Instructor assignment:

Instructor's Directions or Comments:

CHART NO. 15	Cosmetology Program					
Instructor(s)	Date			Student's Name		
SANITATION Examples: SB - Sh. bowls SP - Put away supplies PW - PW rods RC - Recept. area	SB					
TASK (CHAPTER) NAMES						
Psychology of Interpersonal Skills and Retail Sales 33	Read: The Professional Cosmetologist (TPC), John W. Dalton Pages________ Workbook: Study Guide for TPC Pages________ Instr. Init./Date________ Other (AV, Tests, Assignments)________ Written Test Score ________					
Principles of Electricity 34	Read: The Professional Cosmetologist (TPC) Pages________ Workbook: Study Guide for TPC Pages________ Instr. Init./Date________ Other (AV, Tests, Assignments)________ Written Test Score ________					
Chemistry of Cosmetology 35	Read: The Professional Cosmetologist (TPC) Pages________ Workbook: Study Guide for TPC Pages________ Instr. Init./Date________ Other (AV, Tests, Assignments)________ Written Test Score ________					
Anatomy and Physiology in Cosmetology: Bones, Muscles, Nerves 36 + 37	Read: The Professional Cosmetologist (TPC) Pages________ Workbook: Study Guide for TPC Pages________ Instr. Init./Date________ Other (AV, Tests, Assignments)________ Written Test Score ________					

PERFORMANCE CHECKLISTS

1. Performance/Product Checklist (The following 25 checklists sample student mastery).

A. Sanitizing Cosmetology Implements Checklist.

Evaluator's Name____

Student's Name____

Attempt 1: Date________________

Timings________________

Attempt 2: Date________________

Timings________________

Attempt 3: Date________________

Timings________________

Comments:

Note to Evaluator: The performance item numbers preceded by a printer's bullet (•) MUST BE MONITORED and totaled in the space provided. The product items that are not preceded by a bullet need not be monitored step-by-step. They can be totaled in the space provided. With the exception of asterisked items (*), weight each *YES* response one (1).

Supplies Needed: combs, brushes, clippers, rollers, scissors, razor, shampoo bowl, shampoo chair, styling station, hydraulic chair, dryer lounge, plastic container, paper towels, cotton, formalin (or quats), comb and brush cleaner, fumigant tablets, 70 percent ethyl alcohol (or 99 percent isopropyl alcohol), small glass container with ventilated top, and manicure nippers and scissors. (Evaluator will circle supplies student failed to obtain.)

I. Student prepares wet sterilizer.

	Attempt 1 No/Yes	Attempt 2 No/Yes	Attempt 3 No/Yes
•1.* Mixes formalin (or quats) according to label directions.	☐	☐	☐
•2.* Wipes up any sanitizing solution.	☐	☐	☐
•3. Caps and safely stores formalin bottle.	☐	☐	☐
•4.* Does not smell concentrated sanitizing solution, and does not allow it to come in contact with skin.	☐	☐	☐

Subtotal............. ________________

II. Student cleans setting and combing implements.

5. Mixes comb and brush cleaner. ☐ ☐ ☐

6. Combs, brushes, rollers and clips are free from hair, spray and other residue. ☐ ☐ ☐

•7. Leaves all implements in comb and brush cleaner for observation. ☐ ☐ ☐

•8. Rinses implements with clear water. ☐ ☐ ☐

•9. Immerses implements in wet sterilizer and covers container. ☐ ☐ ☐

•10. Removes and rinses implements. ☐ ☐ ☐

•11. Dries implements. ☐ ☐ ☐

•12. Places implements in dry sanitizer. ☐ ☐ ☐

Subtotal. ____________

III. Student prepares dry sanitizer.

13. Two fumigant tablets are placed in a small glass container with ventilated top. ☐ ☐ ☐

14. Glass container is placed in an airtight drawer or student kit. ☐ ☐ ☐

15. Setting and combing implements are placed in dry sanitizer. ☐ ☐ ☐

16. Dry sanitizer is closed. ☐ ☐ ☐

Subtotal ____________

IV. Student sanitizes cutting implements.

•17. Uses cotton saturated with 70 percent alcohol to wipe cutting edges of hair-cutting scissors, tapering shears, manicure nippers and scissors. ☐ ☐ ☐

•18.* Removes guard and razor blade from razor without injury. .... ☐ ☐ ☐

•19. Uses 70 percent alcoholized cotton to wipe blade from razor. .... ☐ ☐ ☐

•20.* Replaces blade and guard in shaper without injury. .... ☐ ☐ ☐

•21. Correctly replaces all implements and supplies. .... ☐ ☐ ☐

Subtotal .... ____________________

TOTAL .... ____________________

At least 17 yes responses are necessary to validate. All asterisked (*) items must be marked *YES*.

B. Sanitizing Salon Equipment.

Evaluator's Name ____

Student's Name ____

Attempt 1: Date ____________________

Timings ____________________

Attempt 2: Date ____________________

Timings ____________________

Attempt 3: Date ____________________

Timings ____________________

Comments:

I. Student sanitizes one piece of each type of equipment.

	Attempt 1 No/Yes	Attempt 2 No/Yes	Attempt 3 No/Yes
1. Styling station.	☐	☐	☐
2. Hydraulic chair.	☐	☐	☐
3. Shampoo bowl.	☐	☐	☐
4. Dryer lounge.	☐	☐	☐

5. Furniture from reception room. .... ☐ ☐ ☐

Subtotal. .... ________________

II. Allows evaluator to check equipment.

6. Styling station is free from hair, hairspray and other residue; mirrors are free from streaks or smudges. .... ☐ ☐ ☐

7. The hydraulic chair base is wiped clean from soil, such as hairspray, hair, dirt, and other foreign substances. .... ☐ ☐ ☐

8. Upholstery on hydraulic chair is wiped free of hair, hairspray, dust, and other foreign substances. .... ☐ ☐ ☐

9. The shampoo bowl is wiped clean of hair, streaks, dust, and other residue. .... ☐ ☐ ☐

10. The dryer lounge is wiped clean of hair, dust, dirt, and other foreign substances. .... ☐ ☐ ☐

11. Reception furniture meets same requirements as item #10. .... ☐ ☐ ☐

12. Sanitizing supplies are properly stored in their respective locations. .... ☐ ☐ ☐

Subtotal .... ________________

TOTAL .... ________________

At least 9 *YES* responses are necessary to validate. This is 75 percent of the total number of questions. This percentage is the level of acceptability for all chapters.

2. Performance/Product Checklist

A. Shampooing the Hair Checklist

Evaluator's Name______________________________

Student's Name______________________________

Attempt 1: Date________________

Timings________________

Attempt 2: Date________________

Timings________________

Attempt 3: Date________________

Timings________________

Comments:

Note to Evaluator: The performance item numbers preceded by a printer's bullet (•) MUST BE MONITORED and totaled in the space provided. The product items that are not preceded by a bullet need not be monitored step-by-step. They can be totaled in the space provided. With the exception of asterisked items (*), weight each *YES* response one (1).

	Attempt 1 No/Yes	Attempt 2 No/Yes	Attempt 3 No/Yes
I. Student prepares client for shampoo service.			
1. Drapes client with shampoo cape and towel.	☐	☐	☐
2.* Identifies type of service client wants.	☐	☐	☐
3. Removes hairpins, bobbi pins, etc.	☐	☐	☐
4. Requests client to remove eyeglasses, earrings, etc.	☐	☐	☐
5.* Examines the condition of the client's scalp and hair.	☐	☐	☐

Starting time: ________________

Subtotal .... ________________

	Attempt 1 No/Yes	Attempt 2 No/Yes	Attempt 3 No/Yes
II. Student brushes client's hair.			
6. Divides hair on the head into sections.	☐	☐	☐
7. Begins on left front of head.	☐	☐	☐

8. Uses horizontal 1/2 - 3/4 inch partings.................................. ☐ ☐ ☐

•9.* Brush is rotated 180° in right hand, while the section of hair is held in the left hand.. ☐ ☐ ☐

•10.* Brush is rotated on the scalp and then into the hair. .... ☐ ☐ ☐

•11.* Subsections are brushed three times thoroughly.................. ☐ ☐ ☐

12. Proceeds to follow the prescribed procedure until entire head of hair has been brushed. .... ☐ ☐ ☐

Subtotal .... ______________

III. Student rinses client's hair thoroughly.

13. Reclines client's head into neckrest of shampoo bowl. .... ☐ ☐ ☐

•14.* Adjusts water temperature before spraying client's head. .... ☐ ☐ ☐

•15.* Checks water temperature with little finger. .... ☐ ☐ ☐

•16.* Saturates client's entire head, starting in crown area............. ☐ ☐ ☐

•17.* Cups hand to protect nape area as the hair is saturated. .... ☐ ☐ ☐

Subtotal .... ______________

IV. Student follows prescribed procedure for shampooing the hair.

•18.* Applies shampoo, massaging firmly but gently through all the hair. .... ☐ ☐ ☐

•19.* Using both hands on each side of the head, manipulates fingertips firmly in a zig-zag pattern from hairline to back of head, 3 times. .... ☐ ☐ ☐

•20.* Lifts client's head, manipulates fingertips firmly in a zig-zag pattern from behind right ear to behind left ear 3 times. .... ☐ ☐ ☐

•21.* Carefully lowers the client's head on neckrest in bowl. .... ☐ ☐ ☐

•22.* Manipulates fingertips firmly across the crown from right to left in a zig-zag pattern 3 times. .... ☐ ☐ ☐

•23.* Manipulates fingertips firmly on the top front hairline to the back crown in a zig-zag pattern 3 times. .... ☐ ☐ ☐

•24.* Rinses entire hairline and head. .... ☐ ☐ ☐

•25.* Repeats procedural steps for second shampoo. .... ☐ ☐ ☐

•26.* Uses thumbs to massage cosmetic hairline, starting at temples to center. .... ☐ ☐ ☐

•27.* Rinses entire hairline and head. .... ☐ ☐ ☐

Subtotal .... ____________________

V. Final evaluation of service.

•28.* No shampoo present or visible on the entire head or hairline. .... ☐ ☐ ☐

•29.* Safety precautions have been followed (shampoo or water have not contacted client's eyes, ears, face or clothing). .... ☐ ☐ ☐

•30.* All supplies and implements are returned to the proper places. .... ☐ ☐ ☐

Subtotal .... ____________________

TOTAL .... ____________________

At least 26 *YES* responses are necessary to validate. Asterisked items MUST be answered *YES*.

3. Performance/Product Checklist

A. Conditioning the Hair Checklist

Evaluator's Name______________________________

Student's Name______________________________

Attempt 1: Date______________

Timings______________

Attempt 2: Date______________

Timings______________

Attempt 3: Date______________

Timings______________

Comments:

Note to Evaluator: The performance item numbers preceded by a printer's bullet (•) MUST BE MONITORED and totaled in the space provided. The product items that are not preceded by a bullet need not be monitored step-by-step. They can be totaled in the space provided. With the exception of the asterisked (*) items, weight each *YES* response one (1).

I. Hair Analysis.

	Attempt 1 No/Yes	Attempt 2 No/Yes	Attempt 3 No/Yes
•1. Analyzes the hair by using the correct steps to determine if it is dry.	☐	☐	☐
•2.* Analyzes the porosity of the hair in the prescribed manner.	☐	☐	☐
•3.* Analyzes elasticity of hair in the prescribed manner.	☐	☐	☐
•4. Asks client what services were done in home or salon.	☐	☐	☐
•5. Determines if shaping (cutting) will improve overall hair condition.	☐	☐	☐

Subtotal .... ______________

II. Student sells conditioner to the client.

•6.* Explains the condition of the hair in easy-to-understand terms to the client. (Explains why a conditioner is needed.) .... ☐ ☐ ☐

•7.* Recommends at least two different kinds of conditioners. .... ☐ ☐ ☐

•8.* Explains the effects (what the product does) and the price of each conditioner to the client. .... ☐ ☐ ☐

9. States the extra time each type of conditioner requires. .... ☐ ☐ ☐

10. Offers the client a choice between at least two conditioners. .... ☐ ☐ ☐

Subtotal .... ______________

TOTAL .... ______________

At least 8 *YES* responses are necessary to validate. All asterisked items MUST be answered *YES*.

4. Performance/Product Checklist

A. Scalp Treatments Checklist

Evaluator's Name____

Student's Name____

Attempt 1: Date________________

Timings________________

Attempt 2: Date________________

Timings________________

Attempt 3: Date________________

Timings________________

Comments:

Note to Evaluator: The performance item numbers preceded by a printer's bullet (•) MUST BE MONITORED and totaled in the space provided. The product items that are not preceded by a bullet need not be monitored step-by-step. They can be totaled in the space provided. With the exception of asterisked items (*), weight each *YES* response one (1).

Supplies Needed: laundered towels, scalp conditioner, electric steamer or heating cap, and plastic undercap. (Evaluator will circle supplies student failed to obtain.)

I. Preparation and safety precautions.

		Attempt 1 No/Yes	Attempt 2 No/Yes	Attempt 3 No/Yes
•1.*	Identifies service to be given according to procedure..........	☐	☐	☐
2.	Follows safety procedures to protect client's clothing.	☐	☐	☐
•3.*	Examines hair and scalp for irregularities............................	☐	☐	☐
4.	Shampoos client's hair..	☐	☐	☐

Subtotal .... ________________

II. Application of conditioning cream.

•5.* Parts hair into four equal sections.

a. Ear to ear across top of head... ☐ ☐ ☐

b. Center front hairline to nape... ☐ ☐ ☐

•6. Applies conditioner cream in 1/2 inch to 1 inch horizontal subdivisions in first section using cushion of fingers. .... ☐ ☐ ☐

7. Applies cream evenly to all four sections, reapplying where necessary.. ☐ ☐ ☐

Subtotal .... ____________________

III. Manipulations

•8.* Standing behind client, places fingers on each side of neck at trapezius muscle and presses four seconds. .... ☐ ☐ ☐

•9. Rotates fingers clockwise and counterclockwise. .... ☐ ☐ ☐

•10. Moves upward at 1 inch intervals over entire scalp until fingers met earlobes. .... ☐ ☐ ☐

11. Continues with manipulations according to directions. .... ☐ ☐ ☐

Subtotal............ ____________________

IV. Completion

12.* Rinses all cream not absorbed from hair and scalp. .... ☐ ☐ ☐

13.* No residue is on scalp, hair, neck, ears or hairline. .... ☐ ☐ ☐

14.* Sanitizes equipment.. ☐ ☐ ☐

15.* Returns supplies and equipment to proper places. .... ☐ ☐ ☐

Subtotal .... ____________________

Total............ ____________________

Ending time: ____________________

5. Performance/Product Checklist

A. Finger Waving the Hair Checklist

Evaluator's Name____

Student's Name____

Attempt 1: Date_______________

Timings_______________

Attempt 2: Date_______________

Timings_______________

Attempt 3: Date_______________

Timings_______________

Comments:

Note to Evaluator: The performance item numbers preceded by a printer's bullet (•) MUST BE MONITORED and totaled in the space provided. The product items that are not preceded by a bullet need not be monitored step-by-step. They can be totaled in the space provided. With the exception of asterisked items (*), weight each *YES* response one (1).

I. Finger waving the top styling section.

		Attempt 1 No/Yes	Attempt 2 No/Yes	Attempt 3 No/Yes
•1.	Makes right side part.	☐ ☐	☐ ☐	☐ ☐
•2.*	Applies finger-waving setting lotion.	☐ ☐	☐ ☐	☐ ☐
•3.	Combs hair from the right front hairline to the left ear.	☐ ☐	☐ ☐	☐ ☐
•4.	Makes clockwise shaping from the front hairline to the back of the part.	☐ ☐	☐ ☐	☐ ☐
•5.	Makes the first ridge parallel to the part.	☐ ☐	☐ ☐	☐ ☐
•6.	Makes ridge by shifting the comb parallel to the part.	☐ ☐	☐ ☐	☐ ☐
•7.*	Secures the ridge between the middle and index finger before rotating.	☐ ☐	☐ ☐	☐ ☐

•8.* Rotates the comb from the index finger after shifting the comb. .... ☐ ☐ ☐

•9.* Combs hair from the scalp to make the wave pattern. .... ☐ ☐ ☐

•10.* Continues finger-wave pattern around through the crown of the head. .... ☐ ☐ ☐

Subtotal .... ________

II. Student finger waves side, crown and nape sections.

11.* Hair in the wave trough is smooth and circular. .... ☐ ☐ ☐

12.* Ridges are parallel to each other. .... ☐ ☐ ☐

13.* Wave troughs have uniform width. .... ☐ ☐ ☐

14.* Ridges are sharp and well-defined. .... ☐ ☐ ☐

15.* Wave patterns follow the natural direction of hair growth.......... ☐ ☐ ☐

16.* Hair is kept wet throughout waving process. .... ☐ ☐ ☐

Subtotal .... ________

TOTAL .... ________

At least 14 *YES* responses are needed to validate. All asterisked items must be answered *YES*.

6. Performance/Product Checklist

A. Setting the Hair with Sculpture Curls Checklist

Evaluator's Name________________________________

Student's Name________________________________

Attempt 1: Date________________

Timings________________

Attempt 2: Date________________

Timings________________

Attempt 3: Date________________

Timings________________

Comments:

Note to Evaluator: The performance item numbers preceded by a printer's bullet (•) MUST BE MONITORED and totaled in the space provided. The product items that are not preceded by a bullet need not be monitored step-by-step. They can be totaled in the space provided. Weight each *YES* response one (1).

I. Student shapes and sets half-stem sculpture curls in the top section of mannequin.

	Attempt 1 No/Yes	Attempt 2 No/Yes	Attempt 3 No/Yes
•1. Selects mannequin with appropriate hair length for setting pattern.	☐	☐	☐
•2. Makes a side part from the front hairline to crown on right side of the head.	☐	☐	☐
•3. Applies enough setting lotion and water to mold hair.	☐	☐	☐
•4. Combs clockwise shaping into hair.	☐	☐	☐
•5. Carves first curl from open end of shaping.	☐	☐	☐
•6. Secures curls with clip across base direction.	☐	☐	☐
•7. Curls follow circular direction of shaping.	☐	☐	☐
•8. Shaping is not disturbed as curls are made.	☐	☐	☐

•9. Circumference of each curl corresponds to the hair length. ☐ ☐ ☐

•10. Shapes hair in counterclockwise direction. ☐ ☐ ☐

•11. Second shaping is parallel to first row of curls. ☐ ☐ ☐

•12. Carves first curl from the open end of the shaping. ☐ ☐ ☐

•13. Secures curls with a clip across the base direction. ☐ ☐ ☐

•14. Curls follow the circular direction of the shaping. ☐ ☐ ☐

•15. Shaping is not disturbed as curls are made. ☐ ☐ ☐

•16. When unwound, the last curl in the first row coordinates with the first curl in the second row. ☐ ☐ ☐

•17. Hair ends are placed on the inside of each curl. ☐ ☐ ☐

•18. All curls are set on a half-stem. ☐ ☐ ☐

Subtotal .... ______________

II. Student shapes and sets half-stem sculpture curls in the right-side section of mannequin.

1. Combs vertically counterclockwise. ☐ ☐ ☐
2. Secures curls with a clip across the base direction. ☐ ☐ ☐
3. The curls follow a circular direction of the shaping. ☐ ☐ ☐
4. The shaping is not disturbed as the curls are made. ☐ ☐ ☐
5. The circumference of each curl corresponds to the hair length. ☐ ☐ ☐
6. Combs vertical clockwise shaping into the hair. ☐ ☐ ☐
7. Secures curls with clip across base direction. ☐ ☐ ☐
8. The curls follow circular direction of shaping. ☐ ☐ ☐
9. The shaping is not disturbed as curls are made. ☐ ☐ ☐

10. The circumferences of each curl corresponds to hair length. ☐ ☐ ☐

11. When unwound, the last curl in the first row corresponds with the first curl in the second row. ☐ ☐ ☐

12. Hair ends are placed on the inside of each curl. ☐ ☐ ☐

13. All curls are set on a half-stem. ☐ ☐ ☐

Subtotal .... ________________

III. Student shapes and sets no-stem sculpture curls in the left-side section of the mannequin.

1. Combs a vertical clockwise shaping into the hair. ☐ ☐ ☐

2. Secures curls with a clip across the base direction. ☐ ☐ ☐

3. The curls follow the circular direction of the shaping. ☐ ☐ ☐

4. The shaping is not disturbed as the curls are made. ☐ ☐ ☐

5. The circumference of each curl corresponds to the hair length. ☐ ☐ ☐

6. Makes a vertical part behind the ear. ☐ ☐ ☐

7. Places a second row of base-directed curls parallel to the first row. ☐ ☐ ☐

8. The curls follow circular direction of shaping. ☐ ☐ ☐

9. The shaping is not disturbed as curls are made. ☐ ☐ ☐

10. The circumference of each curl corresponds to the hair length. ☐ ☐ ☐

11. The hair ends are placed on the inside of each curl. ☐ ☐ ☐

12. All curls are set on a no-stem. ☐ ☐ ☐

Subtotal .... ________________

IV. Student shapes and sets full-stem and no-stem sculpture curls in the back section of the mannequin.

1. Combs 4 alternating horizontal clockwise and counterclockwise shapings into the hair............................... ☐ ☐ ☐
2. Secures curls with a clip across the base direction................ ☐ ☐ ☐
3. The curls follow the circular direction of the shaping. .... ☐ ☐ ☐
4. The shaping is not disturbed as the curls are made............... ☐ ☐ ☐
5. The circumference of each curl corresponds to the hair length.. ☐ ☐ ☐
6. When unwound, the last curl in the first row corresponds with the first curl in the second row (second with third, etc.).. ☐ ☐ ☐
7. The hair ends are placed on the inside of the curl................ ☐ ☐ ☐
8. Row 1 is set on full-stem sculpture curls. .... ☐ ☐ ☐
9. Row 2 is set on half-stem sculpture curls............................ ☐ ☐ ☐
10. Row 3 is set on no-stem sculpture curls.............................. ☐ ☐ ☐
11. Row 4 is set on no-stem sculpture curls.............................. ☐ ☐ ☐

Subtotal .... ____________________

TOTAL .... ____________________

At least 6 *YES* responses are needed to validate in each numbered section.

B. Combing Hair Previously Set in Sculpture Curls.

Evaluator's Name____

Student's Name____

Attempt 1: Date________________

Timings________________

Attempt 2: Date________________

Timings________________

Attempt 3: Date________________

Timings________________

Comments:

Note to Evaluator: The performance item numbers preceded by a printer's bullet (•) MUST BE MONITORED and totaled in the space provided. The product items that are not preceded by a bullet need not be monitored step-by-step. They can be totaled in the space provided. Weight each *YES* response one (1).

	Attempt 1 No/Yes	Attempt 2 No/Yes	Attempt 3 No/Yes
I. Student prepares the mannequin for comb-out.			
1. Removes all clips.	☐	☐	☐
•2. Unfolds the hair into the setting pattern.	☐	☐	☐
•3. Relaxes the hair by using hair brush.	☐	☐	☐
Subtotal	________		
II. Student combs the hair into a wave pattern.			
•4. Combs hair in waves according to the setting pattern.	☐	☐	☐
Subtotal	________		
III. Evaluating the comb-out.			
5. All ridges are definite.	☐	☐	☐
6. All ridges are parallel to each other.	☐	☐	☐
7. Waves are laid close to the head.	☐	☐	☐

8. A definite "5 inch pattern is visible.................................... ☐ ☐ ☐

9. All wave troughs are equal in size. .... ☐ ☐ ☐

Subtotal .... ____________

TOTAL .... ____________

Actual: At least 6 *YES* responses are needed to validate.

7. Performance/Product Checklist

A. Student sets the Hair with Rollers Checklist

Evaluator's Name ____

Student's Name ____

Attempt 1: Date ______________

Timings ______________

Attempt 2: Date ______________

Timings ______________

Attempt 3: Date ______________

Timings ______________

Comments:

	Attempt 1 No/Yes	Attempt 2 No/Yes	Attempt 3 No/Yes
1. Selects a mannequin with appropriate length hair for the setting pattern.	☐	☐	☐
2. Roller sizes correspond to hair length (hair encircles roller at least once but not more than 2 1/2 times).	☐	☐	☐
3. Hair is wound firmly around the rollers (tension is used).	☐	☐	☐
4. Hair is wound smoothly around the rollers.	☐	☐	☐
5. Hair is evenly distributed around the rollers.	☐	☐	☐

6. When the roller is unwound, the ends are placed smoothly around the roller (no fish hooks). .... ☐ ☐ ☐

7. Rollers are secured with clips without disturbing the bases. .... ☐ ☐ ☐

8. All rollers are set on a no-stem or half-stem base. .... ☐ ☐ ☐

9. Partings are straight and uniform. .... ☐ ☐ ☐

10. Width of the subsection is slightly less than the length of the roller. .... ☐ ☐ ☐

11. Length of the subsection is slightly less than the length of the roller. .... ☐ ☐ ☐

12. Circumferences of rollers decreases toward the hairline. .... ☐ ☐ ☐

13. Hair is kept wet with water after initial saturation with setting lotion. .... ☐ ☐ ☐

TOTAL .... ________________

To validate, at least 10 items must have *YES* responses.

8. Performance/Product Checklist

A. Combing Hair Previously Set in Rollers Checklist

Evaluator's Name________________________________

Student's Name________________________________

Attempt 1: Date__________

Timings__________

Attempt 2: Date__________

Timings__________

Attempt 3: Date__________

Timings__________

Comments:

Note to Evaluator: The performance item numbers preceded by a printer's bullet (•) MUST BE MONITORED and totaled in the space provided. The product items that are not preceded by a bullet need not be monitored step-by-step. They can be totaled in the space provided. Weight each *YES* response one (1).

I. Student prepares the mannequin for styling.

	Attempt 1 No/Yes	Attempt 2 No/Yes	Attempt 3 No/Yes
•1. The hair is unfolded and relaxed into a setting pattern.	☐	☐	☐
•2. Backcombing is restricted within the first inches of hair at the scalp.	☐	☐	☐
•3. The hair is backcombed into place according to the setting pattern.	☐	☐	☐
Subtotal	________		

II. Student styles the mannequin.

	Attempt 1 No/Yes	Attempt 2 No/Yes	Attempt 3 No/Yes
4. Smooths hair into place without destroying backcombed base.	☐	☐	☐
5. Sees there are no roller splits.	☐	☐	☐
6. There are no clip marks across the hair.	☐	☐	☐

7. Hair is not overly sprayed with hairspray. ☐ ☐ ☐

8. No backcombing is visible on the top of the hair. ☐ ☐ ☐

9. All sections of hair blend together. ☐ ☐ ☐

10. Design corresponds with setting pattern. ☐ ☐ ☐

11. Maintains balance throughout the hairstyle. ☐ ☐ ☐

Subtotal............. ________________

TOTAL............. ________________

9. Performance/Product Checklist

A. A Basic Hair Shaping Checklist

Evaluator's Name____

Student's Name____

Attempt 1: Date________________

Timings________________

Attempt 2: Date________________

Timings________________

Attempt 3: Date________________

Timings________________

Comments:

Note to Evaluator: The performance item numbers preceded by a printer's bullet (•) MUST BE MONITORED and totaled in the space provided. The product items that are not preceded by a bullet need not be monitored step-by-step. They can be totaled in the space provided. With the exception of asterisked items (*), weight each *YES* response one (1).

I. Student prepares to cut hair.

	Attempt 1 No/Yes	Attempt 2 No/Yes	Attempt 3 No/Yes
1. Collects necessary supplies and implements.	☐	☐	☐
2. Drapes client.	☐	☐	☐
a. Neck strip between cape and neck.	☐	☐	☐

b. Clean towel between cape (or chair cloth) and neck.. ☐ ☐ ☐

3. Thoroughly shampoos or saturates hair with water. .... ☐ ☐ ☐

4. Parts and secures the hair into the five styling sections of the head. .... ☐ ☐ ☐

•5.* Leaves a guideline on nape and side sections that doesn't exceed 1 1/2 inch in width, and leaves hair at least 3 1/2 inch in top/crown sections. .... ☐ ☐ ☐

6. Discusses hanging length with the client. .... ☐ ☐ ☐

Subtotal............. ________________

II. Student cuts the guideline and first section.

•7.* Guideline is cut uniformly and shows a definite line............. ☐ ☐ ☐

•8.* The first section of the upper crepe is combed into guideline. .... ☐ ☐ ☐

•9.* Upper nape section is cut from left toward right side of head. .... ☐ ☐ ☐

•10.* Hair is uniformly cut from one subsection to the next.......... ☐ ☐ ☐

Subtotal .... ________________

III. Cutting the crown and side sections.

11. Hair in the crown section is combed into the guide and evenly cut. .... ☐ ☐ ☐

•12.* Hair in both side sections is combed into the guide and evenly cut. .... ☐ ☐ ☐

Subtotal .... ________________

IV. Cutting the top section.

•13.* The top section is parted down the middle from the face to the crown. ☐ ☐ ☐

•14.* Begins cutting on the right side of the client, from the crown toward the face. ☐ ☐ ☐

•15.* Uses previously cut hair for a guide. ☐ ☐ ☐

•16.* Using hair beneath as a guide, cutting angle is doubled for top section. ☐ ☐ ☐

•17. Keeps razor/scissors in one hand or the other throughout the shaping. ☐ ☐ ☐

a. Does not lay comb or razor on work surface. ☐ ☐ ☐

b. Does not put comb or razor in pocket. ☐ ☐ ☐

•18. Checks haircut for evenness. ☐ ☐ ☐

19. Cleans neckline of hair. ☐ ☐ ☐

Subtotal .... ____________

V. Evaluation of completed shaping.

20. Client has not been cut. ☐ ☐ ☐

21. Lengths of hair are even when combed in vertical or horizontal subsections (according to intent). ☐ ☐ ☐

22. Hanging length displays conformity for desired styling techniques to be applied in the setting and combing procedure. ☐ ☐ ☐

23. Hanging length is even on both sides. ☐ ☐ ☐

24. Hair is swept from the floor immediately after shaping. ☐ ☐ ☐

Subtotal .... ____________

TOTAL .... ________________

At least 15 *YES* responses are necessary for validation. ALL asterisked items MUST be marked *YES*.

10. Performance/Product Checklist

A. Blow Waving the Hair Checklist

Evaluator's Name____

Student's Name____

Attempt 1: Date______________

Timings______________

Attempt 2: Date______________

Timings______________

Attempt 3: Date______________

Timings______________

Comments:

Note to Evaluator: The performance item numbers preceded by a printer's bullet (•) MUST BE MONITORED and totaled in the space provided. The product items that are not preceded by a bullet need not be monitored step-by-step. They can be totaled in the space provided. With the exception of asterisked items (*), weight each *YES* response one (1).

Supplies Needed: shampoo supplies, styling comb, electric blower, round brush, hair spray and blow wave lotion. (Evaluator will circle supplies student failed to obtain.)

I. Student prepares client for blow waving.	Attempt 1 No/Yes	Attempt 2 No/Yes	Attempt 3 No/Yes
1. Drapes client.	☐	☐	☐
2. Shampoos hair.	☐	☐	☐
3. Towel dries hair.	☐	☐	☐
4. Applies blow wave lotion.	☐	☐	☐

TOTAL I .... ________________

II. Follows correct procedure for blow waving.

5. Turns blow waver on and sets temperature. ☐ ☐ ☐

6. Begins at left front side of section. ☐ ☐ ☐

•7.* Directs flow of heat toward base of hair strand. ☐ ☐ ☐

•8.* Does NOT direct flow of air towards scalp, face, ears, or eyes. ☐ ☐ ☐

•9. As the hair dries, slides the brush through the strands. ☐ ☐ ☐

•10. Thoroughly dries and shapes the hair from the front hairline to the center of the ear in both side sections. ☐ ☐ ☐

•11. Rotates the brush to help shape all the hair next to the scalp. ☐ ☐ ☐

•12. Rotates the brush in a vertical, horizontal or diagonal position. ☐ ☐ ☐

•13.* Dries and directs hair ends in the nape, top, crown sections. ☐ ☐ ☐

•14. Arranges ends with a styling comb as needed to complete hairstyling. ☐ ☐ ☐

15. Finishes the style by spraying the hair lightly. ☐ ☐ ☐

TOTAL II .... ______________

III. Procedural steps for air waving.

5.* Turns on air waver and adjusts temperature. ☐ ☐ ☐

6. Subdivides the hair into strands about the same size as used for a roller. ☐ ☐ ☐

7.* Holds the end of the strand with the left hand and places comb close to the scalp. ☐ ☐ ☐

8.* Using circular motion, turns comb attachments against the hair. ☐ ☐ ☐

9.* Slides air comb close to the scalp toward the face at angle of desired wave pattern. ☐ ☐ ☐

10.* Uses left hand to support the hair in the side section while flipping the end. Continues to dry the hair until a diagonal wave is formed. ☐ ☐ ☐

11. Begins drying hair in top section; directs teeth of comb toward the part. ☐ ☐ ☐

12. Continues to form an "S inch pattern in the hair. ☐ ☐ ☐

13.* Checks wave lines for depth, definition and design. ☐ ☐ ☐

TOTAL III .... ________________

Total I and II .... ________________ or

Total I and III .... ________________

At least 9 *YES* responses are necessary to validate (Total I and III). All asterisked items MUST be answered *YES*.

11. Performance/Product Checklist

A. Iron Curling Checklist

Evaluator's Name____

Student's Name____

Attempt 1: Date________________

Timings________________

Attempt 2: Date________________

Timings________________

Attempt 3: Date________________

Timings________________

Comments:

Note to Evaluator: The performance item numbers preceded by a printer's bullet (•) MUST BE MONITORED and totaled in the space provided. The product items that are not preceded by a bullet need not be monitored step-by-step. They can be totaled in the space provided. With the exception of asterisked items (*), weight each *YES* response one (1).

Supplies Needed: shampoo supplies, chair cloth, neck strap, client release form, hard rubber combs or heat resistant combs, curling iron and duck bill clips. (Evaluator will circle supplies student failed to obtain.)

	Attempt 1 No/Yes	Attempt 2 No/Yes	Attempt 3 No/Yes
I. Student prepares client for shampoo.			
1. Drapes the client for shampooing..	☐	☐	☐
2. Brushes the hair according to procedure.	☐	☐	☐
3. Examines the scalp for abrasions and dryness or flakiness..	☐	☐	☐
4.* Applies lanolin creme or oil as needed to protect and condition the hair and scalp before curling with iron............	☐	☐	☐
5. Dries the hair as needed under dryer....................................	☐	☐	☐
Subtotal.............	______		
II. Prepares the client for thermal curling.			
6. Drapes the client with dry styling service using neck strip..	☐	☐	☐
7. Divides the hair into 4 equal sections....................................	☐	☐	☐
8.* Tests the temperature of the iron before using it..................	☐	☐	☐
Subtotal	______		
III. Begins thermal curling of hair in the first section.			
Starting time: ______________________			
•9. Begins at the hairline of the nape or uses school method (at either back section), and curls the hair using 1/2-inch horizontal subdivisions................................	☐	☐	☐
•10. Silks the hair from the nape to the crown............................	☐	☐	☐

•11. Inserts the iron as close to the scalp as possible; yet protects scalp using a comb. .... ☐ ☐ ☐

•12. Rotates the iron against the strand of hair using moderate to firm pressure. .... ☐ ☐ ☐

•13. Allows heat to penetrate through each strand. .... ☐ ☐ ☐

Subtotal .... ______________

IV. Repeats curling procedure for remaining 3 sections of hair.

14.* All the hair appears uniformly curled. .... ☐ ☐ ☐

15.* Hair is not discolored (scorched). .... ☐ ☐ ☐

16.* No broken hairs are visible. .... ☐ ☐ ☐

17.* No broken hairs are on temperature-testing .... ☐ ☐ ☐

18.* Client does not sustain any burns from curling iron. .... ☐ ☐ ☐

19.* Hair feels "soft," not excessively oily or dry. .... ☐ ☐ ☐

Ending time: ______________

Subtotal .... ______________

TOTAL .... ______________

At least 14 *YES* responses are needed to validate. ALL asterisked items MUST be answered *YES*.

12. Performance/Product Checklist

A. Applying a Temporary Color to the Hair Checklist

Evaluator's Name____

Student's Name____

Attempt 1: Date________________

Timings________________

Attempt 2: Date________________

Timings________________

Attempt 3: Date________________

Timings________________

Comments:

Note to Evaluator: The performance item numbers preceded by a printer's bullet (•) MUST BE MONITORED and totaled in the space provided. The product items that are not preceded by a bullet need not be monitored step-by-step. They can be totaled in the space provided. Weight each *YES* response one (1).

	Attempt 1 No/Yes	Attempt 2 No/Yes	Attempt 3 No/Yes
I. Student prepares client for application of rinse.			
1. Drapes client with protective cape.	☐	☐	☐
2. Puts on protective cape.	☐	☐	☐
3. Towel-dries hair.	☐	☐	☐
Subtotal			
II. Prepares for application of rinse.			
4. Applies selected rinse according to manufacturer's directions.	☐	☐	☐
•5. Combs rinse through the hair toward the back of the head.	☐	☐	☐
•6. Lifts head and applies a small amount of color to nape line.	☐	☐	☐

•7. Blots excess color with a clean towel.................................... ☐ ☐ ☐

8. Keeps rinse from dripping on client's neck ____ face ____ ears _____ clothing _____. .... ☐ ☐ ☐
(If the *NO* response is checked, indicate in space which item is incorrect.)

9. Cleans shampoo bowl and surrounding splash area............... ☐ ☐ ☐

10. Recaps bottles and returns supplies to dispensary. .... ☐ ☐ ☐

Subtotal .... ________________

TOTAL .... ________________

At least 8 *YES* responses are needed to validate.

13. Performance/Product Checklist

A. Applying Semipermanent Hair Color Checklist

Evaluator's Name____

Student's Name____

Attempt 1: Date________________

Timings________________

Attempt 2: Date________________

Timings________________

Attempt 3: Date________________

Timings________________

Comments:

Note to Evaluator: The performance item numbers preceded by a printer's bullet (•) MUST BE MONITORED and totaled in the space provided. The product items that are not preceded by a bullet need not be monitored step-by-step. They can be totaled in the space provided. If the procedure is simulated using wave set, the student must still mix at least a half formula of tint. See bottom of last sheet for items to omit. With the exception of asterisked (*) items, weight each *YES* response one (1).

I. Student prepares client for application of semipermanent hair colo:

	Attempt 1 No/Yes	Attempt 2 No/Yes	Attempt 3 No/Yes
1.* Records results of patch test.	☐	☐	☐
2. Drapes client with protective cape.	☐	☐	☐
3. Removes tangles from hair.	☐	☐	☐
4. Divides hair into 4 equal sections.	☐	☐	☐
5. Communicates with client in selection of color desired.	☐	☐	☐
6.* Puts on protective gloves	☐	☐	☐
7. Puts on protective operator's apron.	☐	☐	☐

Subtotal .... ________________

II. Prepares for application of color.

	Attempt 1 No/Yes	Attempt 2 No/Yes	Attempt 3 No/Yes
•8.* Examines scalp for abrasions.	☐	☐	☐
•9.* Mixes color according to manufacturer's directions.	☐	☐	☐

Subtotal .... ________________

III. Student correctly applies semipermanent color to client's head.

	Attempt 1 No/Yes	Attempt 2 No/Yes	Attempt 3 No/Yes
10. Avoids dripping color on client's face or clothing.	☐	☐	☐
11. Doesn't allow color to run onto client's hairline or ears.	☐	☐	☐
12.* Saturates each strand with color.	☐	☐	☐
13. Applies tint to all strands in 5 to 8 minutes.	☐	☐	☐

Subtotal .... ________________

IV. Processes semipermanent color.

	Attempt 1 No/Yes	Attempt 2 No/Yes	Attempt 3 No/Yes
14. Sets timer.	☐	☐	☐

•15. Strand tested. ☐ ☐ ☐

16. Processes according to manufacturer's directions. ☐ ☐ ☐

Subtotal .... ________

V. Removes color from hair and scalp.

17.* Follows manufacturer's directions for removal of color. ☐ ☐ ☐

Subtotal .... ________

VI. Final evaluation of service.

18. Hair color is uniform throughout head. ☐ ☐ ☐

•19. No color is on or behind the ears. ☐ ☐ ☐

•20. No stains are on scalp. ☐ ☐ ☐

21. Hair is tangle-free and easy to comb. ☐ ☐ ☐

22. All supplies and implements are returned to the proper places. ☐ ☐ ☐

23. Client's color card records formula used and results. ☐ ☐ ☐

Subtotal .... ________

TOTAL .... ________

Actual: At least 17 *YES* responses are needed to validate. ALL asterisked items MUST be answered *YES*.

Simulated: Omit items 1, 14, 15, 16, 18, 19, 20. At least 14 *YES* responses are needed to validate.

14. Performance/Product Checklist

A. Applying a Virgin Tint to Lighten Hair Checklist

Evaluator's Name____

Student's Name____

Attempt 1: Date_______________

Timings_______________

Attempt 2: Date_______________

Timings_______________

Attempt 3: Date_______________

Timings_______________

Comments:

Note to Evaluator: The performance item numbers preceded by a printer's bullet (•) MUST BE MONITORED and totaled in the space provided. The product items that are not preceded by a bullet need not be monitored step-by-step. They can be totaled in the space provided. With the exception of asterisked items (*), weight each *YES* response one (1).

	Attempt 1 No/Yes	Attempt 2 No/Yes	Attempt 3 No/Yes
I. Student prepares client for application of tint.			
1.* Records the results of the patch test.	☐	☐	☐
2. Drapes the client with protective cape.	☐	☐	☐
3. Removes tangles from the hair.	☐	☐	☐
4. Divides the hair into 4 equal sections.	☐	☐	☐
5.* Powders and puts on protective cape.	☐	☐	☐
6. Puts on protective operator's apron.	☐	☐	☐
Subtotal			
II. Prepares for application of tint and applies it to first half of the section.			
•7. Examines scalp for lesions.	☐	☐	☐

•8.* Mixes color according to the manufacturer's directions. .... ☐ ☐ ☐

•9.* Begins application one inch from the scalp on the strand in the right top crown section. .... ☐ ☐ ☐

•10. Parts the hair by using the nozzle of bottle. .... ☐ ☐ ☐

Subtotal .... ____________

III. Student correctly applies tint to remaining three sections.

11. Uses 1/4 inch horizontal partings and applies tint from the top to the bottom of section. .... ☐ ☐ ☐

12.* Avoids dripping tint on the client's face or clothing. .... ☐ ☐ ☐

13. Keeps tint from the scalp area in all sections. .... ☐ ☐ ☐

14. Saturates each strand with tint. .... ☐ ☐ ☐

15. Keeps tint from dripping on floor. .... ☐ ☐ ☐

16. Doesn't allow tint to run onto client's hairline or into the client's ears. .... ☐ ☐ ☐

17.* Applies tint to all strands in 15 to 20 minutes. .... ☐ ☐ ☐

Subtotal .... ____________

IV. Processes tint.

18. Uses timer. .... ☐ ☐ ☐

19. Strand-tests the hair. .... ☐ ☐ ☐

20. Processes tint according to manufacturer's directions and results of strand test. .... ☐ ☐ ☐

21. Applies tint to all hair next to the scalp. .... ☐ ☐ ☐

Subtotal .... ____________

V. Color is checked.

•22. Strand test shows color is even from the scalp to the end of the strand. ☐ ☐ ☐

•23. All hair is evenly covered with tint. ☐ ☐ ☐

Subtotal .... ________

VI. Removes tint from the hair and scalp.

24. Uses correct shampoo. ☐ ☐ ☐

25. Uses tint material to remove color stains from the hairline. ☐ ☐ ☐

26. Uses tint remover to erase color stains from the scalp, hairline, and ears. ☐ ☐ ☐

27. Shampoos all tint from the hair and scalp. ☐ ☐ ☐

28. Conditions the hair as needed. ☐ ☐ ☐

Subtotal .... ________

VII. Final evaluation of the service.

•29. Hair color is uniform in three 1/2 inch square strands sampled in different areas of the head. ☐ ☐ ☐

•30. No color is on or behind the ears. ☐ ☐ ☐

•31. No stains are on scalp. ☐ ☐ ☐

•32. No shampoo or tint residue is present on the nape of neck. ☐ ☐ ☐

•33.* There are no visible stains anywhere on the client's clothing. ☐ ☐ ☐

34. Hair is tangle-free and easy to comb. ☐ ☐ ☐

35. All supplies and implements are in the proper places. ☐ ☐ ☐

36. Client's hair color card records formula product used and the end results. .... ☐ ☐ ☐

Subtotal .... ____________

TOTAL .... ____________

Actual: At least 7 *YES* responses are needed to validate. ALL asterisked items MUST be answered *YES*.

Simulated: Omit items 1, 18, 19, 20, 22, 25, 26, 27, 29, 30, and 31. At least 9 *YES* responses on the remaining items are needed to validate. ALL asterisked items must be answered *YES*.

15. Performance/Product Checklist

A. Applying a Retouch Tint Checklist

Evaluator's Name____

Student's Name____

Attempt 1: Date________________

Timings________________

Attempt 2: Date________________

Timings________________

Attempt 3: Date________________

Timings________________

Comments:

Note to Evaluator: The performance item numbers preceded by a printer's bullet (•) MUST BE MONITORED and totaled in the space provided. The product items that are not preceded by a bullet need not be monitored step-by-step. They can be totaled in the space provided. With the exception of asterisked items (*), weight each *YES* response one (1).

I. Student prepares the client for application of the tint.

	Attempt 1 No/Yes	Attempt 2 No/Yes	Attempt 3 No/Yes
1.* Records the results of the patch test.	☐	☐	☐
2. Drapes the client with protective cape.	☐	☐	☐
3. Removes tangles from the hair.	☐	☐	☐

4. Divides the hair into 4 equal sections.................................... ☐ ☐ ☐

5.* Puts on protective gloves.. ☐ ☐ ☐

6. Puts on protective operator's apron. .... ☐ ☐ ☐

Subtotal .... ________________

II. Prepares for application of tint.

•7. Examines scalp for lesions. .... ☐ ☐ ☐

•8.* Mixes color according to the manufacturer's directions. .... ☐ ☐ ☐

•9.* Begins application by outlining the parts with hair color.. ☐ ☐ ☐

•10. Proceeds with the application at the right back section using 1/4 inch partings. .... ☐ ☐ ☐

•11. Parts the hair by using the nozzle of the bottle. .... ☐ ☐ ☐

•12.* Applies tint from the top to the bottom of the section. .... ☐ ☐ ☐

Subtotal .... ________________

III. Student applies tint to remaining 3 sections.

13. Avoids dripping tint on the client's face and clothing............ ☐ ☐ ☐

14. Completely covers new growth with hair tint. .... ☐ ☐ ☐

15. Pulls strands away from the scalp so that the color could oxidize. .... ☐ ☐ ☐

16. Keeps the tint from dripping on the floor............................. ☐ ☐ ☐

17. Doesn't allow tint to run onto client's hairline or into the client's ears. .... ☐ ☐ ☐

18.* Applies tint to entire new growth in 15 to 20 minutes.......... ☐ ☐ ☐

Subtotal .... ________________

IV. Processes tint.

19. Uses timer.. ☐ ☐ ☐

20. Strand-tests the hair. .... ☐ ☐ ☐

21. Processes the tint according to the manufacturer's directions and the results of the strand test. .... ☐ ☐ ☐

22. Applies tint to ends of the hair. .... ☐ ☐ ☐

Subtotal .... ____________

V. Checks color.

•23.* Strand test shows color is even from the scalp to the end of the strand. There is no line of demarcation. .... ☐ ☐ ☐

•24. All the hair is evenly covered with tint. .... ☐ ☐ ☐

Subtotal .... ____________

VI. Removes tint from the hair and scalp.

25. Uses correct shampoo.. ☐ ☐ ☐

26. Uses tint material to remove color stains from the hairline.. ☐ ☐ ☐

27. Uses tint remover to erase color stains from the scalp, hairline, and ears. .... ☐ ☐ ☐

28. Shampoos all tint from the hair and scalp. .... ☐ ☐ ☐

29. Conditions the hair as needed.. ☐ ☐ ☐

Subtotal .... ____________

VII. Final evaluation of the service.

•30. Hair color is uniform in three 1/2 inch square strands sampled in different areas of head.. ☐ ☐ ☐

•31. No color is on or behind the ears. ☐ ☐ ☐

•32. No stains are on the scalp. ☐ ☐ ☐

•33. No shampoo residue is present in the nape of neck. ☐ ☐ ☐

•34.* There are no visible stains anywhere on client's clothing. ☐ ☐ ☐

35. Hair is tangle-free and easy to comb. ☐ ☐ ☐

36. All supplies and implements are in the proper places. ☐ ☐ ☐

37. The formula used and the end results have been recorded on the client's hair color card. ☐ ☐ ☐

Subtotal .... ________________

TOTAL .... ________________

At least 27 *YES* responses are needed to validate. ALL asterisked items MUST be answered *YES*

16. Performance/Product Checklist

A. Applying a virgin lightener Checklist

Evaluator's Name____

Student's Name____

Attempt 1: Date________________

Timings________________

Attempt 2: Date________________

Timings________________

Attempt 3: Date________________

Timings________________

Comments:

Note to Evaluator: The performance item numbers preceded by a printer's bullet (•) MUST BE MONITORED and totaled in the space provided. The product items that are not preceded by a bullet need not be monitored step-by-step. They can be totaled in the space provided. If procedure is simulated using wave set, the student must still mix at least 1/2 formula of bleach. See bottom of last sheet for items to omit. with the exception of asterisked items, weight each *YES* response one (1).

I. Student prepares the client for application of bleach.	Attempt 1 No/Yes	Attempt 2 No/Yes	Attempt 3 No/Yes
1.* Records the results of the patch test.	☐	☐	☐
2. Drapes the client with protective cape.	☐	☐	☐
3. Removes tangles from the hair.	☐	☐	☐
4. Divides the hair into equal sections.	☐	☐	☐
5.* Powders and puts on protective gloves.	☐	☐	☐
6. Puts on protective operator's apron.	☐	☐	☐

Subtotal .... ________________

II. Student prepares for application of bleach and applies it to the first half of the section.	Attempt 1	Attempt 2	Attempt 3
•7. Examines scalp for lesions.	☐	☐	☐

•8.* Mixes bleach according to the manufacturer's directions. ☐ ☐ ☐

•9.* Begins application one inch from the scalp on strand in the right top crown section to one inch from ends. ☐ ☐ ☐

•10. Parts hair using nozzle of bottle. ☐ ☐ ☐

•11 Uses 1/8 inch horizontal partings and applies bleach from the top to the bottom of the section. ☐ ☐ ☐

•12.* Avoids dripping bleach on client's face, ears, or clothing. ☐ ☐ ☐

•13. Uses the nozzle of the bottle to spread the bleach to within one inch of the ends. ☐ ☐ ☐

Subtotal .... ____________

III. Student applies bleach to remaining three sections.

14. Keeps bleach from scalp and ends area in all sections. ☐ ☐ ☐

15. Saturates each strand with bleach. ☐ ☐ ☐

16. Keeps bleach from dripping to floor. ☐ ☐ ☐

17. Doesn't allow bleach to drip onto client's hairline or ears. ☐ ☐ ☐

18.* Applies bleach to all strands in 15 to 20 minutes. ☐ ☐ ☐

Subtotal .... ____________

15. Processes bleach.

19. Uses a timer. ☐ ☐ ☐

20. Strand-tests the hair. ☐ ☐ ☐

21. Processes the bleach according to the manufacturer's directions and desired degree of lightening. ☐ ☐ ☐

22. Applies bleach to all hair ends. .... ☐ ☐ ☐

23. Applies bleach to root area until entire strand is covered from the scalp to the ends. .... ☐ ☐ ☐

Subtotal .... ________________

V. Checks lightener.

•24. Strand test shows that the lightening is even from the scalp to the end of the strand. .... ☐ ☐ ☐

•25. All hair is evenly covered with bleach. .... ☐ ☐ ☐

Subtotal .... ________________

VI. Student removes bleach from the hair and scalp.

26. Uses the correct shampoo. .... ☐ ☐ ☐

27. Removes bleach from the hairline. .... ☐ ☐ ☐

28. Shampoos all bleach from the hair and scalp with tepid water. .... ☐ ☐ ☐

Subtotal .... ________________

VII. Final evaluation of service.

•29. Hair lightening is uniform in three 1/2 inch square strands sampled in different areas of the head. .... ☐ ☐ ☐

•30. No bleach is on or behind the ears. .... ☐ ☐ ☐

•31. No bleach is left on the scalp. .... ☐ ☐ ☐

•32. No shampoo residue is present in the nape of neck. .... ☐ ☐ ☐

•33.* Lightener is even from the scalp to the ends. .... ☐ ☐ ☐

•34. Hair is tangle-free and easy to comb. .... ☐ ☐ ☐

•35. All supplies and implements are in the proper places. .... ☐ ☐ ☐

•36. The bleaching product used, the time required, and the end results have been recorded on the client's hair color card.. ☐ ☐ ☐

Subtotal .... ____________

TOTAL .... ____________

<u>Actual:</u> At least 7 *YES* responses are needed to validate. ALL asterisked items MUST be answered *YES*.

<u>Simulated:</u> 0mit items 1, 19, 20, 24, 26, 27, 29, 30, and 31. At least 9 *YES* responses on the remaining items are needed to validate. ALL asterisked items MUST be answered *YES*.

17. Performance/Product Checklist

A. Permanent Waving - Checklist

Evaluator's Name______________________________

Student's Name______________________________

Attempt 1: Date_______________

Timings_______________

Attempt 2: Date_______________

Timings_______________

Attempt 3: Date_______________

Timings_______________

Comments:

Note to Evaluator: The performance item numbers preceded by a printer's bullet (•) MUST BE MONITORED and totaled in the space provided. The product items that are not preceded by a bullet need not be monitored step-by-step. They can be totaled in the space provided. Weight each *YES* response one (1).

I. Student prepares client and examines scalp.	Attempt 1 No/Yes	Attempt 2 No/Yes	Attempt 3 No/Yes
1. Displays the completed release form.	☐	☐	☐
2. Client is properly draped.	☐	☐	☐
3. Client is asked the kind (type) of wave preferred.	☐	☐	☐
4. Scalp is examined for abrasions and cuts.	☐	☐	☐
5. Hair is not vigorously brushed prior to service.	☐	☐	☐
6. Hair and scalp are not vigorously shampooed prior to service.	☐	☐	☐

Subtotal .... _______________

II. Analyzes the condition of the hair.	Attempt 1 No/Yes	Attempt 2 No/Yes	Attempt 3 No/Yes
•7. Analyzes the porosity of the hair in the prescribed manner.	☐	☐	☐

•8. Analyzes the elasticity of the hair in the prescribed manner. ☐ ☐ ☐

•9. Analyzes the texture of the hair in the prescribed manner. ☐ ☐ ☐

•10. Asks the client about the use of drugstore-purchased coloring and waving products. ☐ ☐ ☐

•11. Determines if the client is in need of a haircut or not. ☐ ☐ ☐

•12. Chooses the permanent wave rods according to the amount of curl requested. ☐ ☐ ☐

•13. Selects the waving lotion strength that corresponds to the condition and texture of the client's hair. ☐ ☐ ☐

•14. Dries hair with towel or dryer according to the manufacturer's directions. ☐ ☐ ☐

Subtotal............. ______________

TOTAL............. ______________

At least 10 *YES* responses are needed to validate.

B. Cold Waving.

Evaluator's Name ______________________________

Student's Name ______________________________

Attempt 1: Date ______________

Timings ______________

Attempt 2: Date ______________

Timings ______________

Attempt 3: Date ______________

Timings ______________

Comments:

Note to Evaluator: The performance item numbers preceded by a printer's bullet (•) MUST BE MONITORED and totaled in the space provided. The product items that are not preceded by a bullet need not be monitored step-by-step. They can be totaled in the space provided. With the exception of asterisked items (*), weight each *YES* response one (1).

I. Student assembles necessary supplies.

	Attempt 1 No/Yes	Attempt 2 No/Yes	Attempt 3 No/Yes
1. Timer	☐	☐	☐
2. End wraps	☐	☐	☐
3. Comb	☐	☐	☐
4. Rods	☐	☐	☐
5. Clips	☐	☐	☐
6. Cotton	☐	☐	☐
7. Plastic applicator bottle	☐	☐	☐
8. Neutralizing bib	☐	☐	☐
9. Wrapping solution	☐	☐	☐

Subtotal .... ____________

II. Divides hair into wrapping sections.

	Attempt 1 No/Yes	Attempt 2 No/Yes	Attempt 3 No/Yes
10.* Length of section is equal to length of rod to be used	☐	☐	☐
11. Parts between sections are clean.	☐	☐	☐
12.* Neck towel is secured around the client's neck.	☐	☐	☐

Subtotal .... ____________

III. Begins wrapping procedure on the first section.

	Attempt 1 No/Yes	Attempt 2 No/Yes	Attempt 3 No/Yes
•13.* The strand to be wrapped is not larger than the rod.	☐	☐	☐
•14.* The width of strand is 1/2 of the diameter of the rod.	☐	☐	☐

•15.* During wrapping, the end wrap extends beyond the end of hair strand. ☐ ☐ ☐

•16.* The hair is evenly spread across the rod as it is wrapped. ☐ ☐ ☐

•17.* Moderate tension is applied to each rod during wrapping. ☐ ☐ ☐

•18.* Elastic secures rod to the head without binding the hair at either end of the rod. ☐ ☐ ☐

•19.* The rod, elastic and lower part are parallel. ☐ ☐ ☐

•20.* The rod is centered on the lower parting. ☐ ☐ ☐

•21.* The wrapping of first section is completed. ☐ ☐ ☐

Subtotal .... ____________

IV. Continues wrapping remaining hair.

22.* Keeps comb in hand during wrapping. ☐ ☐ ☐

23. Tension is evenly applied to the rod during wrapping. ☐ ☐ ☐

24.* The rod circumference decreases according to the length of the hair. ☐ ☐ ☐

25.* When the rod is unwound, there are no fishhook ends. ☐ ☐ ☐

26. Sections are uniformly wrapped according to the head size. ☐ ☐ ☐

27.* All elastics are centered on the rod so hair is not bound at either end. ☐ ☐ ☐

28. The strip is placed around entire hairline including the nape. ☐ ☐ ☐

29.* The hair is wrapped in 45 minutes or less. ☐ ☐ ☐

Subtotal .... ____________

TOTAL............. ____________

Actual: At least 17 *YES* responses are needed to validate. ALL asterisked items MUST be answered *YES*.

C. Processing and Neutralizing

Evaluator's Name ____________________

Student's Name ____________________

Attempt 1: Date ____________

Timings ____________

Attempt 2: Date ____________

Timings ____________

Attempt 3: Date ____________

Timings ____________

Comments:

Note to Evaluator: The performance item numbers preceded by a printer's bullet (•) MUST BE MONITORED and totaled in the space provided. The product items that are not preceded by a bullet need not be monitored step-by-step. They can be totaled in the space provided. With the exception of asterisked items (*), weight each *YES* response one (1).

I. Applies waving lotion to rods.

	Attempt 1 No/Yes	Attempt 2 No/Yes	Attempt 3 No/Yes
1.* Removes cotton from around the hairline.	☐	☐	☐
2.* Blots all excess lotion from the scalp.	☐	☐	☐
3.* Replaces the neck towel when necessary.	☐	☐	☐
4.* Saturates each rod with waving lotion.	☐	☐	☐
5.* Examines the scalp for irritation from the lotion.	☐	☐	☐
6.* Uses correct waving lotion strength.	☐	☐	☐

Subtotal .... ____________

II. Processes chemical wave.

•7. Takes two test curls to determine approximate processing. ☐ ☐ ☐

•8. Places the processing cap over the rods. ☐ ☐ ☐

•9. Avoids tightening the processing cap around the hairline. ☐ ☐ ☐

•10. Sets the timer for 3 minutes, or according to label directions. ☐ ☐ ☐

•11. Returns unused rods and other supplies to proper location. ☐ ☐ ☐

•12.* Takes test curls in each section of the head. ☐ ☐ ☐

Subtotal .... ____________

III. Completes processing according to the size of rod used.

13.* Displayed wave trough from unwound hair is the same size as the rod used. ☐ ☐ ☐

14.* When partially unwound, the wave trough splits to right and left. ☐ ☐ ☐

15. The wave pattern splits and reverses direction in the test strand. ☐ ☐ ☐

16.* The elastic band does not mark the hair. ☐ ☐ ☐

Subtotal .... ____________

IV. Neutralizes chemical wave.

•17. Attaches neutralizing bib around the hairline. ☐ ☐ ☐

•18. Places cotton between the bib fastener and the forehead. ☐ ☐ ☐

•19.* Rinses rods with tepid water for three minutes. ☐ ☐ ☐

•20.* Carefully towel-blots each rod. ☐ ☐ ☐

•21.* Uses neutralizer according to manufacturer's directions. ☐ ☐ ☐

•22.* Applies neutralizer evenly to the top and bottom of each rod. ☐ ☐ ☐

•23.* Applies all neutralizer provided. ☐ ☐ ☐

•24.* Leaves neutralizer on the rods according to the manufacturer's directions. ☐ ☐ ☐

•25.* Rinses or removes rods according to the label directions. ☐ ☐ ☐

•26. Sanitizes immediate work area (shampoo bowl, shampoo chair, etc. and implements). ☐ ☐ ☐

•27. Discards used supplies in a closed refuse container. ☐ ☐ ☐

•28.* Records product used, rods and processing time on the client's chemical-waving card. ☐ ☐ ☐

Subtotal .... ______________

TOTAL .... ______________

At least 20 *YES* responses are needed to validate. ALL asterisked items MUST be answered *YES*

18. Performance/Product Checklist

A. Chemically Relaxing the Hair Checklist

Evaluator's Name____

Student's Name____

Attempt 1: Date________________

Timings________________

Attempt 2: Date________________

Timings________________

Attempt 3: Date________________

Timings________________

Comments:

Note to Evaluator: The performance item numbers preceded by a printer's bullet (•) MUST BE MONITORED and totaled in the space provided. The product items that are not preceded by a bullet need not be monitored step-by-step. They can be totaled in the space provided. If procedure is simulated, the student must still mix at least half of the formula of the relaxer. With the exception of asterisked items, weight each *YES* response one (1).

Supplies Needed: towels, gloves, shampoo cape, combs (rake and rat-tail), timer, relaxing kit, hair conditioner (liquid), hair and scalp conditioner (oil), client's release form and client's chemical service record. (Evaluator will circle supplies student failed to obtain.)

	Attempt 1	Attempt 2	Attempt 3
I. Prepares client for application of base.	No/Yes	No/Yes	No/Yes
1. Drapes the client with protective cape.	☐	☐	☐
2.* Carefully removes tangles from the hair.	☐	☐	☐
3. Divides the hair into four equal sections.	☐	☐	☐
Subtotal.............			
II. Analyzes the hair and scalp.			
•4.* Asks client what other chemicals or services have been applied to the hair.	☐	☐	☐
•5.* Examines scalp for open cuts or irritation.	☐	☐	☐

•6.* Analyzes the hair for porosity and elasticity. ☐ ☐ ☐

•7.* Selects the appropriate relaxer depending on the condition and texture of the hair. ☐ ☐ ☐

Subtotal .... ________________

III. Applies base chemicals as needed.

8.* Applies the base adequately around the hairline including the nape. ☐ ☐ ☐

9.* Applies the base in 1/2-inch horizontal subsections through each of the four large sections. ☐ ☐ ☐

10. Applies the base to all subsections from the scalp through the ends of the hair. ☐ ☐ ☐

11.* Powders and puts on protective gloves. ☐ ☐ ☐

12. Protective apron is put on by student. ☐ ☐ ☐

Subtotal .... ________________

IV. Applies relaxer in one of four main sections.

•13. Mixes relaxer if consistency is not uniform. ☐ ☐ ☐

•14. Begins applying the relaxer in 1/2-inch horizontal partings in the nape section. ☐ ☐ ☐

•15.* Applies the relaxer 1/2-inch from the scalp through the ends of the strand. ☐ ☐ ☐

•16.* Applies the relaxer without pressure to the hair strand. ☐ ☐ ☐

•17.* Applies relaxer with the handle of the rake comb or the regular part of the rat-tail comb. ☐ ☐ ☐

•18.* Systematically applies relaxer in 1/2-inch horizontal subsections from the nape to the crown. ☐ ☐ ☐

Subtotal .... ________________

V. Correctly applies relaxer to remaining three sections.

19.* Applies relaxer so it is visible from both sides of each strand. .... ☐ ☐ ☐

20.* Keeps relaxer from the ears, hairline, (forehead and neck), and client's clothing. .... ☐ ☐ ☐

21.* Doesn't apply enough pressure on hair to activate chemical action of relaxer. .... ☐ ☐ ☐

22.* Keeps relaxer from scalp. .... ☐ ☐ ☐

Subtotal .... ________________

TOTAL .... ________________

At least 16 *YES* responses are necessary to validate. ALL asterisked items MUST be marked *YES*.

B. Processes Relaxer

Evaluator's Name____

Student's Name____

Attempt 1: Date________________

Timings________________

Attempt 2: Date________________

Timings________________

Attempt 3: Date________________

Timings________________

Comments:

Note to Evaluator: The performance item numbers preceded by a printer's bullet (•) MUST BE MONITORED and totaled in the space provided. The product items that are not preceded by a bullet need not be monitored step-by-step. They can be totaled in the space provided. If procedure is SIMULATED, the student must still mix at least half of the formula of relaxer. With the exception of asterisked items, weight each *YES* response one (1).

Attempt 1 Attempt 2 Attempt 3

No/Yes No/Yes No/Yes

I. Correctly processes relaxer.

- •1. Sets timer to determine application time.
- •2. Begins applying pressure to 1/4-inch horizontal strands in nape.
- •3. Applies additional relaxer as needed for correct saturation of each strand.
- •4.* Applies pressure to both sides of each strand with the back of the rat-tail comb.
- •5.* Applies pressure to subsections working from the nape to the crown.
- •6.* Systematically applies pressure to all strands of hair.
- •7. Begins applying more relaxer with the back of the rat-tail comb to first 1/2-inch of hair from the scalp.
- •8. Begins application of relaxer to the scalp in the nape section.
- •9. Evenly distributes relaxer through the first 1/4-inch of hair throughout all four sections.
- •10.* Uses moderate fingertip pressure of both hands to blend the left front section to the left back section.
- •11.* Uses moderate fingertip pressure of both hands to blend the right front section to the right back section.
- •12.* Asks client if any discomfort is present.

Subtotal .... ________________

II. Relaxer is correctly processed before neutralizing.

- 13.* Hair feels soft and pliable.
- 14.* Hair strand appears shiny or silky.

15. There are no single, broken hairs. .... ☐ ☐ ☐

16.* Hair next to scalp is not "puffy" or curly in crown, or around hairline.. ☐ ☐ ☐

Subtotal .... ________________

TOTAL............. ________________

At least 12 *YES* responses are necessary to validate. All asterisked items must be answered *YES*.

C. Chemically Relaxing the Hair (Neutralizes Relaxer)

Evaluator's Name____

Student's Name____

Attempt 1: Date________________

Timings________________

Attempt 2: Date________________

Timings________________

Attempt 3: Date________________

Timings________________

Comments:

I. Student neutralizes chemical action of relaxer.

	Attempt 1 No/Yes	Attempt 2 No/Yes	Attempt 3 No/Yes
•1. Immediately escorts client to shampoo area.	☐	☐	☐
•2. Thoroughly rinses first section to which relaxer is applied with comfortably warm water.	☐	☐	☐
•3.* Continues to thoroughly rinse all relaxer from the hair..	☐	☐	☐
•4.* Continues to rinse the hair until rinse water is clear.	☐	☐	☐
•5.* Checks the ear and nape areas to insure that all relaxer is removed.	☐	☐	☐

•6.* Applies prescribed neutralizing shampoo to harden the cuticle of the hair in the straighter position. ☐ ☐ ☐

•7.* Shampoo manipulations are in a downward direction. ☐ ☐ ☐

•8.* Shampoos hair three or more times as needed. ☐ ☐ ☐

•9. Applies conditioner to the hair according to label directions. ☐ ☐ ☐

•10.* Applies creme rinse and setting lotion according to label directions. ☐ ☐ ☐

•11. Hair condition is good when hair is set. ☐ ☐ ☐

TOTAL .... ____________

At least 8 *YES* responses are necessary to validate. ALL asterisked (*) items MUST be marked *YES*.

19. Performance/Product Checklist

A. Thermal Silking (Pressing) Checklist

Evaluator's Name________________________________

Student's Name________________________________

Attempt 1: Date________________

Timings________________

Attempt 2: Date________________

Timings________________

Attempt 3: Date________________

Timings________________

Comments:

Note to Evaluator: The performance item numbers preceded by a printer's bullet (•) MUST BE MONITORED and totaled in the space provided. The product items that are not preceded by a bullet need not be monitored step-by-step. They can be totaled in the space provided. With the exception of asterisked items (*), weight each *YES* response one (1).

Supplies Needed: shampoo supplies, chair cloth, neck strap, client release form, hard rubber combs (3), pressing combs (2), white tissue, electric heater and duck bill clips. (Evaluator will circle supplies student failed to obtain.)

	Attempt 1 No/Yes	Attempt 2 No/Yes	Attempt No/Yes
I. Student prepares client for shampoo.			
1. Drapes the client for shampooing.	☐	☐	☐
2. Brushes the hair according to procedure.	☐	☐	☐
3. Examines the scalp for abrasions and dryness or flakiness.	☐	☐	☐
4.* Applies lanolin creme or oil as needed to protect the hair and scalp from dryer heat.	☐	☐	☐
5. Dries the hair for 15 minutes under dryer.	☐	☐	☐
Subtotal			
II. Prepares the client for silking.			
6. Drapes the client with chair cloth using neck strap.	☐	☐	☐
7. Divides the hair into 4 equal sections.	☐	☐	☐
8.* Tests the temperature of the pressing comb before using it.	☐	☐	☐
Subtotal			
III. Begins pressing hair in the first section.			
•9. Begins at the hairline of the nape (at either back section), and presses the hair using 1/2-inch horizontal subdivisions.	☐	☐	☐
•10. Silks the hair from the nape to the crown.	☐	☐	☐
•11. Inserts the pressing comb as close to the scalp as possible.	☐	☐	☐
•12. Rotates the pressing comb downward against the strand of hair using moderate to firm pressure.	☐	☐	☐

•13. Presses both sides of each strand... ☐ ☐ ☐

Subtotal .... ________________

IV. Repeats silking procedure for remaining 3 sections of hair.

14.* All the hair appears smooth and straight.............................. ☐ ☐ ☐

15.* Hair is not discolored (scorched). .... ☐ ☐ ☐

16.* No broken hairs are visible.. ☐ ☐ ☐

17.* No broken hairs are on temperature-testing tissue................ ☐ ☐ ☐

18.* Client does not sustain any burns from thermal comb.......... ☐ ☐ ☐

19.* Hair feels "soft," not excessively oily or dry. .... ☐ ☐ ☐

Subtotal .... ________________

TOTAL .... ________________

At least 14 *YES* responses are needed to validate. ALL asterisked items MUST be answered *YES*.

20. Performance/Product Checklist

A. Chemically Recurling the Hair (Soft Curl) Checklist

Evaluator's Name____

Student's Name____

Attempt 1: Date________________

Timings________________

Attempt 2: Date________________

Timings________________

Attempt 3: Date________________

Timings________________

Comments:

Note to Evaluator: The performance item numbers preceded by a printer's bullet (•) MUST BE MONITORED and totaled in the space provided. The product items that are not preceded by a bullet need not be monitored step-by-step. They can be totaled in the space provided. With the exception of asterisked items (*), weight each *YES* response one (1).

	Attempt 1 No/Yes	Attempt 2 No/Yes	Attempt 3 No/Yes
I. Prepares client for application of base and applies it.			
1. Drapes the client with protective cape.	☐	☐	☐
2.* Carefully removes tangles from the hair.	☐	☐	☐
3. Divides the hair into four equal sections.	☐	☐	☐
Subtotal			
II. Analyzes condition of hair and scalp.			
•4.* Asks client what other chemicals or services have been applied to the hair.	☐	☐	☐
•5.* Examines scalp for open cuts or irritation.	☐	☐	☐
•6.* Analyzes the hair for porosity and elasticity.	☐	☐	☐
•7.* Selects the appropriate curl rearranger, depending on the condition and texture of the hair.	☐	☐	☐
Subtotal			
III. Applies scalp condtioner.			
8.* Applies the base adequately around the hairline including the nape if needed.	☐	☐	☐
9.* Applies the base in 1/4 -1/2-inch horizontal subsections through each of the four large sections.	☐	☐	☐
10. Applies the base to all subsections from the scalp through the ends of the hair if needed.	☐	☐	☐
11.* Powders and puts on protective gloves.	☐	☐	☐
12. Protective apron is put on by student.	☐	☐	☐

Subtotal .... ________________

IV. Applies rearranger in one of four main sections.

•13. Begins applying the relaxer in 1/2-inch horizontal partings in the nape section. .... ☐ ☐ ☐

•14.* Applies the rearranger without pressure to the hair strand. .... ☐ ☐ ☐

•15.* Systematically applies rearranger in 1/4 - 1/2-inch horizontal subsections from the nape to the crown. .... ☐ ☐ ☐

Subtotal .... ________________

V. Correctly applies rearranger to remaining three sections.

16.* Applies enough rearranger so it is visible from both sides of each strand. .... ☐ ☐ ☐

17.* Keeps rearranger from the ears, hairline (forehead and neck), and client's clothing. .... ☐ ☐ ☐

Subtotal .... ________________

TOTAL .... ________________

At least 13 *YES* responses are necessary to validate. ALL asterisked items MUST be marked *YES*.

VI. Rearranger is correctly processed before neutralizing.

1.* Hair feels soft and pliable.. ☐ ☐ ☐

2.* Hair strand appears shiny or silky. .... ☐ ☐ ☐

3. There are no single, broken hairs. .... ☐ ☐ ☐

4.* Hair next to scalp is not "puffy" or curly in crown, or around hairline... ☐ ☐ ☐

5. Rearranger is thoroughly rinsed from hair with tepid water. ☐ ☐ ☐

Subtotal .... ________

TOTAL............ ________

At least 4 *YES* responses are necessary to validate. ALL asterisked items MUST be answered *YES*.

B. Chemically Recurling the Hair (Neutralizes Rearranger)

•1.* The strand to be wrapped is not longer than the rod. ☐ ☐ ☐

•2.* The width of strand is 1/2 of the diameter of the rod, or less. ☐ ☐ ☐

•3.* During wrapping, the end wrap extends beyond the end of hair strand. ☐ ☐ ☐

•4.* The hair is evenly spread across the rod as it is wrapped. ☐ ☐ ☐

•5.* Firm tension is applied to each rod during wrapping. ☐ ☐ ☐

•6.* Elastic secures rod to the head without binding the hair at either end of the rod. ☐ ☐ ☐

•7.* The rod, elastic and lower part are parallel. ☐ ☐ ☐

•8.* The rod is centered on the lower parting. ☐ ☐ ☐

•9.* Doesn't drip in/on client's eyes or skin. ☐ ☐ ☐

10.* Completes wrapping all sections. ☐ ☐ ☐

Subtotal .... ________

TOTAL .... ________

At least 7 *YES* responses are necessary to validate. ALL asterisked items MUST be answered *YES*.

VIII. Student processes and neutralizes a recurl.

•1. Takes two test curls to determine approximate processing. ☐ ☐ ☐

•2. Places the processing cap over the rods, and uses hair dryer as needed. ☐ ☐ ☐

•3. Avoids tightening the processing cap around the hairline. ☐ ☐ ☐

•4. Sets the timer for 3 minutes, or according to label directions. ☐ ☐ ☐

•5. Returns unused rods and other supplies to proper locations. ☐ ☐ ☐

•6.* Takes test curls in each section of the head. ☐ ☐ ☐

•7. Attaches neutralizing bib around the hairline. ☐ ☐ ☐

•8. Places cotton between the bib fastener and the forehead. ☐ ☐ ☐

•9. Rinses rods with tepid water for three minutes. ☐ ☐ ☐

•10. Carefully towel-blots each rod. ☐ ☐ ☐

•11. Uses neutralizer according to manufacturer's directions. ☐ ☐ ☐

•12. Applies neutralizer evenly to the top and bottom of each rod. ☐ ☐ ☐

•13. Applies all neutralizer provided. ☐ ☐ ☐

•14. Leaves neutralizer on the rods according to manufacturer's directions. ☐ ☐ ☐

•15. Rinses or removes rods according to the label directions. ☐ ☐ ☐

•16. Sanitizes immediate work area (shampoo bowl, shampoo chair, etc. and implements). ☐ ☐ ☐

•17. Discards used supplies in a closed refuse container.............. ☐ ☐ ☐

•18.* Records product used, rods and processing time on the client's chemical service card. .... ☐ ☐ ☐

Subtotal .... ________________

TOTAL .... ________________

At least 15 *YES* responses are necessary to validate. ALL asterisked items MUST be answered *YES*.

Performance/Product Checklist

A. Facial Checklist

Evaluator's Name____

Student's Name____

Attempt 1: Date________________

Timings________________

Attempt 2: Date________________

Timings________________

Attempt 3: Date________________

Timings________________

Comments:

Note to Evaluator: The performance item numbers preceded by a printer's bullet (•) MUST BE MONITORED and totaled in the space provided. The product items that are not preceded by a bullet need not be monitored step-by-step. They can be totaled in the space provided. With the exception of asterisked items (*), weight each *YES* response one (1).

	Attempt 1 No/Yes	Attempt 2 No/Yes	Attempt 3 No/Yes
I. Student prepares client for application of makeup.			
1. Assembles necessary supplies.	☐	☐	☐
2. Drapes client with protective cape.	☐	☐	☐
3. Secures a towel to cover client's hair.	☐	☐	☐
4. Reclines client in makeup chair.	☐	☐	☐
Subtotal	________		
II. Cleanses client's facial area.			
5. Uses small amount of cleanser.	☐	☐	☐
6.* Works in upward, outward movement.	☐	☐	☐
7. Removes cleanser with damp terry cloth.	☐	☐	☐
Subtotal	________		

III. Application of emollient cream.

•8.* Dispenses emollient from container using spatula. ☐ ☐ ☐

•9.* Distributes emollient over entire facial area in an upward and outward manner. ☐ ☐ ☐

Subtotal .... ________

IV. Manipulates prescribed massage movements.

•10.* Forehead area. ☐ ☐ ☐

•11.* Cheek area. ☐ ☐ ☐

•12.* Nose area. ☐ ☐ ☐

•13.* Chin area. ☐ ☐ ☐

•14.* Neck area. ☐ ☐ ☐

Subtotal .... ________

V. Removes emollient cream.

•15.* Removes emollient using tissue in a mitt form in upward and outward movements. ☐ ☐ ☐

•16.* Applies hot towel to facial area. ☐ ☐ ☐

•17.* Applies cold towel to facial area. ☐ ☐ ☐

•18.* Applies freshener for normal to dry skin or astringent for oily skin. ☐ ☐ ☐

Subtotal............ ________

TOTAL............ ________

At least 15 *YES* responses are needed to validate. ALL asterisked items MUST be answered *YES*.

22. Performance/Product Checklist

A. Applying Makeup Checklist

Evaluator's Name____

Student's Name____

Attempt 1: Date________________

Timings________________

Attempt 2: Date________________

Timings________________

Attempt 3: Date________________

Timings________________

Comments:

	Attempt 1 No/Yes	Attempt 2 No/Yes	Attempt 3 No/Yes
I. Student prepares client for application of makeup.			
1. Assembles necessary supplies.	☐	☐	☐
2. Drapes client with a protective cape.	☐	☐	☐
3. Secures a towel to cover the client's hair.	☐	☐	☐
4. Adjusts client to a reclining position in the makeup chair.	☐	☐	☐
Subtotal			
II. Cleanses the client's facial area.			
5. Uses a small amount of cleanser.	☐	☐	☐
6.* Works in upward, outward movement.	☐	☐	☐
7. Removes cleanser with a damp terry cloth.	☐	☐	☐
8.* Applies freshener for normal to dry skin OR astringent for oily skin.	☐	☐	☐
9. Adds water to the skin after moisturizer application.	☐	☐	☐

Subtotal .... ________________

III. Selects and applies foundation.

10.* Applies contour makeup according to correct guidelines of facial features.. ☐ ☐ ☐

11.* Selects an appropriate shade of foundation........................... ☐ ☐ ☐

12.* Applies foundation with NO demarcation line showing. .... ☐ ☐ ☐

13.* Follows correct guidelines for application of cheek rouge... ☐ ☐ ☐

14. Kneads powder into face. .... ☐ ☐ ☐

15. Dabs a damp terry cloth or sponge over face. .... ☐ ☐ ☐

Subtotal .... ________________

IV. Applies eye and lip makeup.

16.* Uses correct measurements for application of eyebrow pencil. .... ☐ ☐ ☐

17.* Applies eyeshadow in prescribed procedure for day wear. .... ☐ ☐ ☐

18.* Applies eyeliner thinly .... ☐ ☐ ☐

19. Uses upward and outward strokes for application of mascara.. ☐ ☐ ☐

20.* Correctly applies lipstick. .... ☐ ☐ ☐

21. Returns all supplies and implements to proper places. .... ☐ ☐ ☐

Subtotal............ ________________

TOTAL............ ________________

At least 15 *YES* responses are necessary to validate. ALL asterisked items MUST be answered *YES*.

23. Performance/Product Checklist

A. Manicuring the Nails Checklist

Evaluator's Name____

Student's Name____

Attempt 1: Date________________

Timings________________

Attempt 2: Date________________

Timings________________

Attempt 3: Date________________

Timings________________

Comments:

Note to Evaluator: The performance item numbers preceded by a printer's bullet (•) MUST BE MONITORED and totaled in the space provided. The product items that are not preceded by a bullet need not be monitored step-by-step. They can be totaled in the space provided. Weight each *YES* response one (1).

Supplies Needed: towels (2), cotton, sanitizing containers, metal file, emery board, cuticle nipper, pusher (metal), orangewood stick, enamel polish, polish remover, cuticle oil/cream, nail builder, brush and finger bowl. (Evaluator will circle items student failed to obtain.)

	Attempt 1 No/Yes	Attempt 2 No/Yes	Attempt 3 No/Yes
I. Student removes nail polish.			
1. Uses sterile cotton.	☐	☐	☐
2. Removes all traces of polish.	☐	☐	☐
Subtotal			
II. Shapes the nails.			
3. Begins with the little finger of each hand.	☐	☐	☐
4. Shapes the nails from the side to the center.	☐	☐	☐
5. Bevels the free edges of nails.	☐	☐	☐

6. All nails have a uniform oval shape. .... ☐ ☐ ☐

Subtotal .... ____________

III. Conditions the nails and cuticles.

•7. Softens cuticles in warm, soapy water. .... ☐ ☐ ☐

•8. Removes hand from finger bowl and towel dries. .... ☐ ☐ ☐

•9. Applies cuticle remover .... ☐ ☐ ☐

•10. Pushes cuticle back with metal pusher. .... ☐ ☐ ☐

•11. Removes excess cuticle remover with towel. .... ☐ ☐ ☐

•12. Applies nail builder. .... ☐ ☐ ☐

•13. Massages nail builder into cuticles and nails. .... ☐ ☐ ☐

•14. Pushes back cuticle with orangewood stick. .... ☐ ☐ ☐

•15. Nips off excess cuticle with nippers. .... ☐ ☐ ☐

Subtotal .... ____________

IV. Massages the arms and hands.

•16. Applies hand lotion. .... ☐ ☐ ☐

•17. Begins massage at the elbow. .... ☐ ☐ ☐

•18. Uses slow circular motion. .... ☐ ☐ ☐

•19. Massages each finger individually. .... ☐ ☐ ☐

Subtotal .... ____________

V. Cleanses nails.

•20. Scrubs the nails with manicure brush. .... ☐ ☐ ☐

•21. Towel dries nails. .... ☐ ☐ ☐

•22. Applies polish remover to nails.. ☐ ☐ ☐

Subtotal .... ____________________

VI. Applies nail enamel.

•23. Begins with little finger.. ☐ ☐ ☐

24. Applies base coat.. ☐ ☐ ☐

25. Applies colored enamel.. ☐ ☐ ☐

26. Cleanses excess enamel from cuticle and free edge.............. ☐ ☐ ☐

27. Applies sealer. .... ☐ ☐ ☐

28. Sprays quick-dry on nails... ☐ ☐ ☐

Ending time: ____________________

Subtotal .... ____________________

TOTAL .... ____________________

21 *YES* responses are necessary to validate.

24. Performance/Product Checklist

A. Cleaning and Setting a Wig Checklist

Evaluator's Name ____

Student's Name ____

Attempt 1: Date ____________________

Timings ____________________

Attempt 2: Date ____________________

Timings ____________________

Attempt 3: Date ____________________

Timings ____________________

Comments:

Note to Evaluator: The performance item numbers preceded by a printer's bullet (•) MUST BE MONITORED and totaled in the space provided. The product items that are not preceded by a bullet need not be monitored step-by-step. They can be totaled in the space provided. With the exception of asterisked items (*), weight each *YES* response one (1).

I. Procedure for obtaining client's head measurements (using step-by-step procedure for client service form).

	Attempt 1 No/Yes	Attempt 2 No/Yes	Attempt 3 No/Yes
1. Measures distance from the center hairline to the center nape hairline.	☐	☐	☐
2. Measures the distance around the head.	☐	☐	☐
3. Measures each side hairline to the beginning of the crown section.	☐	☐	☐
4. Measures from each side hairline to the beginning of the nape.	☐	☐	☐
5. Measures the width of the nape hairline.	☐	☐	☐
6. Secures the clamp to the styling station.	☐	☐	☐
7. Places the canvas block on the spindle.	☐	☐	☐
8. Secures the plastic cover over the block with T-pins.	☐	☐	☐
•9. Using a tape measure, pencils the client's head measurements onto the plastic cover of the canvas block.	☐	☐	☐

Subtotal .... ____________

II. Procedure for cleaning HUMAN hair wig.

	Attempt 1 No/Yes	Attempt 2 No/Yes	Attempt 3 No/Yes
10. Examines the inside and outside construction of the wig.	☐	☐	☐
11. Obtains dry cleaning fluid.	☐	☐	☐
•12.* Follows safety precautions in the use of the fluid.	☐	☐	☐

•13.* Pours enough dry cleaner into a bowl so the wig is submerged in solution. ☐ ☐ ☐

14. Turns the wig inside-out. ☐ ☐ ☐

•15. Dips the wig up and down in proper solution for four to five minutes. ☐ ☐ ☐

•16. Uses a sanitized manicure brush to clean around hairline. ☐ ☐ ☐

17.* Removes from cleaner and gently towel-blots. ☐ ☐ ☐

•18.* Disposes of cleaning fluid. ☐ ☐ ☐

•19.* Pins the wig to the canvas block matching up measurement pencil marks, inserting pins at 45° angle. ☐ ☐ ☐

•20. Removes tangles. ☐ ☐ ☐

21. Applies setting lotion and/or conditioner. ☐ ☐ ☐

22. Proceeds to set. ☐ ☐ ☐

Subtotal .... ________________

Ending time for HUMAN hair ______________

III. Procedure for cleaning SYNTHETIC wigs.

•10.* Removes tangles from the wig. ☐ ☐ ☐

•11.* Mixes acid-balanced shampoo in lukewarm to cool water. ☐ ☐ ☐

•12. Submerges wig in the shampoo-and-water mixture. ☐ ☐ ☐

13. Scrubs hairline with a small brush. ☐ ☐ ☐

•14.* Using cool water, rinses until the water runs clean. ☐ ☐ ☐

15. Towel-blots gently. ☐ ☐ ☐

•16.* Using T-pins, secures the wig to previously marked canvas block. .... ☐ ☐ ☐

•17.* Inserts T-pins at 45° angle at the ear tabs, the center hairline, and each corner of the nape.................................... ☐ ☐ ☐

•18. After the hair is dry, removed tangles by combing or brushing into the desired style... ☐ ☐ ☐

Subtotal............. ________________

TOTAL............. ________________

Ending time for SYNTHETIC hair __________

At least 13 *YES* responses are needed to validate. ALL asterisked items MUST be answered *YES*.

25. Performance/Product Checklist

A. Giving a High Frequency Scalp Treatment Checklist

Evaluator's Name____

Student's Name____

Attempt 1: Date________________

Timings________________

Attempt 2: Date________________

Timings________________

Attempt 3: Date________________

Timings________________

Comments:

Note to Evaluator: The performance item numbers preceded by a printer's bullet (•) MUST BE MONITORED and totaled in the space provided. The product items that are not preceded by a bullet need not be monitored step-by-step. They can be totaled in the space provided. With the exception of asterisked items (*), weight each *YES* response one (1).

	Attempt 1 No/Yes	Attempt 2 No/Yes	Attempt 3 No/Yes
I. Direct Method.			
•1. Advises client to remove all jewelry.	☐	☐	☐
•2.* Adjusts current to small amount.	☐	☐	☐
•3.* Places finger on electrode before placing on scalp to prevent sparking on skin.	☐	☐	☐
•4. Works from forehead to nape.	☐	☐	☐
•5. Does not break contact with scalp, and follows procedures.	☐	☐	☐
Subtotal			
II. Indirect Method			
•6.* Gives glass electrode to client	☐	☐	☐

•7.* Advises client to hold electrode with both hands.................. ☐ ☐ ☐

•8. Follows school procedures.. ☐ ☐ ☐

•9. Keeps hands in contact with scalp during treatment............. ☐ ☐ ☐

Subtotal .... ____________________

TOTAL .... ____________________

At least 7 *YES* responses are necessary to validate. ALL asterisked items MUST be marked *YES*.

he **Scoring Key** below provides you with a quick method for scoring daily, weekly, or monthly est(s) of your own design. Using the left-hand column for reference, find the number of test items or the test you are administering, then scan across the other three columns to determine the espective percentages for the number of correct/incorrect responses.

alton's Final Tests - There are fifteen tests in this section, and you may wish to select **three or our tests** for your "School Final". For your next class, select a *different* set of questions. The items n these tests - coupled with the use of the State Board Review Questions book - should provide the rospective examinee for licensure with an excellent "sampling" of the types of questions typically sed by state licensing agencies. However, remember that **Dalton's Final Test 1 is also printed in he Theory and Practical Workbook**, so you will probably want to make your selection from alton's Final Tests 2 through 15.

hese testing instruments have used the standard psychometric methodology. Only validated uestions that have proven to be reliable for determining student mastery for the course of osmetology have been used in Dalton's Final Tests. This "core set" of questions has been ransferred from one test to the next to validate each individual test. Of course, we can't tell you which questions make up the core set. However, the core set of items has periodically been edited, nd has evolved and been validated over a fifteen year period. In the author's experience in many osmetology schools, colleges, and programs, students achieving 85% or better on these tests will most likely be successful when taking their licensing examination. One part of the licensing process hat has not been factored into this prediction is your state law test. Some states have a separate law est, while other states combine law examination questions with the theory test.

Scoring Key

(for tests that have between ten and fifty questions)

Possible	Incorrect	Percentage	Correct
10	0	100%	10
10	1	90%	9
10	2	80%	8
10	3	70%	7
10	4	60%	6
10	5	50%	5

Possible	Incorrect	Percentage	Correct
11	0	100%	11
11	1	91%	10
11	2	82%	9
11	3	73%	8
11	4	64%	7
11	5	55%	6

Possible	Incorrect	Percentage	Correct
12	0	100%	12
12	1	92%	11
12	2	83%	10
12	3	75%	9
12	4	67%	8
12	5	58%	7
12	6	50%	6

Possible	Incorrect	Percentage	Correct
13	0	100%	13
13	1	92%	12
13	2	85%	11
13	3	77%	10
13	4	69%	9
13	5	62%	8
13	6	54%	7

Possible	Incorrect	Percentage	Correct
14	0	100%	14
14	1	93%	13
14	2	86%	12
14	3	79%	11
14	4	71%	10
14	5	64%	9
14	6	57%	8

Possible	Incorrect	Percentage	Correct
15	0	100%	15
15	1	93%	14
15	2	87%	13
15	3	80%	12
15	4	73%	11
15	5	67%	10
15	6	60%	9

Possible	Incorrect	Percentage	Correct
16	0	100%	16
16	1	94%	15
16	2	88%	14
16	3	81%	13
16	4	75%	12
16	5	69%	11
16	6	63%	19

Possible	Incorrect	Percentage	Correct
17	0	100%	17
17	1	94%	16
17	2	88%	15
17	3	82%	14
17	4	76%	13
17	5	71%	12
17	6	65%	11

Possible	Incorrect	Percentage	Correct
18	0	100%	18
18	1	94%	17
18	2	89%	16
18	3	83%	15
18	4	78%	14
18	5	72%	13
18	6	67%	12
18	7	61%	11

Possible	Incorrect	Percentage	Correct
19	0	100%	19
19	1	95%	18
19	2	89%	17
19	3	84%	16
19	4	79%	15
19	5	74%	14
19	6	68%	13
19	7	63%	12

Possible	Incorrect	Percentage	Correct
20	0	100%	20
20	1	95%	19
20	2	90%	18
20	3	85%	17
20	4	80%	16
20	5	75%	15
20	6	70%	14
20	7	65%	13

Possible	Incorrect	Percentage	Correct
21	0	100%	21
21	1	95%	20
21	2	90%	19
21	3	86%	18
21	4	81%	17
21	5	76%	16
21	6	71%	15
21	7	67%	14
21	8	62%	13
21	9	57%	12
21	10	52%	11

Possible	Incorrect	Percentage	Correct
22	0	100%	22
22	1	95%	21
22	2	91%	20
22	3	86%	19
22	4	82%	18
22	5	77%	17
22	6	73%	16
22	7	68%	15
22	8	64%	14
22	9	59%	13
22	10	55%	12

Possible	Incorrect	Percentage	Correct
23	0	100%	23
23	1	96%	22
23	2	91%	21
23	3	87%	20
23	4	83%	19
23	5	78%	18
23	6	74%	17
23	7	70%	16
23	8	65%	15
23	9	61%	14
23	10	57%	13

Possible	Incorrect	Percentage	Correct
24	0	100%	24
24	1	96%	23
24	2	92%	22
24	3	88%	21
24	4	83%	20
24	5	79%	19
24	6	75%	18
24	7	71%	17
24	8	67%	16
24	9	63%	15
24	10	58%	14

Possible	Incorrect	Percentage	Correct
25	0	100%	25
25	1	96%	24
25	2	92%	23
25	3	88%	22
25	4	84%	21
25	5	80%	20
25	6	76%	19
25	7	72%	18
25	8	68%	17
25	9	64%	16
25	10	60%	15
25	11	56%	14

Possible	Incorrect	Percentage	Correct
26	0	100%	26
26	1	96%	25
26	2	92%	24
26	3	88%	23
26	4	85%	22
26	5	81%	21
26	6	77%	20
26	7	73%	19
26	8	69%	18
26	9	65%	17
26	10	62%	16
26	11	58%	15

Possible	Incorrect	Percentage	Correct
27	0	100%	27
27	1	96%	26
27	2	93%	25
27	3	89%	24
27	4	85%	23
27	5	81%	22
27	6	78%	21
27	7	74%	20
27	8	70%	19
27	9	67%	18
27	10	63%	17
27	11	59%	16

Possible	Incorrect	Percentage	Correct
28	0	100%	28
28	1	96%	27
28	2	93%	26
28	3	89%	25
28	4	86%	24
28	5	82%	23
28	6	79%	22
28	7	75%	21
28	8	71%	20
28	9	68%	19
28	10	64%	18
28	11	61%	17

Possible	Incorrect	Percentage	Correct
29	0	100%	29
29	1	97%	28
29	2	93%	27
29	3	90%	26
29	4	86%	25
29	5	83%	24
29	6	79%	23
29	7	76%	22
29	8	72%	21
29	9	69%	20
29	10	66%	19
29	11	62%	18

Possible	Incorrect	Percentage	Correct
30	0	100%	30
30	1	97%	29
30	2	93%	28
30	3	90%	27
30	4	87%	26
30	5	83%	25
30	6	80%	24
30	7	77%	23
30	8	73%	22
30	9	70%	21
30	10	67%	20
30	11	63%	19

Possible	Incorrect	Percentage	Correct
31	0	100%	31
31	1	97%	30
31	2	94%	29
31	3	90%	28
31	4	87%	27
31	5	84%	26
31	6	81%	25
31	7	77%	24
31	8	74%	23
31	9	71%	22
31	10	68%	21
31	11	65%	20

Possible	Incorrect	Percentage	Correct
32	0	100%	32
32	1	97%	31
32	2	94%	30
32	3	91%	29
32	4	88%	28
32	5	84%	27
32	6	81%	26
32	7	78%	25
32	8	75%	24
32	9	72%	23
32	10	69%	22
32	11	66%	21

Possible	Incorrect	Percentage	Correct
33	0	100%	33
33	1	97%	32
33	2	94%	31
33	3	91%	30
33	4	88%	29
33	5	85%	28
33	6	82%	27
33	7	79%	26
33	8	76%	25
33	9	73%	24
33	10	70%	23
33	11	67%	22
33	12	64%	21

Possible	Incorrect	Percentage	Correct
34	0	100%	34
34	1	97%	33
34	2	94%	32
34	3	91%	31
34	4	88%	30
34	5	85%	29
34	6	82%	28
34	7	79%	27
34	8	76%	26
34	9	74%	25
34	10	71%	24
34	11	68%	23
34	12	65%	22
34	13	62%	21

Possible	Incorrect	Percentage	Correct
35	0	100%	35
35	1	97%	34
35	2	94%	33
35	3	91%	32
35	4	89%	31
35	5	86%	30
35	6	83%	29
35	7	80%	28
35	8	77%	27
35	9	74%	26
35	10	71%	25
35	11	69%	24
35	12	66%	23
35	13	63%	22

Possible	Incorrect	Percentage	Correct
36	0	100%	36
36	1	97%	35
36	2	94%	34
36	3	92%	33
36	4	89%	32
36	5	86%	31
36	6	83%	30
36	7	81%	29
36	8	78%	28
36	9	75%	27
36	10	72%	26
36	11	69%	25
36	12	67%	24
36	13	64%	23

Possible	Incorrect	Percentage	Correct
37	0	100%	37
37	1	97%	36
37	2	95%	35
37	3	92%	34
37	4	89%	33
37	5	86%	32
37	6	84%	31
37	7	81%	30
37	8	78%	29
37	9	76%	28
37	10	73%	27
37	11	70%	26
37	12	68%	25
37	13	65%	24

Possible	Incorrect	Percentage	Correct
38	0	100%	38
38	1	97%	37
38	2	95%	36
38	3	92%	35
38	4	89%	34
38	5	87%	33
38	6	84%	32
38	7	82%	31
38	8	79%	30
38	9	76%	29
38	10	74%	28
38	11	71%	27
38	12	68%	26
38	13	66%	25

Possible	Incorrect	Percentage	Correct
39	0	100%	39
39	1	97%	38
39	2	95%	37
39	3	92%	36
39	4	90%	35
39	5	87%	34
39	6	85%	33
39	7	82%	32
39	8	79%	31
39	9	77%	30
39	10	74%	29
39	11	72%	28
39	12	69%	27
39	13	67%	26

Possible	Incorrect	Percentage	Correct
40	0	100%	40
40	1	98%	39
40	2	95%	38
40	3	93%	37
40	4	90%	36
40	5	88%	35
40	6	85%	34
40	7	82%	33
40	8	80%	32
40	9	78%	31
40	10	75%	30
40	11	73%	29
40	12	70%	28
40	13	68%	27

Possible	Incorrect	Percentage	Correct
41	0	100%	41
41	1	98%	40
41	2	95%	39
41	3	93%	38
41	4	90%	37
41	5	88%	36
41	6	85%	35
41	7	83%	34
41	8	80%	33
41	9	78%	32
41	10	76%	31
41	11	73%	30
41	12	71%	29
41	13	68%	28

Possible	Incorrect	Percentage	Correct
42	0	100%	42
42	1	98%	41
42	2	95%	40
42	3	93%	39
42	4	90%	38
42	5	88%	37
42	6	86%	36
42	7	83%	35
42	8	81%	34
42	9	79%	33
42	10	76%	32
42	11	74%	31
42	12	71%	30
42	13	69%	29

Possible	Incorrect	Percentage	Correct
43	0	100%	43
43	1	98%	42
43	2	95%	41
43	3	93%	40
43	4	91%	39
43	5	88%	38
43	6	86%	37
43	7	84%	36
43	8	81%	35
43	9	79%	34
43	10	77%	33
43	11	74%	32
43	12	72%	31
43	13	70%	30

Possible	Incorrect	Percentage	Correct
44	0	100%	44
44	1	98%	43
44	2	95%	42
44	3	93%	41
44	4	91%	40
44	5	89%	39
44	6	86%	38
44	7	84%	37
44	8	82%	36
44	9	80%	35
44	10	77%	34
44	11	75%	33
44	12	73%	32
44	13	70%	31

Possible	Incorrect	Percentage	Correct
45	0	100%	45
45	1	98%	44
45	2	96%	43
45	3	93%	42
45	4	91%	41
45	5	89%	40
45	6	87%	39
45	7	84%	38
45	8	82%	37
45	9	80%	36
45	10	78%	35
45	11	76%	34
45	12	73%	33
45	13	71%	32

Possible	Incorrect	Percentage	Correct
46	0	100%	46
46	1	98%	45
46	2	96%	44
46	3	93%	43
46	4	91%	42
46	5	89%	41
46	6	87%	40
46	7	85%	39
46	8	83%	38
46	9	80%	37
46	10	78%	36
46	11	76%	35
46	12	74%	34
46	13	72%	33

Possible	Incorrect	Percentage	Correct
47	0	100%	47
47	1	98%	46
47	2	96%	45
47	3	94%	44
47	4	91%	43
47	5	89%	42
47	6	87%	41
47	7	85%	40
47	8	83%	39
47	9	81%	38
47	10	79%	37
47	11	77%	36
47	12	74%	35
47	13	72%	34

Possible	Incorrect	Percentage	Correct
48	0	100%	48
48	1	98%	47
48	2	96%	46
48	3	94%	45
48	4	92%	44
48	5	90%	43
48	6	88%	42
48	7	85%	41
48	8	83%	40
48	9	81%	39
48	10	79%	38
48	11	77%	37
48	12	75%	36
48	13	73%	35

Possible	Incorrect	Percentage	Correct
49	0	100%	49
49	1	98%	48
49	2	96%	47
49	3	94%	46
49	4	92%	45
49	5	90%	44
49	6	88%	43
49	7	86%	42
49	8	84%	41
49	9	82%	40
49	10	80%	39
49	11	78%	38
49	12	76%	37
49	13	73%	36

Possible	Incorrect	Percentage	Correct
50	0	100%	50
50	1	98%	49
50	2	96%	48
50	3	94%	47
50	4	92%	46
50	5	90%	45
50	6	88%	44
50	7	86%	43
50	8	84%	42
50	9	82%	41
50	10	80%	40
50	11	78%	39
50	12	76%	38
50	13	74%	37

DALTON'S STANDARDIZED FINAL TEST 1

Student Name ______________________________ Score _______ Date ____________

Instructions: Carefully read through each question, then read the answer choices. Write your choice of the word, or the phrase, that correctly completes the statement or answers the question, on the line provided.

___1. The name given to the preservation of personal or public health is

A. hygiene
B. cosmetology
C. chemistry
D. biology

___2. The advantage(s) of being a manager-operator may include the opportunity to learn about

A. overhead expenses
B. accounts payable
C. inventory
D. all of the above

___3. Personal grooming relates to one's

A. daily appearance
B. daily cleanliness
C. hairstyle and voice
D. A and B.

___4. Personal hygiene relates to

A. promoting one's own health
B. preservation of one's health
C. oral care
D. A and B.

___5. Dental care for preserving healthy teeth starts with a daily mouthwash and

A. rinsing and flushing
B. rubbing and scratching
C. rinsing and rubbing
D. brushing and flossing

___6. Ethics is a system that measures human behavior that is

A. voluntary
B. involuntary
C. imposed by local police
D. imposed by the federal government

___7. A professional attitude is

A. natural
B. given when you are licensed
C. acquired in enrollment
D. learned

___8. To equal the strength of 70% ethyl alcohol, you would have to use

A. 20% isopropyl alcohol
B. 39% isopropyl alcohol
C. 50% isopropyl alcohol
D. 70% isopropyl alcohol

___9. A person immune to a disease, but who can infect others is known as a(n)

A. clinical
B. medical
C. agent
D. carrier

___10. To be effective, a solution of quaternary ammonium compound solution requires

A. mixing with alcohol
B. lengthy contact time
C. mixing with peroxide
D. short contact time

___11. If the eye has been chemically burned, what should be done?

A. flush eye with cool water
B. flush eye with boric acid
C. apply alcohol
D. apply quats

___12. To be effective for sanitation, the strength of the quats to be used should be at least

A. 1:200
B. 1:300
C. 1:500
D. 1:1000

___13. Which virus causes the AIDS disease?

A. Rhino virus
B. HIV virus
C. Influenza virus
D. Cold virus

____14. What route of transmission does the AIDS disease follow?

A. injection
B. blood transfusion
C. maternal
D. all of the above

____15. Soiled towels should be stored in a covered

A. linen hamper
B. metal container
C. plastic container
D. laundry basket

____16. A carrier is a person who has a disease that is

A. acute
B. contagious
C. occupational
D. common

____17. What common cosmetology chemical would kill the AIDS virus outside of the body?

A. household bleach
B. water
C. 1% hydrogen peroxide
D. 20% alcohol

____18. What strength hydrogen peroxide would destroy the AIDS virus outside of the body?

A. 1%
B. 2%
C. 3%
D. all of the above

____19. A soapy solution is used to remove foreign particles from

A. brushes
B. thinning shears
C. a razor
D. an ultraviolet sanitizer

____20. What is 100% effective in preventing the spread of the HIV virus?

A. applying water
B. wearing gloves
C. use of a condom
D. abstinence

____21. Hair is an example of

A. hard keratin
B. soft keratin
C. Henle's layer
D. Huxley's layer

____22. The glands in the scalp that naturally lubricate the hair during brushing are called

A. apocrine
B. sebaceous
C. sudoriferous
D. eccrine

____23. Depilatories in the form of a cream, paste, or powder are chemical products used to

A. curl hair
B. remove hair
C. color hair
D. straighten hair

____24. The percentage of the hair shaft represented by the cortex layer is

A. 15%
B. 25%
C. 50%
D. 75%

____25. The technical term applied to the cyclical period when the hair begins to grow is the

A. anagen stage
B. terminal stage
C. telogen stage
D. origin stage

____26. Hypertrichosis is a condition that is also called

A. supercilia hair
B. superfluous hair
C. ringed hair
D. twisted hair

____27. Using a short-wave electrical machine to stop the growth of a hair is called

A. electrolysis
B. trichosis
C. cometose
D. osmosis

____28. The pH of a shampoo indicates the concentration of

A. hydrogen
B. oxygen
C. nitrogen
D. carbon

____29. Peroxide has a pH that is

A. acid
B. alkaline
C. neutral
D. none of the above

____30. Scabies is an infestation of the scalp by

A. the itch mite
B. head lice
C. ringworm
D. tinea

____31. To prevent water from dripping onto the floor from the shampoo bowl, where should you leave the shampoo hose?

A. drain position
B. handle position
C. vacuum breaker position
D. none of the above

____32. The natural lubricant that gives hair a beautiful luster or sheen is called

A. sebum
B. seborrhea
C. seconal
D. permanent color

____33. The extent that hair can be stretched without breaking is known as

A. pressure
B. tone
C. elasticity
D. texture

____34. If damaged hair is going to be given a service that uses strong chemicals the cosmetologist should recommend

A. preconditioning
B. prelightening
C. pre-filling
D. preneutralizing

____35. Semicircular designs combed into the hair are called

A. waves
B. base direction
C. shapings
D. arcs

____36. The main objective in finger waving the hair is to mold even

A. curls and softness
B. waves and ridges
C. shaping and direction
D. parts and shapes

____37. The section of the head that is closest to the neck is the

A. nape section
B. crown section
C. crepe section
D. left side section

____38. After the setting lotion has been applied, should the hair dryout during setting, spray more

A. filler on it
B. conditioner on it
C. water on it
D. setting lotion on it

____39. To get the maximum amount of height or fullness, you should use a

A. no-stem curl
B. half-stem curl
C. long-stem curl
D. tight-stem curl

____40. When setting the hair with rollers, a curved form in the finished hairstyle is achieved by winding hair around the roller

A. 1 turn or less
B. 1-1/2 turns
C. 2 turns
D. none of the above

____41. The profile is the view of the head from the

A. front
B. back
C. side
D. face

____42. For a basic haircut, the cosmetologist would begin cutting the hair in the

A. top
B. side
C. crown
D. nape

____43. Super-curly hair should be cut with a

A. clipper
B. scissors
C. razor
D. thinning shears

___44. Proper storage of cutting implements is important to prevent

A. over-use of implements
B. injury to small children
C. rust from forming
D. the edge from becoming dull

___45. The technique of holding the hair upward toward the crown or top of the head during a hair shaping is called

A. low-elevation
B. high-elevation
C. feather edging
D. stepping

___46. When cutting the hair with a shaper, it is important to

A. cut by using the guard
B. thin toward the scalp
C. use long, sliding strokes
D. blunt all hair

___47. If a razor is used to cut the hair, the hair should be

A. completely dry
B. slightly damp
C. completely wet
D. slightly moist

___48. During a razor cut, as the razor is cutting the hair, the comb is placed in the

A. pocket
B. drawer
C. other hand
D. other section

___49. Hotter air settings on the air waver are generally used on hair that is

A. normal
B. coarse
C. bleached
D. tinted

___50. When doing a tint retouch, apply the tint only to the

A. hair root
B. hair ends
C. cold shaft
D. new growth

___51. Just before applying a hair tint, it would be a good safety precaution to

A. put cotton on the hairline
B. put cotton around the client's neck
C. check again for scalp abrasions
D. clean combs and brushes

___52. A single-application tint is prepared by mixing the required tint with

A. hard water
B. 10-volume peroxide
C. ammonia water
D. 20-volume peroxide

___53. To prevent overlapping on a tint retouch, the tint is applied from the scalp to about

A. 1/16" up to the tinted hair
B. 1/16" over the already tinted hair
C. 1/4" up to the tinted hair
D. 1/2" over the tinted hair

___54. The pH of a semi-permanent color falls in the range of

A. 4 to 6
B. 5 to 6
C. 7 to 9
D. 9 to 10.

___55. Which of the following is the best definition of a permanent toner?

A. an aniline derivative tint in pastel colors
B. an aniline tint having a gold base
C. para-phenylene-diamine dyes
D. color that cannot be removed

___56. The lightest toner can only be applied to hair bleached to the

A. brown stage
B. red-gold stage
C. pale yellow stage
D. red stage

___57. Containers used for mixing bleach should be made of

A. plastic
B. wood
C. metal
D. glass

___58. Applying a normalizing lotion to bleached hair will lower the hair's

A. alkalinity
B. affinity
C. chemistry
D. acidity

___59. Bleach can be kept moist during frostings by using a(n)

A. overcap
B. warm water
C. hot towel
D. dry towel

___60. Pre-bleaching (lightening) is required before the application of a

A. semi-permanent rinse
B. one-process tint
C. permanent toner
D. temporary rinse

___61. Which of the following terms is not used in the text to describe a chemical (cold) wave?

A. body wave
B. support wave
C. structure wave
D. texture wave

___62. To achieve a good curl when permanent waving, how much tension should be applied to the hair during wrapping?

A. very firm tension
B. very little tension
C. moderate-firm, even tension
D. no tension

___63. When sodium bromate fumes and ammonia fumes mix together in an open towel hamper, what could result?

A. a fire
B. a strong acid smell
C. discoloration of towels
D. stain in the hamper

___64. After processing a perm, what can you do to prevent the rods from being forced from the hair during rinsing ?

A. tighten them up
B. use low water pressure
C. put on a hair net
D. rinse with cool water

___65. Cotton is placed around the hairline before applying the cold-waving solution; it should be

A. removed after it is applied
B. allowed to remain until the neutralizer is applied
C. removed following the neutralizer
D. removed when the rods are taken out

___66. To remove dripping cold-waving solution, use a piece of cotton or the corner of a towel saturated with

A. cold water
B. warm water
C. tepid water
D. hot water

___67. When processing the cold wave, the hair tends to swell, or

A. expand
B. contract
C. harden
D. shrink

___68. If a neutralizing bib is used for neutralizing the permanent, where should you place a small piece of cotton?

A. by the ears
B. across the forehead
C. under the eye hook
D. around the nape

___69. A neck towel saturated with waving solution, and left around a client's neck may cause a chemical

A. burn
B. reaction
C. lesion
D. sore

___70. The most often used basic chemical for relaxing super-curly hair is sodium

A. bromate
B. hydroxide
C. bicarbonate
D. sulfur

___71. Before a chemical relaxer, the skin and scalp can be protected from chemical burns by applying a

A. neutralizer
B. stabilizer
C. base
D. jelly

___72. Should a chemical relaxer accidently drip into the client's eye, what should you do?

A. stop action by applying neutralizer to eye
B. flush eye with lots of water
C. blot chemical and apply hot water
D. mist eye with bottle of warm water

___73. The application of a base or no-base relaxer would begin in the

A. nape section
B. left-side section
C. right-side section
D. crown section

___74. After a chemical relaxer, a conditioner should be applied

A. after the hair is set
B. just before the comb-out
C. before the hair is styled with rollers
D. after the comb-out

___75. The process of permanently changing the structural bonds of super-curly hair into a straight position is called

A. bond straightening
B. decurling
C. chemical relaxing
D. uncurling

___76. When applying a chemical relaxer, it is important that you AVOID

A. misting the hair with water
B. using small sections
C. tugging on the hair
D. timing your application

___77. If the client has a little spot on the scalp that is burning during a chemical hair relaxer, what should you do?

A. rinse all relaxer from the hair immediately
B. apply an astringent to the spot
C. apply petrolatum to the spot
D. spray spot with cool water

___78. Thermal pressing usually begins in the

A. nape section
B. crown section
C. side section
D. top section

___79. After the hair is pressed, the thermal iron forms the curl by rotating the iron using a(n)

A. clicking action
B. sliding actions
C. oval action
D. back and forth action

___80. The styling comb used in thermal waving should be made of

A. aluminum
B. steel
C. hard rubber
D. soft rubber

___81. The double-application service in which super-curly hair is straightened, then curled, on permanent wave rods is called a(n)

A. recurl or soft curl
B. structuring
C. Afro-pick
D. none of the above

___82. During a curl reformation the rearranger has been applied, capped, and put under the dryer. When should it be checked?

A. it doesn't need to be checked
B. every 5 minutes
C. every 10 minutes
D. every 15 minutes

___83. Before applying a curl reformation straightener, what should you do?

A. make a client record
B. apply the neutralizer to nape
C. apply a base to hairline
D. give a scalp treatment

___84. What is the name for the product that straightens the hair in the curl reformation service?

A. chemical relaxer
B. chemical rearranger
C. hair straightener
D. hair filler

___85. What is the one thing to watch out for when you are about to give a curl reformation?

A. too many test curls
B. client allergies
C. using too many rods
D. tangled hair

___86. The sweat and oil glands are located in the

A. cuticle layer
B. epidermis layer
C. dermis layer
D. cutis layer

___87. The microscopic study of the skin is called

A. dermatology
B. psychology
C. histology
D. trichology

___88. Another name for miliaria rubra is

A. prickly heat
B. sweat retention
C. anhidrosis
D. a cold sweat

___89. The largest and most efficient organ of the human body is the

A. heart
B. liver
C. pancreas
D. skin

___90. Emollient cream is used in facial massage as a(n)

A. astringent
B. lubricant
C. cleanser
D. toner

___91. To tweeze the eyebrows correctly, this should be done in the direction

A. toward the forehead
B. toward the chin
C. of their natural growth
D. opposite their natural growth

___92. When the foundation makeup protrudes from the surface of the skin, what does this tell you about the skin's alkalinity?

A. high
B. low
C. neutral
D. zero

___93. What effect does the freshener have on the pores of the skin?

A. medicates
B. cleanses
C. opens
D. sanitizes

___94. The symptoms of athlete's foot are white patches between the toes, and

A. flat, oval patches
B. red, inflamed open sores
C. clear, water-filled blisters
D. round, white patches all over the foot

___95. Once a nail becomes infected, it should be treated by a

A. barber
B. cosmetologist
C. manicurist
D. physician

___96. A hairpiece that covers 80 to 100 percent of a client's head is called a

A. wiglet
B. cascade
C. wig
D. toupee

___97. What is at least one factor that society uses to determine the success or failure of a person's career?

A. how tall they are
B. how much money they make
C. what kind of car they drive
D. how they dress

___98. When you are asking the clients questions about their needs, what strategy are you using to provide services or products?

A. grilling
B. discovery
C. anticipation
D. all of the above

___99. What is the term used to describe a new client visiting you for a service as the result of another client sending them?

A. word of mouth
B. a referral
C. lucky to have good friends
D. a random chance

___100. If you use a straight razor, how do you protect yourself and your client from accidental cuts during the shaving service?

A. use of a guard
B. protective spray
C. use of an upward motion
D. being very careful

DALTON'S STANDARDIZED FINAL TEST 2

Student Name ______________________________ Score _______ Date ___________

Instructions: Carefully read through each question, then read the answer choices. Write your choice of the word, or the phrase, that correctly completes the statement or answers the question, on the line provided.

___1. The science that prevents individual disease, and promotes good health is

A. individual development
B. good grooming
C. personal hygiene
D. public sanitation

___2. All full-time employes in a beauty salon must be paid

A. a state or federal minimum commission
B. the state or federal minimum wage
C. for at least one hour of work
D. the company's hourly salary

___3. A salon owner's income may vary according to the

A. number of salons owned
B. size of the salon
C. location of the salon
D. all of the above

___4. Which term fits the job description for a person who specializes in preserving the beauty of the client's face and neck?

A. facial expert
B. esthetician
C. electrologist
D. dermatologist

___5. To communicate, a thought or attitude is conveyed

A. verbally
B. nonverbally
C. person to person
D. all of the above

___6. Dental care for preserving healthy teeth starts with a daily mouthwash and

A. rinsing and flushing
B. rubbing and scratching
C. rinsing and rubbing
D. brushing and flossing

___7. The governing body in most states which is supposed to discipline members that violate professional ethics is the

A. bureau of ethics
B. state legislature
C. state association
D. state board

___8. It is your responsibility to

A. give as much service as needed
B. learn new methods of hairstyling
C. give services based on quality
D. all of the above

___9. Things that may be considered a health hazard are

A. forced air furnaces
B. impure air
C. clean body and clothes
D. hygienic salon practices

___10. The germicidal light used in some dry sanitizers is known as

A. fluorescent light
B. ultra-violet light
C. infrared light
D. incandescent light

___11. Practices in the beauty salon that help preserve the health of the public are called

A. fumigation-deodorization
B. salon grooming
C. cleaning-washing
D. sanitation-sterilization

___12. If the eye has been chemically burned, what should be done?

A. flush eye with cool water
B. flush eye with boric acid
C. apply Vasoline
D. apply calamine lotion

___13. Metal hair-cutting implements are sanitized with

A. 70% alcohol
B. 40% alcohol
C. 30% formalin solution
D. 30% boric acid

___14. Which virus causes the AIDS disease?

A. Rhinovirus
B. HIV virus
C. Influenza virus
D. Cold virus

___15. What route of transmission does the AIDS disease follow?

A. sexual contact
B. injection
C. touching
D. A and B only

___16. Metal electrodes should be sanitized with

A. 2% quats
B. 20% peroxide
C. 70% alcohol
D. 80% ammonium

___17. By law, which of the following must each beauty salon have available?

A. a fire blanket
B. a hot water dispenser
C. an emergency eye wash station
D. a fire extinguisher

___18. A carrier is a person who has a disease that is

A. acute
B. contagious
C. occupational
D. common

___19. Which of the following would destroy the AIDS virus outside the body?

A. water
B. 70% alcohol
C. shampoo
D. hand soap

___20. When giving a service, what should you do if you are exposed to blood?

A. see your doctor
B. wash exposed area with soap and water
C. apply a topical disinfectant
D. B and C only

___21. Hair-cutting implements are sanitized with

A. 30% alcohol
B. 30% formalin solution
C. 40% alcohol
D. 70% alcohol

___22. If the eye has been chemically burned, what should be done?

A. flush eye with cool water
B. flush eye with boric acid
C. apply alcohol
D. apply quats

___23. A common skin antiseptic would be

A. 3% hydrogen peroxide
B. 6% hydrogen peroxide
C. 9% hydrogen peroxide
D. 12% hydrogen peroxide

___24. A hot wax treatment would be used to remove superfluous hair in all of the following areas except one.

A. upper lip
B. lower jaw line
C. eyebrow area
D. underarms

___25. When hair is in its resting cycle, and more likely to fall out, this stage is known as the

A. terminal stage
B. fall-out stage
C. hair loss stage
D. telogen stage

___26. What is the name for the male hair loss due to the aging process?

A. congenital alopecia
B. male-pattern baldness
C. hair thinning
D. routine hair loss

___27. Before applying a chemical depilatory, how should the cosmetologist protect the client?

A. buy only quality depilatories
B. apply gauze to the area to be worked on
C. give the client a skin test
D. ask client to remove jewelry

___28. The layer of the hair in which the coloring pigment is found is the

A. follicle
B. medulla
C. cortex
D. cuticle

____29. Before using a hot wax depilatory, the cosmetologist should

A. apply gauze to the work area
B. give the client instructions
C. check to be sure client is comfortable
D. check the temperature of the wax

____30. What general prefix is used to describe most hair diseases?

A. tricho
B. tricko
C. trio
D. trigo

____31. The skin and hair have a natural pH in a range of

A. 3.5 – 4.5.
B. 4.5 – 5.5.
C. 5.5 – 6.5.
D. 6.5 – 7.5.

____32. Peroxide has a pH that is

A. acid
B. alkaline
C. neutral
D. none of the above

____33. When rinsing the client's hair with hot water, how should you detect temperature changes in the water?

A. watch for steam from the client's scalp
B. little finger of hand held under nozzle of hose
C. the color of the client's scalp turns bright pink
D. the shampoo changes color

____34. How should you protect the client's clothing before shampooing the hair?

A. draping the cape over the back of the chair
B. cover all clothing with towels
C. place plastic clothing protectors
D. place plastic towels across client's shoulder

____35. Hair can be damaged by

A. brush rollers
B. heated rollers
C. thermal curling irons
D. all of the above

____36. When the hair is conditioned using strong chemicals, this is known as

A. pre-treating
B. preconditioning
C. duration conditioning
D. in-process conditioning

____37. Hair can be damaged chemically by

A. improper bleaching
B. wave set
C. shampooing
D. hair cutting

____38. Scalp manipulations should not be given if the hair is going to be

A. cold waved
B. permanently colored
C. chemically lightened
D. all of the above

____39. Before combing out the finger wave, the hair should be

A. thoroughly dried
B. thoroughly lubricated
C. quite damp
D. sprayed with lacquer

____40. For the least amount of tightness when setting sculpture curls, you should use a

A. no-stem curl
B. half-stem curl
C. quarter-stem curl
D. long-stem curl

____41. Set sculpture curls within a shaping should

A. be separate
B. swing down
C. overlap
D. swing over

____42. When putting a shaping into the hair, the hair should be

A. wet
B. damp
C. dry
D. moistened on the ends

____43. To correct a diamond-shaped face, fullness is needed everywhere, except at the

A. cheekbones
B. eyebrows
C. forehead
D. jaw

___44. If too much bulk is removed from coarse hair, it tends to

A. look smooth and natural
B. stick out from the head
C. be super curly
D. set more easily

___45. When razor cutting, strokes that the cosmetologist should use are

A. firm and long
B. smooth and long
C. smooth and short
D. jerky and short

___46. To prevent the electric clipper blades from pulling the hair, what should you do?

A. apply oil to them
B. soak in alcohol
C. apply ammonia to them
D. dip them in peroxide

___47. What is the name given to one or more subsections of hair cut in the hairline or crown of the head that serve as a yardstick for cutting the rest of the hair?

A. trendline
B. radial line
C. bias line
D. guideline

___48. What will happen if you submerge your electric clipper in a wet sanitizer while it is plugged into an outlet?

A. the blades will slide
B. the clipper won't cut correctly
C. you will get an electric shock
D. your clipper will vibrate

___49. Storing your scissors in your uniform pocket may result in

A. a severe cut
B. tarnishing of finish on the scissors
C. dulling of blades of the scissors
D. rust forming on the scissors

___50. The foundation for a good hairstyle is a correct hair

A. setting lotion
B. shaping
C. styling comb
D. brush

___51. The heat from the air waver should be directed

A. away from the scalp
B. toward the scalp
C. at the ends
D. toward the hair root

___52. To prevent overlapping on a tint retouch, the tint is applied from the scalp to about

A. 1/16" up to the tinted hair
B. 1/16" over the already tinted hair
C. 1/4" up to the tinted hair
D. 1/2" over the tinted hair

___53. A predisposition test is required before applying a(n)

A. vegetable derivative tint
B. animal derivative tint
C. metallic derivative tint
D. aniline derivative tint

___54. A client is now in the styling chair for a scheduled virgin tint. After getting the coloring product from the dispensary, you discover there is no developer anywhere in the salon

A. use water for the developer and give the tint
B. use shampoo for developer
C. reschedule the appointment
D. ask the client to leave

___55. Synthetic/organic temporary hair colors are found in

A. vegetable tints
B. aniline derivative tints
C. certified vegetable tints
D. metallic tints

___56. By law, a predisposition test must be given before each

A. oxidation tint
B. bleach
C. temporary rinse
D. conditioning treatment

___57. How many stages does black hair go through to become pale blonde?

A. four
B. five
C. six
D. seven

___58. Lightening the hair begins with the application of a

A. stripping agent
B. toning agent
C. moisturizing agent
D. bleaching agent

___59. When the proper stage of streaking is reached, which shampoo is BEST to remove bleach?

A. mild
B. medicated (alkaline)
C. non-stripping (acid)
D. alkaline

___60. Removing artificial color from the hair requires the use of a

A. stripper
B. steamer
C. dye solvent
D. bleach

___61. If bleach drips onto the skin, the bleach should be removed using

A. cold-cool water
B. tepid-hot water
C. hot water only
D. very hot water

___62. When giving a virgin bleach to medium brown hair, the cosmetologist should begin applying the lightener

A. 1/2" from scalp up through ends
B. from scalp to ends
C. from ends to scalp
D. center of hair shaft to ends

___63. If the elastic strap of the cold wave rod is twisted, or stretched too tightly across the base of the hair, it may cause

A. hair breakage
B. curl relaxation
C. frizzy curls
D. straight curls

___64. Before a cold wave is wrapped the hair is usually dried using a

A. blow comb
B. hand dryer
C. towel
D. rat-tail comb

___65. When permanent waving the hair, how many turns must the hair be wound around the rod to achieve a curl pattern?

A. once
B. twice
C. four turns
D. five turns

___66. In which of the following conditions should the cosmetologist REFUSE to give the client a cold wave?

A. a scar on the scalp
B. cranial surgical wound
C. a scalp freckle
D. an ulna surgical wound

___67. During a wrapping procedure using waving solution, breakages can occur if too much tension is placed on the

A. hair
B. comb
C. end wrap
D. rod

___68. When wrapping a ponytail cold wave, it is better to begin wrapping in the

A. bottom section
B. top section
C. middle section
D. front section

___69. Two basic chemicals used in cold-waving solution are

A. ammonia and formalin
B. sulfuric acid and ammonia
C. carbolic acid and formalin
D. thioglycolic acid and ammonia

___70. A neck towel saturated with waving solution, and left around a client's neck may cause a chemical

A. burn
B. reaction
C. lesion
D. sore

___71. Chemical relaxers are also called

A. curl straighteners
B. thermal pressures
C. perms
D. presses

____72. As in cold waving, chemical relaxers work faster on hair that is

A. wiry
B. coarse
C. porous
D. non-porous

____73. The difference between a base and no-base relaxer is that the no-base

A. does not require application of the base
B. always requires the use of protective gloves
C. is safer to use, but requires more time
D. is more dangerous to use, but requires more time

____74. After a sodium hydroxide relaxer has processed, but before it is shampooed, the hair should be thoroughly

A. combed
B. conditioned
C. rinsed
D. brushed

____75. The neutralizing shampoo used in the chemical relaxing service is also called a

A. stabilizer
B. cleaner
C. conditioner
D. filler

____76. Hair is chemically straightened with thio, or

A. sodium hydroxide
B. hydrogen peroxide
C. borax
D. formalin

____77. When rinsing the chemical relaxer from the hair, to avoid tangling, it is important to use

A. low to medium water pressure
B. high water pressure
C. hot water at all times
D. an alkaline shampoo

____78. One of the most important things to remember about the processing of a chemical relaxer is

A. apply it slowly and evenly
B. never leave the client unattended
C. never serve coffee during processing
D. brush the hair before neutralizing

____79. The metal part of a pressing comb is made of

A. aluminum and iron
B. copper and brass
C. brass and pewter
D. aluminum and stainless steel

____80. As the iron is rolled toward the scalp, what does the cosmetologist use to protect the client's scalp?

A. cotton
B. towel
C. comb
D. an end paper

____81. Before thermal waving super-curly hair, the cosmetologist should

A. color it
B. press it
C. shape it
D. comb it

____82. To be successful, what size rod subsections should the cosmetologist use when doing a curl reformation?

A. small subsections
B. medium subsections
C. large subsections
D. none of the above

____83. Before applying the neutralizer to the rods when doing a curl reformation, the hair should be rinsed with

A. conditioner
B. hot water
C. tepid water
D. cold water

____84. During a curl reformation, how much tension is used to wrap the hair on the rods?

A. no tension
B. moderate tension
C. slight tension
D. firm tension

____85. The double-application service in which super-curly hair is straightened, then curled, on permanent wave rods is called a(n)

A. recurl or soft curl
B. structuring or rebuilding
C. Afro-pick
D. none of the above

___86. When giving a curl reformation, it is very important to wear

A. a hair net
B. an operator apron
C. protective shoes
D. none of the above

___87. The uppermost layer of skin that protects the body is the

A. epidermis
B. dermis
C. corium
D. cutis

___88. The outermost (top) layer of the skin is the

A. epidermis
B. corium
C. subcutaneous tissue
D. adipose tissue

___89. The thinnest layer of the skin is the

A. epidermis
B. corium
C. subcutaneous tissue
D. adipose tissue

___90. Cold cream is used on the face as a

A. foundation
B. base
C. emollient
D. cleanser

___91. To maintain sanitation, color applied to the lips should be done with a sanitized

A. pledget
B. brush
C. crayon
D. cotton ball

___92. Small eyes can be made to appear larger. What type of makeup is applied to create this illusion?

A. contour
B. foundation
C. lip
D. white

___93. What type of movement should be used when tweezing the eyebrows?

A. slow, sliding movement
B. quick movement
C. circular movement
D. zig-zag movement

___94. The eponychium is the

A. skin that surrounds the entire nail
B. outside point where the skin overlaps the nail
C. inside point where the nail enters the skin
D. deep fold of skin where the nail root is imbedded

___95. If hangnails are neglected, they may become

A. brittle
B. fragile
C. infected
D. loose

___96. If a minor cut should occur during a manicure, apply powdered styptic, or a(n)

A. shampoo
B. antiseptic
C. creme rinse
D. disinfectant

___97. What is the common goal set between you and your client before you have done anything to their hair, nails, or face?

A. improve their appearance
B. make money
C. buy a house
D. make their hair shinier

___98. Talking with your clients about the possible solutions to some of their appearance problems is known as a

A. meeting
B. consultation
C. conversation
D. revelation

___99. How do stylists provide additional money for themselves in addition to the money earned for providing services?

A. retail sales
B. rebook client before they leave the salon
C. steal clients from co-workers
D. hog phoned-in appointments

___100. What is the name for the stone used to sharpen a straight razor?

A. hone
B. whetstone
C. strop
D. crop

DALTON'S STANDARDIZED FINAL TEST 3

Student Name ______________________________ Score _______ Date ___________

Instructions: Carefully read through each question, then read the answer choices. Write your choice of the word, or the phrase, that correctly completes the statement or answers the question, on the line provided.

___1. Personal hygiene is defined as the daily routine followed to preserve and promote the well being of the

A. town
B. individual
C. society
D. community

___2. The advantage(s) of being a manager-operator may include the opportunity to learn about

A. overhead expenses
B. accounts payable
C. inventory
D. all of the above

___3. Personal grooming relates to one's

A. daily appearance
B. daily cleanliness
C. hairstyle and voice
D. A and B.

___4. Personal hygiene relates to

A. promoting one's own health
B. preservation of one's health
C. oral care
D. A and B.

___5. Dental care for preserving healthy teeth starts with a daily mouthwash and

A. rinsing and flushing
B. rubbing and scratching
C. rinsing and rubbing
D. brushing and flossing

___6. Ethics is a system that measures human behavior that is

A. voluntary
B. involuntary
C. imposed by local police
D. imposed by the federal government

___7. A professional attitude is

A. natural
B. given when you are licensed
C. acquired in enrollment
D. learned

___8. To equal the strength of 70% ethyl alcohol, you would have to use

A. 20% isopropyl alcohol
B. 39% isopropyl alcohol
C. 85% isopropyl alcohol
D. 99% isopropyl alcohol

___9. A person immune to a disease, but who can infect others is known as a(n)

A. clinical
B. medical
C. agent
D. carrier

___10. Another name for public hygiene is

A. grooming
B. hair care
C. sanitation
D. community

___11. If the eye has been chemically burned, what should be done?

A. flush eye with cool water
B. flush eye with boric acid
C. apply alcohol
D. apply quats

___12. When removing implements from a wet sanitizer you should wear

A. an operator apron
B. a hair net
C. rubber gloves
D. neutralizing bib

___13. Which virus causes the AIDS disease?

A. Rhino virus
B. HIV virus
C. Influenza virus
D. Cold virus

___14. What route of transmission does the AIDS disease follow?

A. injection
B. blood transfusion
C. maternal
D. all of the above

___15. Soiled towels should be stored in a covered

A. linen hamper
B. metal container
C. plastic container
D. laundry basket

___16. A carrier is a person who has a disease that is

A. acute
B. contagious
C. occupational
D. common

___17. What common cosmetology chemical would kill the AIDS virus outside of the body?

A. household bleach
B. water
C. 1% hydrogen peroxide
D. 20% alcohol

___18. What strength hydrogen peroxide would destroy the AIDS virus outside of the body?

A. 1%
B. 2%
C. 3%
D. all of the above

___19. If you accidently cut your client's neck and it bleeds, what should you do?

A. put on disposable rubber gloves
B. wash area with soap and water
C. apply topical disinfectant to area
D. all of the above

___20. Hair-cutting implements are sanitized with

A. 30% alcohol
B. 30% formalin solution
C. 40% alcohol
D. 70% alcohol

___21. A 5 percent formalin solution is used mainly to sanitize a(n)

A. ultraviolet sanitizer
B. tweezers
C. cuticle scissors
D. styling chair

___22. If the eye has been chemically burned, what should be done?

A. flush eye with cool water
B. flush eye with boric acid
C. apply alcohol
D. apply quats

___23. Hair is not found on the

A. forearm and wrists
B. forearm and nose
C. knuckles of the hands
D. soles of the feet

___24. Hair is an example of

A. hard keratin
B. soft keratin
C. Henle's layer
D. Huxley's layer

___25. Scalp hair usually grows at a monthly rate of

A. 1/4"
B. 1/2"
C. 3/4"
D. 1"

___26. Which of the following would a dermatologist prescribe for men for regular hair loss?

A. vitamin A
B. minoxidal
C. medicated shampoo
D. creme rinse

___27. Hair is made up of a hard protein substance called

A. carbon
B. hydrogen
C. keratin
D. sulfur

___28. The percentage of the hair shaft represented by the cortex layer is

A. 15%
B. 25%
C. 50%
D. 75%

___29. The technical term applied to the cyclical period when the hair begins to grow is the

A. anagen stage
B. terminal stage
C. telogen stage
D. origin stage

___30. Hypertrichosis is a condition that is also called

A. supercilia hair
B. superfluous hair
C. ringed hair
D. twisted hair

___31. Shampoos with a pH greater than seven (7) are called

A. acid
B. alkaline
C. mild
D. neutral

___32. Peroxide has a pH that is

A. acid
B. alkaline
C. neutral
D. none of the above

___33. An overly oily scalp is a disorder medically referred to as

A. steatoma
B. seborrhea
C. asteatosis
D. tinea

___34. To prevent water from dripping onto the floor from the shampoo bowl, where should you leave the shampoo hose?

A. drain position
B. handle position
C. vacuum breaker position
D. none of the above

___35. The natural lubricant that gives hair a beautiful luster or sheen is called

A. sebum
B. seborrhea
C. seconal
D. permanent color

___36. The basic protein found in the hair shaft is

A. cuticle
B. medulla
C. sebum
D. keratin

___37. Very small bits of protein applied to the hair are called

A. macro-proteins
B. micro-proteins
C. poultry proteins
D. substantive proteins

___38. Semicircular designs combed into the hair are called

A. waves
B. base direction
C. shapings
D. arcs

___39. The main objective in finger waving the hair is to mold even

A. curls and softness
B. waves and ridges
C. shaping and direction
D. parts and shapes

___40. The section of the head that is closest to the neck is the

A. nape section
B. crown section
C. crepe section
D. left side section

___41. A large stand-up curl could also be called a barrel curl or

A. skip-curl
B. cascade curl
C. closed-end curl
D. clockwise curl

___42. To get the maximum amount of height or fullness, you should use a

A. no-stem curl
B. half-stem curl
C. long-stem curl
D. tight-stem curl

___43. When setting the hair with rollers, a curved form in the finished hairstyle is done by winding hair around the roller

A. 1 turn or less
B. 1-1/2 turns
C. 2 turns
D. none of the above

___44. The standard or ideal facial shape is

A. oblong
B. round
C. oval
D. square

____45. What draping supply is recommended for the client that is about to have a hair shaping only?

A. towel shampoo cape
B. shampoo cape
C. comb-out cape
D. chair cloth

____46. Super-curly hair should be cut with a

A. clipper
B. scissors
C. razor
D. thinning shears

____47. Proper storage of cutting implements is important to prevent

A. over-use of implements
B. injury to small children
C. rust from forming
D. the edge from becoming dull

____48. You should not use an electric clipper if

A. the client wants a trim
B. the set screw has been adjusted
C. it is noisy
D. any teeth are broken

____49. When cutting the hair with a shaper, it is important to

A. cut by using the guard
B. thin toward the scalp
C. use long, sliding strokes
D. blunt all hair

____50. During a razor cut, as the razor is cutting the hair, the comb is placed in the

A. pocket
B. drawer
C. other hand
D. other section

____51. The hanging length cut around the hairline from which the rest of the hair is shaped is called the

A. high-sign
B. cutting length
C. guideline
D. form

____52. To ensure safety, all hair wavers and blow dryers must be

A. set at low temperature settings
B. used on damp to dry hair
C. Underwriters Laboratories approved
D. inspected at time of purchase

____53. A one-process permanent tint contains

A. aniline derivative dye
B. metallic dye
C. vegetable dye
D. henna dye

____54. One of the main chemicals in aniline derivative tints is

A. sulfonated oils
B. ammonium thioglycolate
C. cystine disulfide
D. para-phenylene-diamine

____55. The name for a chemical reaction of mixing hydrogen peroxide and an aniline derivative tint is

A. hydrolization
B. oxidation
C. softening
D. filling

____56. To prevent overlapping on a tint retouch, the tint is applied from the scalp to about

A. 1/16" up to the tinted hair
B. 1/16" over the already tinted hair
C. 1/4" up to the tinted hair
D. 1/2" over the tinted hair

____57. To prevent a line of demarcation during a tint retouch, it is important to avoid

A. rotating a bottle
B. overlapping the tint
C. mixing tint
D. rubbing the scalp

____58. Which of the following is the best definition of a permanent toner?

A. an aniline derivative tint in pastel colors
B. an aniline tint having a gold base
C. para-phenylene-diamine dyes
D. color that cannot be removed

____59. Decolorization takes place in which layer of the hair?

A. cuticle
B. cortex
C. medulla
D. all of the above

___60. When lightening and toning the hair, you should wear

A. protective shoes
B. a hair net
C. an operator apron
D. protective gloves

___61. A retouch hair lightener is applied to the

A. new growth of hair
B. entire hair shaft
C. the ends only
D. cold shaft only

___62. When hydrogen peroxide is mixed with sulfonated oil (sodium persulfates) the result is an oil

A. lightener
B. rinse
C. relaxer
D. neutralizer

___63. The removal of a penetrating tint from the hair is called

A. relaxing
B. soap cap
C. stripping
D. tinting

___64. If too much tension is used during cold wave wrapping, this may cause the processing time to be

A. stopped
B. increased
C. retarded
D. accelerated

___65. Better saturation of the cold-waving solution into the hair is achieved when it is

A. wrapped correctly
B. analyzed accurately
C. curled properly
D. pressed thoroughly

___66. Before cold waving the entire head, the degree to which the hair will curl can be determined by using

A. concave curls
B. convex curls
C. test curls
D. pin curls

___67. Cotton is placed around the hairline before applying the cold-waving solution; it should be

A. removed after it is applied
B. allowed to remain until the neutralizer is applied
C. removed following the neutralizer
D. removed when the rods are taken out

___68. To remove dripping cold-waving solution, use a piece of cotton or the corner of a towel saturated with

A. cold water
B. warm water
C. tepid water
D. hot water

___69. The action of cold waving solution on the hair is one of

A. softening
B. hardening
C. shrinking
D. contracting

___70. During the winding process in cold waving, the physical bonds in the hair shaft that are broken are called

A. amino
B. cysteine
C. hydrogen
D. salt

___71. A neck towel saturated with waving solution, and left around a client's neck may cause a chemical

A. burn
B. reaction
C. lesion
D. sore

___72. The base in a no-base chemical relaxer is used to

A. straighten the hair
B. protect the scalp
C. protect the hair
D. neutralize the relaxer

___73. If the client has a little spot on the scalp that is burning during a chemical hair relaxer, what should you do?

A. rinse all relaxer from hair immediately
B. apply an astringent to the spot
C. apply petrolatum to the spot
D. spray spot with cool water

____74. Before giving a retouch chemical relaxer, what should be applied to the previously relaxed hair first?

A. water
B. protective conditioner
C. presoftening rinse
D. prerelax shampoo

____75. If you use all of a particular relaxer, but are in need of more to complete the service, it is best to

A. add water to what is on the hair
B. add water to what is left in the jar, then apply to the hair
C. add a relaxer made by another company
D. neutralize the hair and continue when there is enough material to finish

____76. After a chemical relaxer, a conditioner should be applied

A. after the hair is set
B. just before the comb-out
C. before the hair is styled with rollers
D. after the comb-out

____77. Cosmetologists avoid giving a chemical relaxer when the scalp examination reveals the presence of

A. firm, tight scalp
B. abrasions and scratches
C. oily scalp and hair
D. loose, pliable scalp

____78. The actions of chemical hair straightener cause the hair to

A. soften and swell
B. shape and curl
C. shift and mold
D. shrink and harden

____79. During the processing and neutralizing of a chemical relaxer service, what can be done to minimize neck irritation?

A. applying cotton coil
B. changing towel frequently
C. keeping the client's neck against the bowl
D. applying neutralizing cream

____80. During pressing, the hair is protected by

A. foil
B. cap
C. oil
D. gel

____81. After a thermal wave, the hair is brushed and combed into a hairstyle

A. after the lanolin has been applied
B. while the hair is still hot
C. when the hair has been cooled
D. while the hair is lukewarm

____82. What is the name for the service in which the hair is pressed twice on the top of the strand, and once on the underside?

A. one press
B. light press
C. comb press
D. soft press

____83. When giving a curl reformation, it is very important to wear

A. a hair net
B. an operator apron
C. protective shoes
D. none of the above

____84. How often should facial sponges be sanitized

A. immediately after use
B. disposed of in a container
C. boiled for immediately
D. put in an autoclave the next day

____85. During a curl reformation the rearranger has been applied, capped, and put under the dryer. When should it be checked?

A. every 5 minutes
B. every 10 minutes
C. every 15 minutes
D. it doesn't need to be checked

____86. Before applying the neutralizer to the rods when doing a curl reformation, the hair should be

A. conditioned
B. rinsed with hot water
C. rinsed with tepid water
D. rinsed with cold water

____87. During a curl reformation, the hair dries out while you are wrapping the hair on the rods. What should you do?

A. apply more waving solution
B. apply water to dry strands
C. use spray-on conditioner
D. use two end wraps

___88. Dry, or oily skin is related to activity of the

A. renal glands
B. lymph glands
C. sudoriferous glands
D. sebaceous glands

___89. Another name for miliaria rubra is

A. prickly heat
B. sweat retention
C. anhidrosis
D. a cold sweat

___90. The effleurage massage movement is done lightly and slowly, so it is

A. stimulating
B. soothing
C. exciting
D. irritating

___91. If base makeup is applied correctly, the cosmetologist should be able to conceal

A. eye lids
B. blemishes
C. wrinkles
D. facial hair

___92. When the foundation makeup protrudes from the surface of the skin, what does this tell you about the skin's alkalinity?

A. high
B. low
C. neutral
D. zero

___93. When applying semi-permanent lashes, dip the end of the lash in adhesive, stroke the client's lash, then

A. remove it
B. attach it
C. slip it over
D. slide it onto the lid

___94. Tinea(onychomycosis) is a disturbance of nail growth due to a vegetable fungi that is

A. very common
B. contagious
C. noncontagious
D. beneficial

___95. Once a nail becomes infected, it should be treated by a

A. barber
B. cosmetologist
C. manicurist
D. physician

___96. The most expensive type of hair from which hairgoods are made is

A. synthetic hair
B. yak hair
C. angora hair
D. human hair

___97. How does the cosmetologist obtain personal satisfaction and financial gain from working in the salon?

A. scheduling a lot of appointments
B. answering the phone frequently
C. helping others
D. taking risks

___98. When a cosmetologist has so many appointments that it is difficult to fit in new clients, what is this called?

A. booked solid
B. full book
C. booked-up
D. booked to the hilt

___99. If you are at a social event, such as a party, what would be an effective way to let fellow party goers know what kind of work you do, and where you can be contacted for cosmetology services?

A. write your phone number on a napkin
B. ask them to look you up in the book
C. pass out business cards
D. ask your fiends to copy your number and pass it on

___100. When shaving, what purpose does the application of lather serve?

A. softens the skin
B. smoothes the beard
C. softens the beard
D. feels soothing

DALTON'S STANDARDIZED FINAL TEST 4

Student Name ______________________________ Score ________ Date ____________

Instructions: Carefully read through each question, then read the answer choices. Write your choice of the word, or the phrase, that correctly completes the statement or answers the question, on the line provided.

___1. The easiest way to keep the body clean is to use

A. perfume sprays
B. body powder
C. deodorant sprays
D. soap and water

___2. A salon owner's income may vary according to the

A. number of salons owned
B. size of the salon
C. location of the salon
D. all of the above

___3. Which term fits the job description for a person who specializes in preserving the beauty of the client's face and neck?

A. facial expert
B. esthetician
C. electrologist
D. dermatologist

___4. To communicate, a thought or attitude is conveyed

A. verbally
B. nonverbally
C. person to person
D. all of the above

___5. Dental care for preserving healthy teeth starts with a daily mouthwash and

A. rinsing and flushing
B. rubbing and scratching
C. rinsing and rubbing
D. brushing and flossing

___6. The governing body in most states which is supposed to discipline members that violate professional ethics is the

A. bureau of ethics
B. state legislature
C. state association
D. state board

___7. It is your responsibility to

A. give as much service as needed
B. learn new methods of hairstyling
C. give services based on quality
D. all of the above

___8. If cosmetology implements are aseptic, then they are

A. free from bacteria
B. unsanitary
C. soiled
D. covered

___9. Things that may be considered a health hazard are

A. forced air furnaces
B. impure air
C. clean body and clothes
D. hygienic salon practices

___10. The germicidal light used in some dry sanitizers is known as

A. fluorescent light
B. ultra-violet light
C. infrared light
D. incandescent light

___11. Practices in the beauty salon that help preserve the health of the public are called

A. fumigation-deodorization
B. salon grooming
C. cleaning-washing
D. sanitation-sterilization

___12. If the eye has been chemically burned, what should be done?

A. flush eye with cool water
B. flush eye with boric acid
C. apply alcohol
D. apply quats

___13. To be effective for sanitation, the strength of the quats to be used should be at least

A. 1:200
B. 1:200
C. 1:500
D. 1:1000

___14. Hair-cutting implements are sanitized with

A. 70% alcohol
B. 40% alcohol
C. 30% formalin solution
D. 30% alcohol

___15. Which virus causes the AIDS disease?

A. Rhinovirus
B. HIV virus
C. Influenza virus
D. Cold virus

___16. What route of transmission does the AIDS disease follow?

A. sexual contact
B. injection
C. touching
D. A and B only

___17. Metal electrodes should be sanitized with

A. 2% quats
B. 20% peroxide
C. 70% alcohol
D. 80% ammonium

___18. By law, which of the following must each beauty salon have available?

A. a fire blanket
B. a hot water dispenser
C. an emergency eye wash station
D. a fire extinguisher

___19. A carrier is a person who has a disease that is

A. acute
B. contagious
C. occupational
D. common

___20. Which of the following would destroy the AIDS virus outside the body?

A. water
B. 70% alcohol
C. shampoo
D. hand soap

___21. When giving a service, what should you do if you are exposed to blood?

A. see your doctor
B. wash exposed area with soap and water
C. apply a topical disinfectant
D. B and C only

___22. A common skin antiseptic would be

A. 3% hydrogen peroxide
B. 6% hydrogen peroxide
C. 9% hydrogen peroxide
D. 12% hydrogen peroxide

___23. A hot wax treatment would be used to remove superfluous hair in all of the following areas except one.

A. upper lip
B. lower jaw line
C. eyebrow area
D. underarms

___24. When hair is in its resting cycle, and more likely to fall out, this stage is known as the

A. terminal stage
B. fall-out stage
C. hair loss stage
D. telogen stage

___25. What is the name for the male hair loss due to the aging process?

A. congenital alopecia
B. male-pattern baldness
C. hair thinning
D. routine hair loss

___26. Depilatories in the form of a cream, paste, or powder are chemical products used to

A. curl hair
B. remove hair
C. color hair
D. straighten hair

___27. The layer of the hair in which the coloring pigment is found is the

A. follicle
B. medulla
C. cortex
D. cuticle

___28. Before using a hot wax depilatory, the cosmetologist should

A. apply gauze to the work area
B. give the client instructions
C. check to be sure client is comfortable
D. check the temperature of the wax

____29. When alopecia appears in the head, it looks like

A. red, circular bald patches
B. scaly, rectangular bald patches
C. non-inflamed, oval bald patches
D. oily scales and oval bald patches

____30. Using a short-wave electrical machine to stop the growth of a hair is called

A. electrolysis
B. trichosis
C. cometose
D. osmosis

____31. The pH of a shampoo indicates the concentration of

A. hydrogen
B. oxygen
C. nitrogen
D. carbon

____32. Peroxide has a pH that is

A. acid
B. alkaline
C. neutral
D. none of the above

____33. When rinsing the client's hair with hot water, how should you detect temperature changes in the water?

A. watch for steam from the client's scalp
B. little finger of hand held under nozzle of hose
C. the color of the client's scalp turns bright pink
D. the shampoo changes color

____34. How should you protect the client's clothing before shampooing the hair?

A. draping the cape over the back of the chair
B. cover all clothing with towels
C. place in plastic clothing protectors
D. place plastic towels across client's shoulder

____35. To preserve the hairstyle against humidity in the air, the conditioner should contain a(n)

A. barrier coat
B. shield cover
C. wetting agent
D. antihumectant

____36. The extent that hair can be stretched without breaking is known as

A. pressure
B. tone
C. elasticity
D. texture

____37. When the hair is conditioned using strong chemicals, this is known as

A. pre-treating
B. preconditioning
C. duration conditioning
D. in-process conditioning

____38. Scalp manipulations should not be given if the hair is going to be

A. cold waved
B. permanently colored
C. chemically lightened
D. all of the above

____39. The shaping between two finger-wave ridges is called the wave

A. direction
B. trough
C. arc
D. curl

____40. After the setting lotion has been applied, should the hair dry out during setting, spray more

A. filler on it
B. conditioner on it
C. water on it
D. setting lotion on it

____41. When putting a shaping into the hair, the hair should be

A. wet
B. damp
C. dry
D. moistened on the ends

____42. The profile is the view of the head from the

A. front
B. back
C. side
D. face

___43. For a basic haircut, the cosmetologist would begin cutting the hair in the

A. top
B. side
C. crown
D. nape

___44. When razor cutting, strokes that the cosmetologist should use are

A. firm and long
B. smooth and long
C. smooth and short
D. jerky and short

___45. To prevent the electric clipper blades from pulling the hair, what should you do?

A. apply oil to them
B. soak in alcohol
C. apply ammonia to them
D. dip them in peroxide

___46. What is the name given to one or more subsections of hair cut in the hairline or crown of the head that serve as a yardstick for cutting the rest of the hair?

A. trendline
B. radial line
C. bias line
D. guideline

___47. What will happen if you submerge your electric clipper in a wet sanitizer while it is plugged into an outlet?

A. the blades will slide
B. the clipper won't cut correctly
C. you will get an electric shock
D. your clipper will vibrate

___48. Storing your scissors in your uniform pocket may result in

A. a severe cut
B. tarnishing of finish on the scissors
C. dulling of blades of the scissors
D. rust forming on the scissors

___49. The foundation for a good hairstyle is a correct hair

A. setting lotion
B. shaping
C. styling comb
D. brush

___50. Hotter air settings on the air waver are generally used on hair that is

A. normal
B. coarse
C. bleached
D. tinted

___51. Before applying an aniline derivative tint, omit the

A. hair brushing
B. patch test
C. strand test
D. metallic salt test

___52. Just before applying a hair tint, it would be a good safety precaution to

A. put cotton on the hairline
B. put cotton around the client's neck
C. check again for scalp abrasions
D. clean combs and brushes

___53. A client is now in the styling chair for a scheduled virgin tint. After getting the coloring product from the dispensary, the cosmetologist discovers there is no developer anywhere in the salon

A. use water for the developer and give the tint
B. use shampoo for developer
C. reschedule the appointment
D. ask the client to leave

___54. Synthetic/organic temporary hair colors are found in

A. vegetable tints
B. aniline derivative tints
C. certified vegetable tints
D. metallic tints

___55. The pH of a semi-permanent color falls in the range of

A. 4 to 6
B. 5 to 6
C. 7 to 9
D. 9 to 10.

___56. If you overlap bleach when doing a bleach retouch, it will result in

A. more elasticity
B. less elasticity
C. breakage
D. hair yellowing

____57. The lightest toner can only be applied to hair bleached to the

A. brown stage
B. red-gold stage
C. pale yellow stage
D. red stage

____58. Containers used for mixing bleach should be made of

A. plastic
B. wood
C. metal
D. glass

____59. Before giving a lightener retouch, what should you do?

A. a predisposition test
B. brush the hair vigorously
C. examine the scalp for cuts and abrasions
D. give the client a strand test

____60. When changing the color of the hair to a much lighter color, it is required that the hair be

A. pre-neutralized
B. pre-lightened
C. pre-hardened
D. pre-shaded

____61. To equalize the porosity of the hair, use a

A. steamer
B. stripper
C. filler
D. equalizer

____62. The most successful cold wave can only be given to hair that has been properly

A. lubricated
B. brightened
C. lightened
D. shaped

____63. When sodium bromate fumes and ammonia fumes mix together in an open towel hamper, what could result?

A. a fire
B. a strong acid smell
C. discoloration of towels
D. stain in the hamper

____64. After processing a perm, what can you do to prevent the rods from being forced from the hair during rinsing ?

A. tighten them up
B. use low water pressure
C. put on a hair net
D. rinse with cool water

____65. In which of the following conditions should the cosmetologist REFUSE to give the client a cold wave?

A. a scar on the scalp
B. cranial surgical wound
C. a scalp freckle
D. an ulna surgical wound

____66. If a couple of small areas of the hair do not have enough curl one week after the wave process, you should give the client

A. a refund check
B. another cosmetologist
C. some pickup curls
D. another chemical wave

____67. Cold waving resistant hair would usually require a

A. longer processing time
B. shorter processing time
C. conditioner
D. toner

____68. Cold waving hair involves a physical action, and a

A. medical process
B. mineral process
C. chemical process
D. legal process

____69. A neck towel saturated with waving solution, and left around a client's neck may cause a chemical

A. burn
B. reaction
C. lesion
D. sore

____70. The straightening action is stopped during a chemical relaxer by using a

A. stabilizing creme
B. neutralizing creme
C. neutralizing shampoo
D. stabilizing rinse

___71. If you live in a very warm climate and your client arrives perspiring before having a chemical hair relaxer, what should you do?

A. thoroughly shampoo the hair
B. place client under cool dryer
C. wait while client cools off
D. blot moisture from scalp before starting

___72. Should a chemical relaxer accidently drip into the client's eye, what should you do?

A. stop action by applying neutralizer to eye
B. flush eye with lots of water
C. blot chemical and apply hot water
D. mist eye with bottle of warm water

___73. After chemically relaxing the hair for a client with super-curly hair, what service should NOT be given to the client?

A. roller set
B. regular electric curling iron set
C. pressing comb/thermal iron set
D. pick out style after hair has been dried

___74. The neutralizing shampoo used in the chemical relaxing service is also called a

A. stabilizer
B. cleaner
C. conditioner
D. filler

___75. When giving a chemical relaxer, the cosmetologist must wear

A. a coverall apron
B. safety glasses
C. protective gloves
D. thick soled shoes

___76. Before applying a chemical relaxer, analyze the hair for porosity, texture, and elasticity; then, examine the

A. relaxing kit
B. hairline
C. scalp
D. fingernails

___77. One of the most important things to remember about the processing of a chemical relaxer is

A. apply it slowly and evenly
B. never leave the client unattended
C. never serve coffee during processing
D. brush the hair before neutralizing

___78. Round curling involves winding the hair strand from the

A. ends to the scalp
B. mid-strand to the ends
C. ends to the mid-strand
D. scalp to the ends

___79. When thermal waving the hair, fine, short hairs around the hairline are best curled with

A. some pin curls
B. a smaller iron
C. a crimper
D. some perm rods

___80. The styling comb used in thermal waving should be made of

A. aluminum
B. steel
C. hard rubber
D. soft rubber

___81. What is the main chemical used in the neutralizer of most curl reformation products?

A. hydrogen peroxide
B. sodium bromate
C. ammonium thioglycolate
D. sodium chloride

___82. Before applying the neutralizer to the rods when doing a curl reformation, the hair should be rinsed with

A. conditioner
B. hot water
C. tepid water
D. cold water

___83. During a curl reformation, how much tension is used to wrap the hair on the rods?

A. no tension
B. moderate tension
C. slight tension
D. firm tension

___84. Before applying the neutralizer to the rods when doing a curl reformation, the hair should be

A. conditioned
B. rinsed with hot water
C. rinsed with tepid water
D. rinsed with cold water

____85. When giving a curl reformation, it is very important to wear

A. a hair net
B. an operator apron
C. protective shoes
D. none of the above

____86. During which hours should you AVOID sitting out to sun bathe?

A. 2:00 – 4:00 P.M.
B. 3:00 – 5:00 P.M.
C. 1:00 – 5:00 P.M.
D. 10:00 A.M. – 2:00 P.M.

____87. A sun block lotion would have what SPF rating number?

A. 5.
B. 8.
C. 12.
D. 15.

____88. The largest and most efficient organ of the human body is the

A. heart
B. liver
C. pancreas
D. skin

____89. The massage movement that uses a kneading technique is called

A. petrissage
B. effleurage
C. friction
D. vibration

____90. Knowledge of facial structure is important for the application of makeup to achieve the most attractive facial shape which is

A. round
B. square
C. diamond
D. oval

____91. To blend in facial scars and blemishes, what kind of makeup stick should be used?

A. contour
B. rouge
C. corrective
D. powder

____92. After strip lashes are correctly positioned, the outside and inside ends are held in place for

A. one minute
B. two minutes
C. three minutes
D. four minutes

____93. Nail growth can be decreased or slowed down because of

A. illness
B. old age
C. poor nutrition
D. all of the above

____94. Once a nail becomes infected, it should be treated by a

A. barber
B. cosmetologist
C. manicurist
D. physician

____95. When selecting a hairpiece for a client, you will be able to match the color more easily by using a

A. pH color chart
B. color triangle
C. JL color ring
D. color comparison chart

____96. When alopecia appears in the head, it looks like

A. red, circular bald patches
B. scaly, rectangular bald patches
C. non-inflamed, oval bald patches
D. oily scales and oval bald patches

____97. When the stylist and the client have developed a common set of thoughts, what is the term used to describe this relationship?

A. rapport
B. charisma
C. charm
D. poise

____98. If a client is booked for a permanent wave, which of the following would be classified as an extra service?

A. haircut
B. frosting
C. protein conditioner
D. all of the above

___99. What percentage of your business should come from friends recommending your services to friends?

A. 1 – 2%
B. 2 – 3%
C. 4 – 6%
D. all of the above

___100. If you should accidently draw blood when giving the client a shave, what should you do first?

A. apply pressure to stop the bleeding
B. put on rubber gloves
C. apply antiseptic
D. put styptic on wound

DALTON'S STANDARDIZED FINAL TEST 5

Student Name ______________________________ Score _______ Date __________

Instructions: Carefully read through each question, then read the answer choices. Write your choice of the word, or the phrase, that correctly completes the statement or answers the question, on the line provided.

___1. All full-time employes in a beauty salon must be paid

A. a state or federal minimum commission
B. the state or federal minimum wage
C. for at least one hour of work
D. the company's hourly salary

___2. The advantage(s) of being a manager-operator may include the opportunity to learn about

A. overhead expenses
B. accounts payable
C. inventory
D. all of the above

___3. Personal grooming relates to one's

A. daily appearance
B. daily cleanliness
C. hairstyle and voice
D. A and B.

___4. Personal hygiene relates to

A. promoting one's own health
B. preservation of one's health
C. oral care
D. A and B.

___5. Dental care for preserving healthy teeth starts with a daily mouthwash and

A. rinsing and flushing
B. rubbing and scratching
C. rinsing and rubbing
D. brushing and flossing

___6. Ethics is a system that measures human behavior that is

A. voluntary
B. involuntary
C. imposed by local police
D. imposed by the federal government

___7. A professional attitude is

A. natural
B. given when you are licensed
C. acquired in enrollment
D. learned

___8. What practice is 100% effective for preventing the spread of the HIV virus?

A. soap
B. use of a condom
C. wearing of gloves
D. abstinence

___9. The germicidal light used in some dry sanitizers is known as

A. fluorescent light
B. ultra-violet light
C. infrared light
D. incandescent light

___10. Uncleanliness can produce germs that cause

A. good health
B. local canities
C. disease
D. malnutrition

___11. Disease is caused mainly from the lack of

A. cleanliness
B. deodorizers
C. cold water
D. hairspray

___12. If the eye has been chemically burned, what should be done?

A. flush eye with cool water
B. flush eye with boric acid
C. apply alcohol
D. apply quats

___13. Which virus causes the AIDS disease?

A. Rhinovirus
B. HIV virus
C. Influenza virus
D. Cold virus

___14. What route of transmission does the AIDS disease follow?

A. injection
B. blood transfusion
C. maternal
D. all of the above

___15. Soiled towels should be stored in a covered

A. linen hamper
B. metal container
C. plastic container
D. laundry basket

___16. A carrier is a person who has a disease that is

A. acute
B. contagious
C. occupational
D. common

___17. What common cosmetology chemical would kill the AIDS virus outside of the body?

A. household bleach
B. water
C. 1% hydrogen peroxide
D. 20% alcohol

___18. What strength hydrogen peroxide would destroy the AIDS virus outside of the body?

A. 1%
B. 2%
C. 3%
D. all of the above

___19. Hair-cutting implements are sanitized with

A. 30% alcohol
B. 30% formalin solution
C. 40% alcohol
D. 70% alcohol

___20. A 5 percent formalin solution is used mainly to sanitize a(n)

A. ultraviolet sanitizer
B. tweezers
C. cuticle scissors
D. styling chair

___21. The function of the hair is to

A. adorn the body
B. protect the skin
C. adorn the head
D. all of the above

___22. A hot wax treatment would be used to remove superfluous hair in all of the following areas except one.

A. upper lip
B. lower jaw line
C. eyebrow area
D. underarms

___23. Hair is an example of

A. hard keratin
B. soft keratin
C. Henle's layer
D. Huxley's layer

___24. The glands in the scalp that naturally lubricate the hair during brushing are called

A. apocrine
B. sebaceous
C. sudoriferous
D. eccrine

___25. Before applying a chemical depilatory, how should the cosmetologist protect the client?

A. buy only quality depilatories
B. apply gauze to the area to be worked on
C. give the client a skin test
D. ask client to remove jewelry

___26. The percentage of the hair shaft represented by the cortex layer is

A. 15%
B. 25%
C. 50%
D. 75%

___27. The technical term applied to the cyclical period when the hair begins to grow is the

A. anagen stage
B. terminal stage
C. telogen stage
D. origin stage

___28. What general prefix is used to describe most hair diseases?

A. tricho
B. tricko
C. trio
D. trigo

___29. The skin and hair have a natural pH in a range of

A. 3.5 – 4.5.
B. 4.5 – 5.5.
C. 5.5 – 6.5.
D. 6.5 – 7.5.

___30. Peroxide has a pH that is

A. acid
B. alkaline
C. neutral
D. none of the above

____31. Scabies is an infestation of the scalp by

A. the itch mite
B. head lice
C. ringworm
D. tinea

____32. To prevent water from dripping onto the floor from the shampoo bowl, where should you leave the shampoo hose?

A. drain position
B. handle position
C. vacuum breaker position
D. none of the above

____33. The natural lubricant that gives hair a beautiful luster or sheen is called

A. sebum
B. seborrhea
C. seconal
D. permanent color

____34. If damaged hair is going to be given a service that uses strong chemicals the cosmetologist should recommend

A. preconditioning
B. prelightening
C. pre-filling
D. preneutralizing

____35. Hair can be damaged chemically by

A. improper bleaching
B. wave set
C. shampooing
D. hair cutting

____36. Semicircular designs combed into the hair are called

A. waves
B. base direction
C. shapings
D. arcs

____37. Before combing out the finger wave, the hair should be

A. thoroughly dried
B. thoroughly lubricated
C. quite damp
D. sprayed with lacquer

____38. The main objective in finger waving the hair is to mold even

A. curls and softness
B. waves and ridges
C. shaping and direction
D. parts and shapes

____39. For the least amount of tightness when setting sculpture curls, you should use a

A. no-stem curl
B. half-stem curl
C. quarter-stem curl
D. long-stem curl

____40. Set sculpture curls within a shaping should

A. be separate
B. swing down
C. overlap
D. swing over

____41. To get the maximum amount of height or fullness you should use a

A. no-stem curl
B. half-stem curl
C. long-stem curl
D. tight-stem curl

____42. When setting the hair with rollers, a curved form in the finished hairstyle is done by winding hair around the roller

A. 1 turn or less
B. 1-1/2 turns
C. 2 turns
D. none of the above

____43. The problem with a diamond-shaped face is that it is narrow at the chin and

A. eyebrows
B. cheekbones
C. jaws
D. forehead

____44. What draping supply is recommended for the client that is about to have a hair shaping only?

A. towel shampoo cape
B. shampoo cape
C. comb-out cape
D. chair cloth

___45. Super-curly hair should be cut with a

A. clipper
B. scissors
C. razor
D. thinning shears

___46. Proper storage of cutting implements is important to prevent

A. over-use of implements
B. injury to small children
C. rust from forming
D. the edge from becoming dull

___47. The technique of holding the hair upward toward the crown or top of the head during a hair shaping is called

A. low-elevation
B. high-elevation
C. feather edging
D. stepping

___48. When cutting the hair with a shaper, it is important to

A. cut by using the guard
B. thin toward the scalp
C. use long, sliding strokes
D. blunt all hair

___49. If a razor is used to cut the hair, the hair should be

A. completely dry
B. slightly damp
C. completely wet
D. slightly moist

___50. During a razor cut, as the razor is cutting the hair, the comb is placed in the

A. pocket
B. drawer
C. other hand
D. other section

___51. The heat from the air waver should be directed

A. away from the scalp
B. toward the scalp
C. at the ends
D. toward the hair root

___52. When doing a tint retouch, apply the tint only to the

A. hair root
B. hair ends
C. cold shaft
D. new growth

___53. A predisposition test is required before applying a(n)

A. vegetable derivative tint
B. animal derivative tint
C. metallic derivative tint
D. aniline derivative tint

___54. The name given to the process that explains the chemical reaction of mixing hydrogen peroxide and an aniline derivative tint is

A. hydrolization
B. oxidation
C. softening
D. filling

___55. A predisposition test is required before applying a(n)

A. vegetable derivative tint
B. animal derivative tint
C. metallic derivative tint
D. aniline derivative tint

___56. When coloring the hair terms such as cool, drab, and warm, describe

A. tones of a hair color
B. shades of a hair color
C. brightness of a hair color
D. depth of a hair color

___57. By law, a predisposition test must be given before each

A. oxidation tint
B. bleach
C. temporary rinse
D. conditioning treatment

___58. How many stages does black hair go through to become pale blonde?

A. four
B. five
C. six
D. seven

___59. Decolorization takes place in which layer of the hair?

A. cuticle
B. cortex
C. medulla
D. all of the above

____60. When the proper stage of streaking is reached, which shampoo is BEST to remove bleach?

A. mild
B. medicated (alkaline)
C. non-stripping (acid)
D. alkaline

____61. A retouch hair lightener is applied to the

A. new growth of hair
B. entire hair shaft
C. the ends only
D. cold shaft only

____62. Which bleach is recommended for frosting and streaking?

A. creme
B. paste
C. oil
D. powder

____63. When giving a virgin bleach to medium brown hair, the cosmetologist should begin applying the lightener

A. 1/2" from scalp up through ends
B. from scalp to ends
C. from ends to scalp
D. center of hair shaft to ends

____64. The pH range for acid waves is

A. 2.5 – 4.5.
B. 5.8 – 6.8.
C. 7.9 – 8.8.
D. 9.0 – 9.7.

____65. To achieve a good curl when permanent waving, how much tension should be applied to the hair as it is wound on the rods?

A. very firm tension
B. very little tension
C. moderate-firm, even tension
D. no tension

____66. Before a cold wave is wrapped the hair is usually dried using a

A. blow comb
B. hand dryer
C. towel
D. rat-tail comb

____67. When permanent waving the hair, how many turns must the hair be wound around the rod to achieve a curl pattern?

A. once
B. twice
C. four turns
D. five turns

____68. To remove dripping cold-waving solution, use a piece of cotton or the corner of a towel saturated with

A. cold water
B. warm water
C. tepid water
D. hot water

____69. If a plastic cap is used to cover the permanent waving rods during processing, what should you be careful NOT to do?

A. allow too much heat to collect
B. tighten the cap too much
C. allow too much air to escape
D. clip the cap in the front section

____70. The action of the cold waving solution is stopped, and the curl is fixed with a

A. developer
B. curler
C. shaper
D. neutralizer

____71. The process of chemically straightening super-curly hair is called chemical hair

A. normalizing
B. relaxing
C. crimping
D. stabilizing

____72. As in cold waving, chemical relaxers work faster on hair that is

A. wiry
B. coarse
C. porous
D. non-porous

____73. The difference between a base and no-base relaxer is that the no-base

A. does not require application of the base
B. always requires the use of protective gloves
C. is safer to use, but requires more time
D. is more dangerous to use, but requires more time

____74. Hair should be conditioned after a sodium hydroxide relaxer to prevent

A. breakage during combing and setting
B. dry, scaly scalp
C. red, irritated scalp
D. breakage during thermal pressing

____75. After a chemical relaxer, a conditioner should be applied

A. after the hair is set
B. just before the comb-out
C. before the hair is styled with rollers
D. after the comb-out

____76. Just before applying the relaxer, the hair is subdivided into

A. two sections
B. four sections
C. six sections
D. eight sections

____77. Before a chemical hair straightener, the cosmetologist would not

A. read label directions
B. examine the scalp
C. analyze the hair
D. brush the hair

____78. If the client has a little spot on the scalp that is burning during a chemical hair relaxer, what should you do?

A. rinse all relaxer from the hair immediately
B. apply an astringent to the spot
C. apply petrolatum to the spot
D. spray spot with cool water

____79. Poker curls are made in a spiral fashion from the

A. ends to the scalp
B. mid-strand to the ends
C. ends to the mid-strand
D. scalp to the ends

____80. After the hair is pressed, the thermal iron forms the curl by rotating the iron using a(n)

A. clicking action
B. sliding actions
C. oval action
D. back and forth action

____81. Before thermal waving super-curly hair, the cosmetologist should

A. color it
B. press it
C. shape it
D. comb it

____82. If the client is scheduled for a curl reformation and tells you that he/she had a chemical hair relaxer last month, what should you do?

A. give the service
B. condition the hair, then give the service
C. give the service, then condition the hair
D. refuse to give the service

____83. During a curl reformation the rearranger has been applied, capped, and put under the dryer. When should it be checked?

A. every 5 minutes
B. every 10 minutes
C. every 15 minutes
D. it doesn't need to be checked

____84. Before applying a curl reformation straightener, what should you do?

A. make a client record
B. apply the neutralizer to nape
C. apply a base to hairline
D. give a scalp treatment

____85. The double-application service in which super-curly hair is straightened, then curled, on permanent wave rods is called a(n)

A. recurl or soft curl
B. structuring or rebuilding
C. Afro-pick
D. none of the above

____86. What is the one thing to watch out for when you are about to give a curl reformation?

A. too many test curls
B. client allergies
C. using too many rods
D. tangled hair

____87. Continued friction on the skin may cause a

A. stain
B. pimple
C. wart
D. callus

____88. The outermost (top) layer of the skin is the

A. epidermis
B. corium
C. subcutaneous tissue
D. adipose tissue

____89. The thinnest layer of the skin is the

A. epidermis
B. corium
C. subcutaneous tissue
D. adipose tissue

____90. When the petrissage massage movement is used, it has a(n)

A. soothing effect
B. relaxing effect
C. invigorating effect
D. mellowing effect

____91. Removal of unsightly matter on the facial area can be best achieved with a(n)

A. cleanser
B. astringent
C. freshener
D. emollient creme

____92. Small eyes can be made to appear larger. What type of makeup is applied to create this illusion?

A. contour
B. foundation
C. lip
D. white

____93. What effect does the freshener have on the pores of the skin?

A. medicates
B. cleanses
C. opens
D. sanitizes

____94. The basic nail shapes are oval or pointed, and

A. square or round
B. round or ridged
C. all of the above

____95. If hangnails are neglected, they may become

A. brittle
B. fragile
C. infected
D. loose

____96. To prevent a canvas block from becoming unsanitary and giving off an odor, it is advisable to cover it with a

A. nylon cap
B. synthetic fiber
C. plastic bag
D. rubber sheet

____97. Given two students with identical training, what factors determine why one student will graduate from school and earn a lot more money than their classmate?

A. the greater money earner gives many free services
B. the one making more money treats their clients better
C. the student earning less money can't do the work
D. the student earning less didn't attend regularly

____98. How is a stylist usually paid for the sale of retail products in the salon to their clients?

A. $2.00 per item
B. $3.00 per item
C. $5.00 per item
D. a commission

____99. What is the term used for describing the relationship between you and your client that keeps them coming back into the salon?

A. client retention
B. bonding
C. referral
D. client communications

____100. Which of the following should be used to put a finishing edge on your straight razor?

A. towel
B. strop
C. hone
D. comb

DALTON'S STANDARDIZED FINAL TEST 6

Student Name ______________________________ Score _______ Date ___________

Instructions: Carefully read through each question, then read the answer choices. Write your choice of the word, or the phrase, that correctly completes the statement or answers the question, on the line provided.

___1. Hairstyles are judged in a contest for

A. originality
B. adaptability
C. trend
D. all of the above

___2. Nonverbal communication refers to

A. listening to what is said
B. communicating with body movements
C. communicating with your hands
D. keeping steady eye contact during conversation

___3. A salon owner's income may vary according to the

A. number of salons owned
B. size of the salon
C. location of the salon
D. all of the above

___4. Which term fits the job description for a person who specializes in preserving the beauty of the client's face and neck?

A. facial expert
B. esthetician
C. electrologist
D. dermatologist

___5. To communicate, a thought or attitude is conveyed

A. verbally
B. nonverbally
C. person to person
D. all of the above

___6. Dental care for preserving healthy teeth starts with a daily mouthwash and

A. rinsing and flushing
B. rubbing and scratching
C. rinsing and rubbing
D. brushing and flossing

___7. The governing body in most states which is supposed to discipline members that violate professional ethics is the

A. bureau of ethics
B. state legislature
C. state association
D. state board

___8. It is your responsibility to

A. give as much service as needed
B. learn new methods of hairstyling
C. give services based on quality
D. all of the above

___9. A person immune to a disease, but who can infect others is known as a(n)

A. clinical
B. medical
C. agent
D. carrier

___10. Another name for public hygiene is

A. grooming
B. hair care
C. sanitation
D. community

___11. Practices in the beauty salon that help preserve the health of the public are called

A. fumigation-deodorization
B. salon grooming
C. cleaning-washing
D. sanitation-sterilization

___12. If the eye has been chemically burned, what should be done?

A. flush eye with cool water
B. flush eye with boric acid
C. apply alcohol
D. apply quats

___13. When removing implements from a wet sanitizer you should wear

A. an operator apron
B. a hair net
C. rubber gloves
D. neutralizing bib

___14. Hair-cutting implements are sanitized with

A. 70% alcohol
B. 40% alcohol
C. 30% formalin solution
D. 30% alcohol

___15. Which virus causes the AIDS disease?

A. Rhino virus
B. HIV virus
C. Influenza virus
D. Cold virus

___16. What route of transmission does the AIDS disease follow?

A. sexual contact
B. injection
C. touching
D. A and B only

___17. Metal electrodes should be sanitized with

A. 2% quats
B. 20% peroxide
C. 70% alcohol
D. 80% ammonium

___18. By law, which of the following must each beauty salon have available?

A. a fire blanket
B. a hot water dispenser
C. an emergency eye wash station
D. a fire extinguisher

___19. A carrier is a person who has a disease that is

A. acute
B. contagious
C. occupational
D. common

___20. Which of the following would destroy the AIDS virus outside the body?

A. water
B. 70% alcohol
C. shampoo
D. hand soap

___21. When giving a service, what should you do if you are exposed to blood?

A. see your doctor
B. wash exposed area with soap and water
C. apply a topical disinfectant
D. B and C only

___22. If you accidently cut your client's neck and it bleeds, what should you do?

A. put on disposable rubber gloves
B. wash area with soap and water
C. apply topical disinfectant to area
D. all of the above

___23. Hair is not found on the

A. forearm and wrists
B. forearm and nose
C. knuckles of the hands
D. soles of the feet

___24. When hair is in its resting cycle, and more likely to fall out, this stage is known as the

A. terminal stage
B. fall-out stage
C. hair loss stage
D. telogen stage

___25. What is the name for the male hair loss due to the aging process?

A. congenital alopecia
B. male-pattern baldness
C. hair thinning
D. routine hair loss

___26. Hair is made up of a hard protein substance called

A. carbon
B. hydrogen
C. keratin
D. sulfur

___27. The layer of the hair in which the coloring pigment is found is the

A. follicle
B. medulla
C. cortex
D. cuticle

___28. Before using a hot wax depilatory, the cosmetologist should

A. apply gauze to the work area
B. give the client instructions
C. check to be sure client is comfortable
D. check the temperature of the wax

___29. Hypertrichosis is a condition that is also called

A. supercilia hair
B. superfluous hair
C. ringed hair
D. twisted hair

___30. Shampoos with a pH greater than seven (7) are called

A. acid
B. alkaline
C. mild
D. neutral

___31. Peroxide has a pH that is

A. acid
B. alkaline
C. neutral
D. none of the above

___32. An overly oily scalp is a disorder medically referred to as

A. steatoma
B. seborrhea
C. asteatosis
D. tinea

___33. How should you protect the client's clothing before shampooing the hair?

A. draping the cape over the back of the chair
B. cover all clothing with towels
C. place plastic clothing protectors
D. place plastic towels across client's shoulder

___34. Hair can be damaged by

A. brush rollers
B. heated rollers
C. thermal curling irons
D. all of the above

___35. The basic protein found in the hair shaft is

A. cuticle
B. medulla
C. sebum
D. keratin

___36. When the hair is conditioned using strong chemicals, this is known as

A. pre-treating
B. preconditioning
C. duration conditioning
D. in-process conditioning

___37. Scalp manipulations should not be given if the hair is going to be

A. cold waved
B. permanently colored
C. chemically lightened
D. all of the above

___38. The shaping between two finger-wave ridges is called the wave

A. direction
B. trough
C. arc
D. curl

___39. The section of the head that is closest to the neck is the

A. nape section
B. crown section
C. crepe section
D. left side section

___40. A large stand-up curl could also be called a barrel curl or

A. skip-curl
B. cascade curl
C. closed-end curl
D. clockwise curl

___41. When putting a shaping into the hair, the hair should be

A. wet
B. damp
C. dry
D. moistened on the ends

___42. The standard or ideal facial shape is

A. oblong
B. round
C. oval
D. square

___43. If too much bulk is removed from coarse hair, it tends to

A. look smooth and natural
B. stick out from the head
C. be super curly
D. set more easily

___44. When razor cutting, strokes that the cosmetologist should use are

A. firm and long
B. smooth and long
C. smooth and short
D. jerky and short

___45. To prevent the electric clipper blades from pulling the hair, what should you do?

A. apply oil to them
B. soak in alcohol
C. apply ammonia to them
D. dip them in peroxide

___46. What is the name given to one or more subsections of hair cut in the hairline or crown of the head that serve as a yardstick for cutting the rest of the hair?

A. trendline
B. radial line
C. bias line
D. guideline

___47. What will happen if you submerge your electric clipper in a wet sanitizer while it is plugged into an outlet?

A. the blades will slide
B. the clipper won't cut correctly
C. you will get an electric shock
D. your clipper will vibrate

___48. The hanging length cut around the hairline from which the rest of the hair is shaped is called the

A. high-sign
B. cutting length
C. guideline
D. form

___49. The foundation for a good hairstyle is a correct hair

A. setting lotion
B. shaping
C. styling comb
D. brush

___50. To ensure safety, all hair wavers and blow dryers must be

A. set at low temperature settings
B. used on damp to dry hair
C. Underwriters Laboratories approved
D. inspected at time of purchase

___51. To prevent overlapping on a tint retouch, the tint is applied from the scalp to about

A. 1/16" up to the tinted hair
B. 1/16" over the already tinted hair
C. 1/4" up to the tinted hair
D. 1/2" over the tinted hair

___52. One of the main chemicals in aniline derivative tints is

A. sulfonated oils
B. ammonium thioglycolate
C. cystine disulfide
D. para-phenylene-diamine

___53. A single-application tint is prepared by mixing th required tint with

A. hard water
B. 10-volume peroxide
C. ammonia water
D. 20-volume peroxide

___54. A client is now in the styling chair for a schedule virgin tint. After getting the coloring product fro the dispensary, the cosmetologist discovers there is no developer anywhere in the salon

A. use water for the developer and give the tint
B. use shampoo for developer
C. reschedule the appointment
D. ask the client to leave

___55. To prevent overlapping on a tint retouch, the tint is applied from the scalp to about

A. 1/16" up to the tinted hair
B. 1/16" over the already tinted hair
C. 1/4" up to the tinted hair
D. 1/2" over the tinted hair

___56. To prevent a line of demarcation during a tint retouch, it is important to avoid

A. rotating a bottle
B. overlapping the tint
C. mixing tint
D. rubbing the scalp

___57. If you overlap bleach when doing a bleach retouch, it will result in

A. more elasticity
B. less elasticity
C. breakage
D. hair yellowing

___58. Lightening the hair begins with the application of a

A. stripping agent
B. toning agent
C. moisturizing agent
D. bleaching agent

___59. Containers used for mixing bleach should be made of

A. plastic
B. wood
C. metal
D. glass

___60. Before giving a lightener retouch, what should you do?

A. a predisposition test
B. brush the hair vigorously
C. examine the scalp for cuts and abrasions
D. give the client a strand test

___61. The alkalinity of bleach is neutralized by applying a

A. rinse
B. normalizer
C. conditioner
D. neutralizer

___62. The removal of a penetrating tint from the hair is called

A. relaxing
B. soap cap
C. stripping
D. tinting

___63. One disadvantage of an acid wave is that it is

A. difficult to time
B. slow processing
C. harder on the skin
D. drying to the hair

___64. Better saturation of the cold-waving solution into the hair is achieved when it is

A. wrapped correctly
B. analyzed accurately
C. curled properly
D. pressed thoroughly

___65. Before cold waving the entire head, the degree to which the hair will curl can be determined by using

A. concave curls
B. convex curls
C. test curls
D. pin curls

___66. Cotton is placed around the hairline before applying the cold-waving solution; it should be

A. removed after it is applied
B. allowed to remain until the neutralizer is applied
C. removed following the neutralizer
D. removed when the rods are taken out

___67. In which of the following conditions should the cosmetologist REFUSE to give the client a cold wave?

A. a scar on the scalp
B. cranial surgical wound
C. a scalp freckle
D. an ulna surgical wound

___68. If a couple of small areas of the hair do not have enough curl one week after the wave process, you should give the client

A. a refund check
B. another cosmetologist
C. some pickup curls
D. another chemical wave

___69. When relaxing a permanent wave that is too curly, where should you begin your application?

A. the nape section
B. the top section
C. the side section
D. the crown section

___70. The cold waving solution is applied to the

A. rod, hair, and scalp
B. rod and hair
C. scalp and neutralizer
D. hair and scalp

___71. If cold waving hair that is bleached (lightened), it is best to select rods that are

A. large
B. small
C. midget
D. of any size

____72. When cold waving, the size of the curl or wave pattern will be controlled by the

A. cold-wave solution
B. type of neutralizer
C. size of the rod
D. size of the end papers

____73. The actions of chemical hair straightener cause the hair to

A. shrink and harden
B. shift and mold
C. shape and curl
D. soften and swell

____74. If the client has a little spot on the scalp that is burning during a chemical hair relaxer, what should you do?

A. rinse all relaxer from hair immediately
B. apply an astringent to the spot
C. apply petrolatum to the spot
D. spray spot with cool water

____75. The application of a base or no-base relaxer would begin in the

A. nape section
B. left-side section
C. right-side section
D. crown section

____76. The neutralizing shampoo used in the chemical relaxing service is also called a

A. stabilizer
B. cleaner
C. conditioner
D. filler

____77. When subsectioning the hair around the face for application of the relaxer, it is best to part the hair

A. horizontally
B. vertically
C. up and down
D. diagonally

____78. When rinsing the chemical relaxer from the hair, to avoid tangling, it is important to use

A. low to medium water pressure
B. high water pressure
C. hot water at all times
D. an alkaline shampoo

____79. During the processing and neutralizing of a chemical relaxer service, what can be done to minimize neck irritation?

A. applying cotton coil
B. changing towel frequently
C. keeping the client's neck against the bowl
D. applying neutralizing cream

____80. The marcel iron was developed by a Frenchman named Marcel

A. Pierson
B. Jenereaux
C. Dalton
D. Grateau

____81. As the iron is rolled toward the scalp, what does the cosmetologist use to protect the client's scalp?

A. cotton
B. towel
C. comb
D. an end paper

____82. What is the name for the service in which the hair is pressed twice on the top of the strand, and once on the underside?

A. one press
B. light press
C. comb press
D. soft press

____83. Which of the following is part of the curl reformation service?

A. place cap over hair during processing
B. test curl strand
C. apply curl booster
D. all of the above

____84. Before applying the neutralizer to the rods when doing a curl reformation, the hair should be rinsed with

A. conditioner
B. hot water
C. tepid water
D. cold water

____85. During a curl reformation, how much tension is used to wrap the hair on the rods?

A. no tension
B. moderate tension
C. slight tension
D. firm tension

___86. During a curl reformation, the hair dries out while you are wrapping the hair on the rods. What should you do?

A. apply more waving solution
B. apply water to dry strands
C. use spray-on conditioner
D. use two end wraps

___87. Nevus flameus is the technical name for a(n)

A. mole
B. wart
C. birthmark
D. acne

___88. A sun block lotion would have what SPF rating number?

A. 5.
B. 8.
C. 12.
D. 15.

___89. One way to penetrate unbroken skin is through the

A. adipose tissue
B. papilla
C. corium
D. follicle

___90. Tapotement is a massage movement that uses a

A. kneading technique
B. pinching technique
C. stroking technique
D. tapping technique

___91. Foundation makeup is applied to the facial area to enhance the client's skin tone and

A. protect it
B. dampen it
C. blend it
D. cleanse it

___92. When the foundation makeup protrudes from the surface of the skin, what does this tell you about the skin's alkalinity?

A. high
B. low
C. neutral
D. zero

___93. What type of movement should be used when tweezing the eyebrows?

A. slow, sliding movement
B. quick movement
C. circular movement
D. zig-zag movement

___94. The average daily growth rate of the nail is

A. .7 mm
B. .5 mm
C. .3 mm
D. .1 mm

___95. Once a nail becomes infected, it should be treated by a

A. barber
B. cosmetologist
C. manicurist
D. physician

___96. If a minor cut should occur during a manicure, apply powdered styptic, or a(n)

A. shampoo
B. antiseptic
C. creme rinse
D. disinfectant

___97. What is at least one factor that society uses to determine the success or failure of a person's career?

A. how tall they are
B. how much money they make
C. what kind of car they drive
D. how they dress

___98. What can be done to make clients want to come into the salon?

A. make them feel good about their salon experience
B. sell them products they don't need
C. always call them by their first names
D. all of the above

___99. What is the term used to describe a new client visiting you for a service as the result of another client sending them?

A. word of mouth
B. a referral
C. lucky to have good friends
D. a random chance

___100. What should be used to sanitize a straight razor?

A. wet sanitizer
B. soap and water
C. 70 % alcohol
D. towel

DALTON'S STANDARDIZED FINAL TEST 7

Student Name ______________________________ Score _______ Date ___________

Instructions: Carefully read through each question, then read the answer choices. Write your choice of the word, or the phrase, that correctly completes the statement or answers the question, on the line provided.

___1. Participation as a platform artist will help build

A. recognition
B. a large clientele
C. a good income
D. all of the above

___2. The advantage(s) of being a manager-operator may include the opportunity to learn about

A. overhead expenses
B. accounts payable
C. inventory
D. all of the above

___3. Personal grooming relates to one's

A. daily appearance
B. daily cleanliness
C. hairstyle and voice
D. A and B.

___4. Personal hygiene relates to

A. promoting one's own health
B. preservation of one's health
C. oral care
D. A and B.

___5. Dental care for preserving healthy teeth starts with a daily mouthwash and

A. rinsing and flushing
B. rubbing and scratching
C. rinsing and rubbing
D. brushing and flossing

___6. Ethics is a system that measures human behavior that is

A. voluntary
B. involuntary
C. imposed by local police
D. imposed by the federal government

___7. A professional attitude is

A. natural
B. given when you are licensed
C. acquired in enrollment
D. learned

___8. To equal the strength of 6% hydrogen peroxide, you would have to use

A. 1 volume hydrogen peroxide
B. 2 volume hydrogen peroxide
C. 10 volume hydrogen peroxide
D. 20 volume hydrogen peroxide

___9. If cosmetology implements are aseptic, then they are

A. free from bacteria
B. unsanitary
C. soiled
D. covered

___10. The germicidal light used in some dry sanitizers is known as

A. fluorescent light
B. ultra-violet light
C. infrared light
D. incandescent light

___11. If the eye has been chemically burned, what should be done?

A. flush eye with cool water
B. flush eye with boric acid
C. apply alcohol
D. apply quats

___12. To be effective for sanitation, the strength of the quats to be used should be at least

A. 1:200
B. 1:200
C. 1:500
D. 1:1000

___13. Which virus causes the AIDS disease?

A. Rhino virus
B. HIV virus
C. Influenza virus
D. Cold virus

___14. What route of transmission does the AIDS disease follow?

A. injection
B. blood transfusion
C. maternal
D. all of the above

___15. Soiled towels should be stored in a covered

A. linen hamper
B. metal container
C. plastic container
D. laundry basket

___16. A carrier is a person who has a disease that is

A. acute
B. contagious
C. occupational
D. common

___17. What common cosmetology chemical would kill the AIDS virus outside of the body?

A. household bleach
B. water
C. 1% hydrogen peroxide
D. 20% alcohol

___18. What strength hydrogen peroxide would destroy the AIDS virus outside of the body?

A. 1%
B. 2%
C. 3%
D. all of the above

___19. A 5 percent formalin solution is used mainly to sanitize a(n)

A. ultraviolet sanitizer
B. tweezers
C. cuticle scissors
D. styling chair

___20. A common skin antiseptic would be

A. 3% hydrogen peroxide
B. 6% hydrogen peroxide
C. 9% hydrogen peroxide
D. 12% hydrogen peroxide

___21. The protein cross-bonds of the hair are called

A. polypeptide bonds
B. monopeptide bonds
C. hydrogen bonds
D. cystine bonds

___22. Hair is an example of

A. hard keratin
B. soft keratin
C. Henle's layer
D. Huxley's layer

___23. Scalp hair usually grows at a monthly rate of

A. 1/4"
B. 1/2"
C. 3/4"
D. 1"

___24. Which of the following would a dermatologist prescribe for men for regular hair loss?

A. vitamin A
B. minoxidal
C. medicated shampoo
D. creme rinse

___25. Before applying a chemical depilatory, how should the cosmetologist protect the client?

A. buy only quality depilatories
B. apply gauze to the area to be worked on
C. give the client a skin test
D. ask client to remove jewelry

___26. The percentage of the hair shaft represented by the cortex layer is

A. 15%
B. 25%
C. 50%
D. 75%

___27. The technical term applied to the cyclical period when the hair begins to grow is the

A. anagen stage
B. terminal stage
C. telogen stage
D. origin stage

___28. When alopecia appears in the head, it looks like

A. red, circular bald patches
B. scaly, rectangular bald patches
C. non-inflamed, oval bald patches
D. oily scales and oval bald patches

___29. The pH of a shampoo indicates the concentration of

A. hydrogen
B. oxygen
C. nitrogen
D. carbon

___30. Peroxide has a pH that is

A. acid
B. alkaline
C. neutral
D. none of the above

___31. When rinsing the client's hair with hot water, how should you detect temperature changes in the water?

A. watch for steam from the client's scalp
B. little finger of hand held under nozzle of hose
C. the color of the client's scalp turns bright pink
D. the shampoo changes color

___32. To prevent water from dripping onto the floor from the shampoo bowl, where should you leave the shampoo hose?

A. drain position
B. handle position
C. vacuum breaker position
D. none of the above

___33. The natural lubricant that gives hair a beautiful luster or sheen is called

A. sebum
B. seborrhea
C. seconal
D. permanent color

___34. Very small bits of protein applied to the hair are called

A. macro-proteins
B. micro-proteins
C. poultry proteins
D. substantive proteins

___35. Hair can be damaged chemically by

A. improper bleaching
B. wave set
C. shampooing
D. hair cutting

___36. Semicircular designs combed into the hair are called

A. waves
B. base direction
C. shapings
D. arcs

___37. The main objective in finger waving the hair is to mold even

A. curls and softness
B. waves and ridges
C. shaping and direction
D. parts and shapes

___38. The section of the head that is closest to the neck is the

A. nape section
B. crown section
C. crepe section
D. left side section

___39. After the setting lotion has been applied, should the hair dry out during setting, spray more

A. filler on it
B. conditioner on it
C. water on it
D. setting lotion on it

___40. To get the maximum amount of height or fullness, you should use a

A. no-stem curl
B. half-stem curl
C. long-stem curl
D. tight-stem curl

___41. When setting the hair with rollers, a curved form in the finished hairstyle is done by winding hair around the roller

A. 1 turn or less
B. 1-1/2 turns
C. 2 turns
D. none of the above

___42. To correct a diamond-shaped face, fullness is needed everywhere, except at the

A. cheekbones
B. eyebrows
C. forehead
D. jaw

___43. For a basic haircut, the cosmetologist would begin cutting the hair in the

A. top
B. side
C. crown
D. nape

___44. Super-curly hair should be cut with a

A. clipper
B. scissors
C. razor
D. thinning shears

___45. Proper storage of cutting implements is important to prevent

A. over-use of implements
B. injury to small children
C. rust from forming
D. the edge from becoming dull

___46. You should not use an electric clipper if

A. the client wants a trim
B. the set screw has been adjusted
C. it is noisy
D. any teeth are broken

___47. When cutting the hair with a shaper, it is important to

A. cut by using the guard
B. thin toward the scalp
C. use long, sliding strokes
D. blunt all hair

___48. If a razor is used to cut the hair, the hair should be

A. completely dry
B. slightly damp
C. completely wet
D. slightly moist

___49. During a razor cut, as the razor is cutting the hair, the comb is placed in the

A. pocket
B. drawer
C. other hand
D. other section

___50. Extra care must be taken when blow waving long hair because it

A. may become hard to manage and curl
B. may dry too quickly and become oily
C. may be drawn into the air intake of the dryer
D. could stick to the brush and become straight

___51. A one-process permanent tint contains

A. aniline derivative dye
B. metallic dye
C. vegetable dye
D. henna dye

___52. A predisposition test is required before applying a(n)

A. vegetable derivative tint
B. animal derivative tint
C. metallic derivative tint
D. aniline derivative tint

___53. The general term used to describe a lightener and toner is

A. separate application
B. single application
C. double application
D. triple application

___54. A predisposition test is required before applying a(n)

A. vegetable derivative tint
B. animal derivative tint
C. metallic derivative tint
D. aniline derivative tint

___55. The pH of a semi-permanent color falls in the range of

A. 4 to 6
B. 5 to 6
C. 7 to 9
D. 9 to 10.

___56. Which of the following is the best definition of a permanent toner?

A. an aniline derivative tint in pastel colors
B. an aniline tint having a gold base
C. para-phenylene-diamine dyes
D. color that cannot be removed

___57. Decolorization takes place in which layer of the hair?

A. cuticle
B. cortex
C. medulla
D. all of the above

___58. When lightening and toning the hair, you should wear

A. protective shoes
B. a hair net
C. an operator apron
D. protective gloves

___59. A retouch hair lightener is applied to the

A. new growth of hair
B. entire hair shaft
C. the ends only
D. cold shaft only

___60. An effect achieved by placing a plastic or rubber cap on the client's hair and pulling strands through the cap is known as

A. painting
B. streaking
C. frosting
D. tipping

___61. Pre-bleaching (lightening) is required before the application of a

A. semi-permanent rinse
B. one-process tint
C. permanent toner
D. temporary rinse

___62. A self-timing permanent wave is one in which the manufacturer recommends that you

A. test curl every 3 minutes
B. towel blot each rod
C. process for a set period of time
D. place client under a dryer

___63. Before a cold wave is wrapped the hair is usually dried using a

A. blow comb
B. hand dryer
C. towel
D. rat-tail comb

___64. After processing a perm, what can you do to prevent the rods from being forced from the hair during rinsing ?

A. tighten them up
B. use low water pressure
C. put on a hair net
D. rinse with cool water

___65. During a wrapping procedure using waving solution, breakages can occur if too much tension is placed on the

A. hair
B. comb
C. end wrap
D. rod

___66. When rinsing a permanent wave, what can you do to prevent water from running down the client's neck and back?

A. ask the client to raise their head
B. use low water pressure
C. use a neutralizing bib
D. place foil around the neck

___67. If a neutralizing bib is used for neutralizing the permanent, where should you place a small piece of cotton?

A. by the ears
B. across the forehead
C. under the eye hook
D. around the nape

___68. If cold waving hair that is bleached (lightened), it is best to select rods that are

A. large
B. small
C. midget
D. of any size

___69. When cold waving, the size of the curl or wave pattern will be controlled by the

A. cold-wave solution
B. type of neutralizer
C. size of the rod
D. size of the end papers

___70. Before applying a chemical relaxer, analyze the hair for porosity, texture, and elasticity; then examine the

A. fingernails
B. scalp
C. hairline
D. relaxing kit

___71. If you live in a very warm climate and your client arrives perspiring before having a chemical hair relaxer, what should you do?

A. thoroughly shampoo the hair
B. place client under cool dryer
C. wait while client cools off
D. blot moisture from scalp before starting

___72. Before giving a retouch chemical relaxer, what should be applied to the previously relaxed hair first?

A. water
B. protective conditioner
C. presoftening rinse
D. prerelax shampoo

___73. After a sodium hydroxide relaxer has processed, but before it is shampooed, the hair should be thoroughly

A. combed
B. conditioned
C. rinsed
D. brushed

___74. After a chemical relaxer, a conditioner should be applied

A. after the hair is set
B. just before the comb-out
C. before the hair is styled with rollers
D. after the comb-out

___75. If too much pressure is applied during the relaxing service, the hair will

A. break
B. dissolve
C. stretch
D. revert to curl

___76. When applying a chemical relaxer, it is important that you AVOID

A. misting the hair with water
B. using small sections
C. tugging on the hair
D. timing your application

___77. One of the most important things to remember about the processing of a chemical relaxer is

A. apply it slowly and evenly
B. never leave the client unattended
C. never serve coffee during processing
D. brush the hair before neutralizing

___78. A pressing comb is heated using a(n)

A. electric heater
B. oil heater
C. solar heater
D. core heater

___79. After a thermal wave, the hair is brushed and combed into a hairstyle

A. after the lanolin has been applied
B. while the hair is still hot
C. when the hair has been cooled
D. while the hair is lukewarm

___80. Before pressing the hair, it should be

A. combed and brushed
B. shampooed and dried
C. shampooed and marcelled
D. dried and curled

___81. During a curl reformation, how much tension is used to wrap the hair on the rods?

A. no tension
B. moderate tension
C. slight tension
D. firm tension

___82. During a curl reformation the rearranger has been applied, capped, and put under the dryer. When should it be checked?

A. every 5 minutes
B. every 10 minutes
C. every 15 minutes
D. it doesn't need to be checked

___83. During a curl reformation the rearranger has been applied, capped, and put under the dryer. When should it be checked?

A. every 5 minutes
B. every 10 minutes
C. every 15 minutes
D. it doesn't need to be checked

___84. What is the name for the product that straightens the hair in the curl reformation service?

A. chemical relaxer
B. chemical rearranger
C. hair straightener
D. hair filler

___85. When giving a curl reformation, it is very important to wear

A. a hair net
B. an operator apron
C. protective shoes
D. none of the above

___86. The skin can be protected from the sun by applying

A. baby oil
B. lotion with PABA.
C. moisturizing lotion
D. coconut oil

___87. Another name for miliaria rubra is

A. prickly heat
B. sweat retention
C. anhidrosis
D. a cold sweat

___88. The three main divisions of the skin are the epidermis, subcutaneous tissue, and the

A. dermis
B. cutis
C. sebaceous
D. basal

___89. The main purpose of a massage is to stimulate and strengthen

A. nerve branches
B. fatty tissue
C. muscle tone
D. cartilage

___90. Which of the following should be applied to remove cleansing creme from oily skin?

A. soap
B. astringent
C. toner
D. cream

___91. To blend in facial scars and blemishes, what kind of makeup stick should be used?

A. contour
B. rouge
C. corrective
D. powder

___92. When applying semi-permanent lashes, dip the end of the lash in adhesive, stroke the client's lash, then

A. remove it
B. attach it
C. slip it over
D. slide it onto the lid

___93. The inner part of the nail that affects the nail's shape, size, regeneration, and growth is

A. nail wall
B. matrix
C. lunula
D. nail root

___94. Once a nail becomes infected, it should be treated by a

A. barber
B. cosmetologist
C. manicurist
D. physician

___95. To prevent a canvas block from becoming unsanitary and giving off an odor, it is advisable to cover it with a

A. nylon cap
B. synthetic fiber
C. plastic bag
D. rubber sheet

___96. When alopecia appears in the head, it looks like

A. red, circular bald patches
B. scaly, rectangular bald patches
C. non-inflamed, oval bald patches
D. oily scales and oval bald patches

___97. What is the common goal set between you and your client before you have done anything to their hair, nails, or face?

A. improve their appearance
B. to make money
C. buy a house
D. make their hair shinier

___98. Today, salon stylists should think of themselves as

A. salespersons
B. helpers
C. educators
D. all of the above

___99. How do stylists provide additional money for themselves in addition to the money earned for providing services?

A. retail sales
B. rebook client before they leave the salon
C. steal clients from co-workers
D. hog phoned-in appointments

___100. What type of motion should be used when applying lather to the face before shaving?

A. circular
B. back and forth
C. zig zag
D. up and down

DALTON'S STANDARDIZED FINAL TEST 8

Student Name ____ Score _______ Date ___________

Instructions: Carefully read through each question, then read the answer choices. Write your choice of the word, or the phrase, that correctly completes the statement or answers the question, on the line provided.

___1. A good manager - operator should have

A. 2 to 3 years work experience
B. some bookkeeping experience
C. skill in all basic salon services
D. some experience in supply purchasing

___2. The educational requirement for entry into a registered beauty school in some states is at least

A. an eighth-grade education
B. a twelfth-grade education
C. a four-year college education
D. variable from city to city

___3. A salon owner's income may vary according to the

A. number of salons owned
B. size of the salon
C. location of the salon
D. all of the above

___4. Which term fits the job description for a person who specializes in preserving the beauty of the client's face and neck?

A. facial expert
B. esthetician
C. electrologist
D. dermatologist

___5. To communicate, a thought or attitude is conveyed

A. verbally
B. nonverbally
C. person to person
D. all of the above

___6. Dental care for preserving healthy teeth starts with a daily mouthwash and

A. rinsing and flushing
B. rubbing and scratching
C. rinsing and rubbing
D. brushing and flossing

___7. The governing body in most states which is supposed to discipline members that violate professional ethics is the

A. bureau of ethics
B. state legislature
C. state association
D. state board

___8. It is your responsibility to

A. give as much service as needed
B. learn new methods of hairstyling
C. give services based on quality
D. all of the above

___9. Things that may be considered a health hazard are

A. forced air furnaces
B. impure air
C. clean body and clothes
D. hygienic salon practices

___10. Uncleanliness can produce germs that cause

A. good health
B. local canities
C. disease
D. malnutrition

___11. Disease is caused mainly from the lack of

A. cleanliness
B. deodorizers
C. cold water
D. hairspray

___12. The electrical device that removes stale air from the salon is called a(n)

A. humidifier
B. ceiling fan
C. exhaust fan
D. de-humidifier

___13. Practices in the beauty salon that help preserve the health of the public are called

A. fumigation-deodorization
B. salon grooming
C. cleaning-washing
D. sanitation-sterilization

____14. If the eye has been chemically burned, what should be done?

A. flush eye with cool water
B. flush eye with boric acid
C. apply alcohol
D. apply quats

____15. Hair-cutting implements are sanitized with

A. 70% alcohol
B. 40% alcohol
C. 30% formalin solution
D. 30% alcohol

____16. Which virus causes the AIDS disease?

A. Rhino virus
B. HIV virus
C. Influenza virus
D. Cold virus

____17. What route of transmission does the AIDS disease follow?

A. sexual contact
B. injection
C. touching
D. A and B only

____18. Metal electrodes should be sanitized with

A. 2% quats
B. 20% peroxide
C. 70% alcohol
D. 80% ammonium

____19. By law, which of the following must each beauty salon have available?

A. a fire blanket
B. a hot water dispenser
C. an emergency eye wash station
D. a fire extinguisher

____20. A carrier is a person who has a disease that is

A. acute
B. contagious
C. occupational
D. common

____21. Which of the following would destroy the AIDS virus outside the body?

A. water
B. 70% alcohol
C. shampoo
D. hand soap

____22. When giving a service, what should you do if you are exposed to blood?

A. see your doctor
B. wash exposed area with soap and water
C. apply a topical disinfectant
D. B and C only

____23. The protein cross-bonds of the hair are called

A. polypeptide bonds
B. monopeptide bonds
C. hydrogen bonds
D. cystine bonds

____24. When hair is in its resting cycle, and more likely to fall out, this stage is known as the

A. terminal stage
B. fall-out stage
C. hair loss stage
D. telogen stage

____25. What is the name for the male hair loss due to the aging process?

A. congenital alopecia
B. male-pattern baldness
C. hair thinning
D. routine hair loss

____26. Depilatories in the form of a cream, paste, or powder are chemical products used to

A. curl hair
B. remove hair
C. color hair
D. straighten hair

____27. The layer of the hair in which the coloring pigment is found is the

A. follicle
B. medulla
C. cortex
D. cuticle

____28. Before using a hot wax depilatory, the cosmetologist should

A. apply gauze to the work area
B. give the client instructions
C. check to be sure client is comfortable
D. check the temperature of the wax

___29. What general prefix is used to describe most hair diseases?

A. tricho
B. tricko
C. trio
D. trigo

___30. Shampoos with a pH greater than seven (7) are called

A. acid
B. alkaline
C. mild
D. neutral

___31. Peroxide has a pH that is

A. acid
B. alkaline
C. neutral
D. none of the above

___32. When rinsing the client's hair with hot water, how should you detect temperature changes in the water?

A. watch for steam from the client's scalp
B. little finger of hand held under nozzle of hose
C. the color of the client's scalp turns bright pink
D. the shampoo changes color

___33. How should you protect the client's clothing before shampooing the hair?

A. draping the cape over the back of the chair
B. cover all clothing with towels
C. place in plastic clothing protectors
D. place plastic towels across client's shoulder

___34. To preserve the hairstyle against humidity in the air, the conditioner should contain a(n)

A. barrier coat
B. shield cover
C. wetting agent
D. antihumectant

___35. The extent that hair can be stretched without breaking is known as

A. pressure
B. tone
C. elasticity
D. texture

___36. When the hair is conditioned using strong chemicals, this is known as

A. pre-treating
B. preconditioning
C. duration conditioning
D. in-process conditioning

___37. Scalp manipulations should not be given if the hair is going to be

A. cold waved
B. permanently colored
C. chemically lightened
D. all of the above

___38. Before combing out the finger wave, the hair should be

A. thoroughly dried
B. thoroughly lubricated
C. quite damp
D. sprayed with lacquer

___39. For the least amount of tightness when setting sculpture curls, you should use a

A. no-stem curl
B. half-stem curl
C. quarter-stem curl
D. long-stem curl

___40. Set sculpture curls within a shaping should

A. be separate
B. swing down
C. overlap
D. swing over

___41. When putting a shaping into the hair, the hair should be

A. wet
B. damp
C. dry
D. moistened on the ends

___42. What draping supply is recommended for the client that is about to have a hair shaping only?

A. towel shampoo cape
B. shampoo cape
C. comb-out cape
D. chair cloth

___43. When razor cutting, strokes that the cosmetologist should use are

A. firm and long
B. smooth and long
C. smooth and short
D. jerky and short

___44. To prevent the electric clipper blades from pulling the hair, what should you do?

A. apply oil to them
B. soak in alcohol
C. apply ammonia to them
D. dip them in peroxide

___45. What is the name given to one or more subsections of hair cut in the hairline or crown of the head that serve as a yardstick for cutting the rest of the hair?

A. trendline
B. radial line
C. bias line
D. guideline

___46. What will happen if you submerge your electric clipper in a wet sanitizer while it is plugged into an outlet?

A. the blades will slide
B. the clipper won't cut correctly
C. you will get an electric shock
D. your clipper will vibrate

___47. Storing your scissors in your uniform pocket may result in

A. a severe cut
B. tarnishing of finish on the scissors
C. dulling of blades of the scissors
D. rust forming on the scissors

___48. The foundation for a good hairstyle is a correct hair

A. setting lotion
B. shaping
C. styling comb
D. brush

___49. The heat from the air waver should be directed

A. away from the scalp
B. toward the scalp
C. at the ends
D. toward the hair root

___50. Before applying an aniline derivative tint, omit the

A. hair brushing
B. patch test
C. strand test
D. metallic salt test

___51. Just before applying a hair tint, it would be a good safety precaution to

A. put cotton on the hairline
B. put cotton around the client's neck
C. check again for scalp abrasions
D. clean combs and brushes

___52. A client is now in the styling chair for a scheduled virgin tint. After getting the coloring product from the dispensary, you discover there is no developer anywhere in the salon

A. use water for the developer and give the tint
B. use shampoo for developer
C. reschedule the appointment
D. ask the client to leave

___53. Synthetic/organic temporary hair colors are found in

A. vegetable tints
B. aniline derivative tints
C. certified vegetable tints
D. metallic tints

___54. To prevent a line of demarcation during a tint retouch, it is important to avoid

A. rotating a bottle
B. overlapping the tint
C. mixing tint
D. rubbing the scalp

___55. How many stages does black hair go through to become pale blonde?

A. four
B. five
C. six
D. seven

___56. The lightest toner can only be applied to hair bleached to the

A. brown stage
B. red-gold stage
C. pale yellow stage
D. red stage

____57. Containers used for mixing bleach should be made of

A. plastic
B. wood
C. metal
D. glass

____58. Before giving a lightener retouch, what should you do?

A. a predisposition test
B. brush the hair vigorously
C. examine the scalp for cuts and abrasions
D. give the client a strand test

____59. When an aniline toner is used, what test must be given first?

A. shampoo
B. strand
C. patch
D. elasticity

____60. The removal of a penetrating tint from the hair is called

A. relaxing
B. soap cap
C. stripping
D. tinting

____61. The strength of the cold-waving solution to be used is determined by the hair texture and

A. color
B. condition
C. density
D. viscosity

____62. When sodium bromate fumes and ammonia fumes mix together in an open towel hamper, what could result?

A. a fire
B. a strong acid smell
C. discoloration of towels
D. stain in the hamper

____63. When permanent waving the hair, how many turns must the hair be wound around the rod to achieve a curl pattern?

A. once
B. twice
C. four turns
D. five turns

____64. In which of the following conditions should the cosmetologist REFUSE to give the client a cold wave?

A. a scar on the scalp
B. cranial surgical wound
C. a scalp freckle
D. an ulna surgical wound

____65. When rinsing a permanent wave, what can you do to prevent water from running down the client's neck and back?

A. ask the client to raise their head
B. use low water pressure
C. use a neutralizing bib
D. place foil around the neck

____66. A self-timing permanent wave is one in which the manufacturer recommends that you

A. test curl every 3 minutes
B. towel blot each rod
C. process for a set period of time
D. place client under a dryer

____67. If cold waving hair that is bleached (lightened), it is best to select rods that are

A. large
B. small
C. midget
D. of any size

____68. When cold waving, the size of the curl or wave pattern will be controlled by the

A. cold-wave solution
B. type of neutralizer
C. size of the rod
D. size of the end papers

____69. For chemically straightening the hair, use a chemical relaxer, and a(n)

A. conditioner
B. pre-creme
C. stabilizer
D. setting lotion

____70. As in cold waving, chemical relaxers work faster on hair that is

A. wiry
B. coarse
C. porous
D. non-porous

___71. The difference between a base and no-base relaxer is that the no-base

A. does not require application of the base
B. always requires the use of protective gloves
C. is safer to use, but requires more time
D. is more dangerous to use, but requires more time

___72. Hair should be conditioned after a sodium hydroxide relaxer to prevent

A. breakage during combing and setting
B. dry, scaly scalp
C. red, irritated scalp
D. breakage during thermal pressing

___73. The neutralizing shampoo used in the chemical relaxing service is also called a

A. stabilizer
B. cleaner
C. conditioner
D. filler

___74. During neutralizing, the hair should be shampooed at least how many times?

A. 1 to 2
B. 2 to 3
C. 3 to 4
D. as many as needed

___75. Before a chemical hair straightener, the cosmetologist would not

A. read label directions
B. examine the scalp
C. analyze the hair
D. brush the hair

___76. One of the most important things to remember about the processing of a chemical relaxer is

A. apply it slowly and evenly
B. never leave the client unattended
C. never serve coffee during processing
D. brush the hair before neutralizing

___77. The roller technique of curling hair involves winding the hair strand from the

A. ends to the scalp
B. mid-strand to ends
C. ends to mid-strand
D. scalp to the ends

___78. When thermal waving the hair, fine, short hairs around the hairline are best curled with

A. some pin curls
B. a smaller iron
C. a crimper
D. some perm rods

___79. The styling comb used in thermal waving should be made of

A. aluminum
B. steel
C. hard rubber
D. soft rubber

___80. What is the name for the product that straightens the hair in the curl reformation service?

A. chemical relaxer
B. chemical rearranger
C. hair straightener
D. hair filler

___81. Before applying the neutralizer to the rods when doing a curl reformation, the hair should be rinsed with

A. conditioner
B. hot water
C. tepid water
D. cold water

___82. During a curl reformation, how much tension is used to wrap the hair on the rods?

A. no tension
B. moderate tension
C. slight tension
D. firm tension

___83. To be successful, what size rod subsections should the cosmetologist use when doing a curl reformation?

A. small subsections
B. medium subsections
C. large subsections
D. none of the above

___84. What is the one thing to watch out for when you are about to give a curl reformation?

A. too many test curls
B. client allergies
C. using too many rods
D. tangled hair

___85. The silhouette, shape, or contour of the body is affected by bone structure, and amount of

A. adipose tissue
B. nerve tissue
C. follicle tissue
D. shaft tissue

___86. The outermost (top) layer of the skin is the

A. epidermis
B. corium
C. subcutaneous tissue
D. adipose tissue

___87. An esthetician is a person who is mainly concerned with the promoting and preserving of health and beauty of the

A. fingernails
B. toenails
C. eyebrows
D. skin

___88. The three main divisions of the skin are the epidermis, subcutaneous tissue, and the

A. dermis
B. cutis
C. sebaceous
D. basal

___89. In the presence of severe acne, the cosmetologist should

A. avoid facial massage
B. use tapotement massage
C. use kneading massage
D. avoid use of emollient cream

___90. Lash and brow tint is applied with, then against, the natural direction of the hair's

A. insertion
B. growth
C. follicle
D. strand

___91. Powder is applied over foundation makeup to

A. black it out
B. set it
C. cover it
D. blend it

___92. After strip lashes are correctly positioned, the outside and inside ends are held in place for

A. one minute
B. two minutes
C. three minutes
D. four minutes

___93. The nail root is located

A. at each side of the nail wall
B. beneath the skin at the base of the nail
C. beyond the end of the fingertip
D. near the skin directly beneath the nail's free edge

___94. If hangnails are neglected, they may become

A. brittle
B. fragile
C. infected
D. loose

___95. The most expensive type of hair from which hairgoods are made is

A. synthetic hair
B. yak hair
C. angora hair
D. human hair

___96. To prevent a canvas block from becoming unsanitary and giving off an odor, it is advisable to cover it with a

A. nylon cap
B. synthetic fiber
C. plastic bag
D. rubber sheet

___97. How does the cosmetologist obtain personal satisfaction and financial gain from working in the salon?

A. scheduling a lot of appointments
B. answering the phone frequently
C. helping others
D. taking risks

___98. What is the greatest fear faced by people in sales-related jobs?

A. which clothes to wear
B. what to do with the client's hair
C. what to do with the client's face
D. how to overcome rejection

___99. If you are at a social event, such as a party, what would be an effective way to let fellow party goers know what kind of work you do, and where you can be contacted for cosmetology services?

A. write your phone number on a napkin
B. ask them to look you up in the book
C. pass out business cards
D. ask your fiends to copy your number and pass it on

___100. How should an ingrown hair be removed from the skin?

A. dig it out with a needle
B. scrap it to the surface
C. apply a drying lotion
D. use a tweezers

DALTON'S STANDARDIZED FINAL TEST 9

Student Name ________________________________ Score _______ Date ___________

Instructions: Carefully read through each question, then read the answer choices. Write your choice of the word, or the phrase, that correctly completes the statement or answers the question, on the line provided.

___1. Personal grooming relates to one's

A. daily appearance
B. daily cleanliness
C. hairstyle and voice
D. A and B.

___2. Personal hygiene relates to

A. promoting one's own health
B. preservation of one's health
C. oral care
D. A and B.

___3. Dental care for preserving healthy teeth starts with a daily mouthwash and

A. rinsing and flushing
B. rubbing and scratching
C. rinsing and rubbing
D. brushing and flossing

___4. Ethics is a system that measures human behavior that is

A. voluntary
B. involuntary
C. imposed by local police
D. imposed by the federal government

___5. A professional attitude is

A. natural
B. given when you are licensed
C. acquired in enrollment
D. learned

___6. To equal the strength of 6% hydrogen peroxide, you would have to use

A. 1 volume hydrogen peroxide
B. 2 volume hydrogen peroxide
C. 10 volume hydrogen peroxide
D. 20 volume hydrogen peroxide

___7. If cosmetology implements are aseptic, then they are

A. free from bacteria
B. unsanitary
C. soiled
D. covered

___8. A person immune to a disease, but who can infect others is known as a(n)

A. clinical
B. medical
C. agent
D. carrier

___9. The germicidal light used in some dry sanitizers is known as

A. fluorescent light
B. ultra-violet light
C. infrared light
D. incandescent light

___10. Another name for public hygiene is

A. grooming
B. hair care
C. sanitation
D. community

___11. If the eye has been chemically burned, what should be done?

A. flush eye with cool water
B. flush eye with boric acid
C. apply alcohol
D. apply quats

___12. When removing implements from a wet sanitizer you should wear

A. an operator apron
B. a hair net
C. rubber gloves
D. neutralizing bib

___13. How is the disease AIDS transmitted from one person to another?

A. blood
B. semen
C. vaginal secretions
D. all of the above

___14. What route of transmission does the AIDS disease follow?

A. injection
B. blood transfusion
C. maternal
D. all of the above

___15. Soiled towels should be stored in a covered

A. linen hamper
B. metal container
C. plastic container
D. laundry basket

___16. A carrier is a person who has a disease that is

A. acute
B. contagious
C. occupational
D. common

___17. What common cosmetology chemical would kill the AIDS virus outside of the body?

A. household bleach
B. water
C. 1% hydrogen peroxide
D. 20% alcohol

___18. What strength hydrogen peroxide would destroy the AIDS virus outside of the body?

A. 1%
B. 2%
C. 3%
D. all of the above

___19. If you accidently cut your client's neck and it bleeds, what should you do?

A. put on disposable rubber gloves
B. wash area with soap and water
C. apply topical disinfectant to area
D. all of the above

___20. Hair is not found on the

A. forearm and wrists
B. forearm and nose
C. knuckles of the hands
D. soles of the feet

___21. Hair is an example of

A. hard keratin
B. soft keratin
C. Henle's layer
D. Huxley's layer

___22. Scalp hair usually grows at a monthly rate of

A. 1/4″
B. 1/2″
C. 3/4″
D. 1″

___23. The glands in the scalp that naturally lubricate the hair during brushing are called

A. apocrine
B. sebaceous
C. sudoriferous
D. eccrine

___24. Which of the following would a dermatologist prescribe for men for regular hair loss?

A. vitamin A
B. minoxidal
C. medicated shampoo
D. creme rinse

___25. Before applying a chemical depilatory, how should the cosmetologist protect the client?

A. buy only quality depilatories
B. apply gauze to the area to be worked on
C. give the client a skin test
D. ask client to remove jewelry

___26. The percentage of the hair shaft represented by the cortex layer is

A. 15%
B. 25%
C. 50%
D. 75%

___27. The technical term applied to the cyclical period when the hair begins to grow is the

A. anagen stage
B. terminal stage
C. telogen stage
D. origin stage

___28. Hypertrichosis is a condition that is also called

A. supercilia hair
B. superfluous hair
C. ringed hair
D. twisted hair

___29. The skin and hair have a natural pH in a range of

A. 3.5 – 4.5.
B. 4.5 – 5.5.
C. 5.5 – 6.5.
D. 6.5 – 7.5.

____30. Peroxide has a pH that is

A. acid
B. alkaline
C. neutral
D. none of the above

____31. An overly oily scalp is a disorder medically referred to as

A. steatoma
B. seborrhea
C. asteatosis
D. tinea

____32. To prevent water from dripping onto the floor from the shampoo bowl, where should you leave the shampoo hose?

A. drain position
B. handle position
C. vacuum breaker position
D. none of the above

____33. The amount of water the hair can absorb is called

A. porosity
B. tension
C. elasticity
D. tone

____34. The basic protein found in the hair shaft is

A. cuticle
B. medulla
C. sebum
D. keratin

____35. Very small bits of protein applied to the hair are called

A. macro-proteins
B. micro-proteins
C. poultry proteins
D. substantive proteins

____36. Semicircular designs combed into the hair are called

A. waves
B. base direction
C. shapings
D. arcs

____37. The main objective in finger waving the hair is to mold even

A. curls and softness
B. waves and ridges
C. shaping and direction
D. parts and shapes

____38. A large stand-up curl could also be called a barre curl or

A. skip-curl
B. cascade curl
C. closed-end curl
D. clockwise curl

____39. To get the maximum amount of height or fullness you should use a

A. no-stem curl
B. half-stem curl
C. long-stem curl
D. tight-stem curl

____40. When setting the hair with rollers, a curved form in the finished hairstyle is done by winding hair around the roller

A. 1 turn or less
B. 1-1/2 turns
C. 2 turns
D. none of the above

____41. The standard or ideal facial shape is

A. oblong
B. round
C. oval
D. square

____42. If too much bulk is removed from coarse hair, it tends to

A. look smooth and natural
B. stick out from the head
C. be super curly
D. set more easily

____43. When dry, super-curly hair should be shortened using a

A. clipper
B. scissors
C. razor
D. thinning shears

____44. Proper storage of cutting implements is important to prevent

A. over-use of implements
B. injury to small children
C. rust from forming
D. the edge from becoming dull

___45. You should not use an electric clipper if

A. the client wants a trim
B. the set screw has been adjusted
C. it is noisy
D. any teeth are broken

___46. When cutting the hair with a shaper, it is important to

A. cut by using the guard
B. thin toward the scalp
C. use long, sliding strokes
D. blunt all hair

___47. During a razor cut, as the razor is cutting the hair, the comb is placed in the

A. pocket
B. drawer
C. other hand
D. other section

___48. The hanging length cut around the hairline from which the rest of the hair is shaped is called the

A. high-sign
B. cutting length
C. guideline
D. form

___49. Extra care must be taken when blow waving long hair because it

A. may become hard to manage and curl
B. may dry too quickly and become oily
C. may be drawn into the air intake of the dryer
D. could stick to the brush and become straight

___50. To prevent overlapping on a tint retouch, the tint is applied from the scalp to about

A. 1/16" up to the tinted hair
B. 1/16" over the already tinted hair
C. 1/4" up to the tinted hair
D. 1/2" over the tinted hair

___51. One of the main chemicals in aniline derivative tints is

A. sulfonated oils
B. ammonium thioglycolate
C. cystine disulfide
D. para-phenylene-diamine

___52. The general term used to describe a lightener and toner is

A. separate application
B. single application
C. double application
D. triple application

___53. After tweezing the client's eyebrows, what should be applied to the skin?

A. antiseptic
B. disinfectant
C. fumigant
D. neutralizer

___54. The pH of a semi-permanent color falls in the range of

A. 4 to 6
B. 5 to 6
C. 7 to 9
D. 9 to 10.

___55. If you overlap bleach when doing a bleach retouch, it will result in

A. more elasticity
B. less elasticity
C. breakage
D. hair yellowing

___56. Lightening the hair begins with the application of a

A. stripping agent
B. toning agent
C. moisturizing agent
D. bleaching agent

___57. When lightening and toning the hair, you should wear

A. protective shoes
B. a hair net
C. an operator apron
D. protective gloves

___58. A retouch hair lightener is applied to the

A. new growth of hair
B. entire hair shaft
C. the ends only
D. cold shaft only

___59. The chemical process of bleaching hair is (known as)

A. stimulation
B. neutralization
C. evaporation
D. oxidation

___60. To equalize the porosity of the hair, use a

A. steamer
B. stripper
C. filler
D. equalizer

___61. Cold-waving solution causes the hair shaft to

A. soften and contract
B. soften and swell
C. harden and contract
D. harden and swell

___62. Better saturation of the cold-waving solution into the hair is achieved when it is

A. wrapped correctly
B. analyzed accurately
C. curled properly
D. pressed thoroughly

___63. Before cold waving the entire head, the degree to which the hair will curl can be determined by using

A. concave curls
B. convex curls
C. test curls
D. pin curls

___64. Cotton is placed around the hairline before applying the cold-waving solution; it should be

A. removed after it is applied
B. allowed to remain until the neutralizer is applied
C. removed following the neutralizer
D. removed when the rods are taken out

___65. To remove dripping cold-waving solution, use a piece of cotton or the corner of a towel saturated with

A. cold water
B. warm water
C. tepid water
D. hot water

___66. When rinsing a permanent wave, what can you do to prevent water from running down the client's neck and back?

A. ask the client to raise their head
B. use low water pressure
C. use a neutralizing bib
D. place foil around the neck

___67. When applying the waving solution as part of the permanent waving process, the cosmetologist sees that there is a purple discoloration of the solution on the client's towel What should the cosmetologist do?

A. stop and rinse the hair with water
B. apply neutralizer immediately
C. continue to give the permanent
D. apply a different waving solution

___68. Two basic chemicals used in cold-waving solution are

A. ammonia and formalin
B. sulfuric acid and ammonia
C. carbolic acid and formalin
D. thioglycolic acid and ammonia

___69. If cold waving hair that is bleached (lightened), it is best to select rods that are

A. large
B. small
C. midget
D. of any size

___70. When cold waving, the size of the curl or wave pattern will be controlled by the

A. cold-wave solution
B. type of neutralizer
C. size of the rod
D. size of the end papers

___71. Before a chemical hair straightener, the cosmetologist would not

A. brush the hair
B. analyze the hair
C. examine the scalp
D. read label directions

___72. Before a chemical relaxer, the skin and scalp can be protected from chemical burns by applying a

A. neutralizer
B. stabilizer
C. base
D. jelly

___73. Should a chemical relaxer accidently drip into the client's eye, what should you do?

A. stop action by applying neutralizer to eye
B. flush eye with lots of water
C. blot chemical and apply hot water
D. mist eye with bottle of warm water

___74. After chemically relaxing the hair for a client with super-curly hair, what service should NOT be given to the client?

A. roller set
B. regular electric curling iron set
C. pressing comb/thermal iron set
D. pick-out style after hair has been dried

___75. After a chemical relaxer, a conditioner should be applied

A. after the hair is set
B. just before the comb-out
C. before the hair is styled with rollers
D. after the comb-out

___76. The suggested implement to use for cutting wet hair that has been chemically relaxed is the

A. scissors
B. razor
C. thinning shears
D. electric clipper

___77. The actions of chemical hair straightener cause the hair to

A. soften and swell
B. shape and curl
C. shift and mold
D. shrink and harden

___78. During the processing and neutralizing of a chemical relaxer service, what can be done to minimize neck irritation?

A. applying cotton coil
B. changing towel frequently
C. keeping the client's neck against the bowl
D. applying neutralizing cream

___79. Croquingnole curling involves winding the hair strand from the

A. ends to the scalp
B. mid-strand to ends
C. ends to mid-strand
D. scalp to ends

___80. After the hair is pressed, the thermal iron forms the curl by rotating the iron using a(n)

A. clicking action
B. sliding actions
C. oval action
D. back and forth action

___81. Before thermal waving super-curly hair, the cosmetologist should

A. color it
B. press it
C. shape it
D. comb it

___82. When giving a curl reformation, how many turns is the rod unwound in order to test curl the strand?

A. 1-1/2 – 2 turns
B. 2-1/2 – 3 turns
C. 3-1/2 – 4 turns
D. 4-1/2 – 5 turns

___83. During a curl reformation the rearranger has been applied, capped, and put under the dryer. When should it be checked?

A. every 5 minutes
B. every 10 minutes
C. every 15 minutes
D. it doesn't need to be checked

___84. After a facial has been given, what should be done with the tweezers?

A. sanitized and stored in dry sanitizer
B. wiped clean for reuse
C. discarded
D. rinsed and put on station

___85. To be successful, what size rod subsections should the cosmetologist use when doing a curl reformation?

A. small subsections
B. medium subsections
C. large subsections
D. none of the above

___86. During a curl reformation, the hair dries out while you are wrapping the hair on the rods. What should you do?

A. apply more waving solution
B. apply water to dry strands
C. use spray-on conditioner
D. use two end wraps

____87. Body temperature is regulated by the blood (98.6), and the

A. thyroid gland
B. adrenal glands
C. sebaceous glands
D. sweat glands

____88. A sun block lotion would have what SPF rating number?

A. 5.
B. 8.
C. 12.
D. 15.

____89. The three main divisions of the skin are the epidermis, subcutaneous tissue, and the

A. dermis
B. cutis
C. sebaceous
D. basal

____90. Of all the light from the sun, infrared rays make up about

A. 20% of it
B. 40% of it
C. 60% of it
D. 80% of it

____91. When applying corrective or contour makeup, the rule is "lights in the valley, shadows on the hills". This means that indentations should be filled, and protrusions should be

A. shadowed
B. lightened
C. toned up
D. highlighted

____92. Small eyes can be made to appear larger. What type of makeup is applied to create this illusion?

A. contour
B. foundation
C. lip
D. white

____93. What type of movement should be used when tweezing the eyebrows?

A. slow, sliding movement
B. quick movement
C. circular movement
D. zig-zag movement

____94. That portion of the skin directly beneath the nail's free edge is the

A. mantle
B. eponychium
C. hyponychium
D. nail groove

____95. Once a nail becomes infected, it should be treated by a

A. barber
B. cosmetologist
C. manicurist
D. physician

____96. If a minor cut should occur during a manicure, apply powdered styptic, or a(n)

A. shampoo
B. antiseptic
C. creme rinse
D. disinfectant

____97. When the stylist and the client have developed a common set of thoughts, what is the term used to describe this relationship?

A. rapport
B. charisma
C. charm
D. poise

____98. What is the first step in becoming a successful cosmetologist?

A. styling the hair well
B. answering the phone well
C. realizing you are a salesperson
D. knowing that you can help all clients

____99. What percentage of your business should come from friends recommending your services to friends?

A. 1 – 2%
B. 2 – 3%
C. 4 – 6%
D. all of the above

____100. In which area of the neck should you be extra careful?

A. Adam's apple
B. base of the chin
C. jaw line
D. base of neck

DALTON'S STANDARDIZED FINAL TEST 10

Student Name ______________________________ Score _______ Date ___________

Instructions: Carefully read through each question, then read the answer choices. Write your choice of the word, or the phrase, that correctly completes the statement or answers the question, on the line provided.

___1. A research technician

A. tests newly developed products
B. works at a cosmetic manufacturing company
C. must be at least twenty-five years old
D. A and B

___2. A salon owner's income may vary according to the

A. number of salons owned
B. size of the salon
C. location of the salon
D. all of the above

___3. Which term fits the job description for a person who specializes in preserving the beauty of the client's face and neck?

A. facial expert
B. esthetician
C. electrologist
D. dermatologist

___4. To communicate, a thought or attitude is conveyed

A. verbally
B. nonverbally
C. person to person
D. all of the above

___5. Dental care for preserving healthy teeth starts with a daily mouthwash and

A. rinsing and flushing
B. rubbing and scratching
C. rinsing and rubbing
D. brushing and flossing

___6. The governing body in most states which is supposed to discipline members that violate professional ethics is the

A. bureau of ethics
B. state legislature
C. state association
D. state board

___7. It is your responsibility to

A. give as much service as needed
B. learn new methods of hairstyling
C. give services based on quality
D. all of the above

___8. Practices in the beauty salon that help preserve the health of the public are called

A. fumigation-deodorization
B. salon grooming
C. cleaning-washing
D. sanitation-sterilization

___9. If the eye has been chemically burned, what should be done?

A. flush eye with cool water
B. flush eye with boric acid
C. apply alcohol
D. apply quats

___10. To be effective for sanitation, the strength of the quats to be used should be at least

A. 1:200
B. 1:200
C. 1:500
D. 1:1000

___11. Hair-cutting implements are sanitized with

A. 70% alcohol
B. 40% alcohol
C. 30% formalin solution
D. 30% alcohol

___12. How is the disease AIDS transmitted from one person to another?

A. blood
B. semen
C. vaginal secretions
D. all of the above

___13. What route of transmission does the AIDS disease follow?

A. sexual contact
B. injection
C. touching
D. A and B only

____14. Metal electrodes should be sanitized with

A. 2% quats
B. 20% peroxide
C. 70% alcohol
D. 80% ammonium

____15. By law, which of the following must each beauty salon have available?

A. a fire blanket
B. a hot water dispenser
C. an emergency eye wash station
D. a fire extinguisher

____16. A carrier is a person who has a disease that is

A. acute
B. contagious
C. occupational
D. common

____17. Which of the following would destroy the AIDS virus outside the body?

A. water
B. 70% alcohol
C. shampoo
D. hand soap

____18. When giving a service, what should you do if you are exposed to blood?

A. see your doctor
B. wash exposed area with soap and water
C. apply a topical disinfectant
D. B and C only

____19. The function of the hair is to

A. adorn the body
B. protect the skin
C. adorn the head
D. all of the above

____20. The physical wrapping of the hair during cold wave breaks the

A. hydrogen bonds
B. cystine bonds
C. atomic bonds
D. molecular bonds

____21. Hair is an example of

A. hard keratin
B. soft keratin
C. Henle's layer
D. Huxley's layer

____22. When hair is in its resting cycle, and more likely to fall out, this stage is known as the

A. terminal stage
B. fall-out stage
C. hair loss stage
D. telogen stage

____23. The glands in the scalp that naturally lubricate the hair during brushing are called

A. apocrine
B. sebaceous
C. sudoriferous
D. eccrine

____24. What is the name for the male hair loss due to the aging process?

A. congenital alopecia
B. male-pattern baldness
C. hair thinning
D. routine hair loss

____25. Hair is made up of a hard protein substance called

A. carbon
B. hydrogen
C. keratin
D. sulfur

____26. The layer of the hair in which the coloring pigment is found is the

A. follicle
B. medulla
C. cortex
D. cuticle

____27. Before using a hot wax depilatory, the cosmetologist should

A. apply gauze to the work area
B. give the client instructions
C. check to be sure client is comfortable
D. check the temperature of the wax

____28. What general prefix is used to describe most hair diseases?

A. tricho
B. tricko
C. trio
D. trigo

____29. The pH of a shampoo indicates the concentration of

A. hydrogen
B. oxygen
C. nitrogen
D. carbon

____30. Peroxide has a pH that is

A. acid
B. alkaline
C. neutral
D. none of the above

____31. Scabies is an infestation of the scalp by

A. the itch mite
B. head lice
C. ringworm
D. tinea

____32. How should you protect the client's clothing before shampooing the hair?

A. draping the cape over the back of the chair
B. cover all clothing with towels
C. place in plastic clothing protectors
D. place plastic towels across client's shoulder

____33. The natural lubricant that gives hair a beautiful luster or sheen is called

A. sebum
B. seborrhea
C. seconal
D. permanent color

____34. If damaged hair is going to be given a service that uses strong chemicals the cosmetologist should recommend

A. preconditioning
B. prelightening
C. pre-filling
D. preneutralizing

____35. Hair can be damaged chemically by

A. improper bleaching
B. wave set
C. shampooing
D. hair cutting

____36. Scalp manipulations should not be given if the hair is going to be

A. cold waved
B. permanently colored
C. chemically lightened
D. all of the above

____37. The shaping between two finger-wave ridges is called the wave

A. direction
B. trough
C. arc
D. curl

____38. After the setting lotion has been applied, should the hair dry out during setting, spray more

A. filler on it
B. conditioner on it
C. water on it
D. setting lotion on it

____39. When putting a shaping into the hair, the hair should be

A. wet
B. damp
C. dry
D. moistened on the ends

____40. To correct a diamond-shaped face, fullness is needed everywhere, except at the

A. cheekbones
B. eyebrows
C. forehead
D. jaw

____41. For a basic haircut, the cosmetologist would begin cutting the hair in the

A. top
B. side
C. crown
D. nape

____42. When razor cutting, strokes that the cosmetologist should use are

A. firm and long
B. smooth and long
C. smooth and short
D. jerky and short

____43. To prevent the electric clipper blades from pulling the hair, what should you do?

A. apply oil to them
B. soak in alcohol
C. apply ammonia to them
D. dip them in peroxide

___44. The technique of holding the hair upward toward the crown or top of the head during a hair shaping is called

A. low-elevation
B. high-elevation
C. feather edging
D. stepping

___45. What will happen if you submerge your electric clipper in a wet sanitizer while it is plugged into an outlet?

A. the blades will slide
B. the clipper won't cut correctly
C. you will get an electric shock
D. your clipper will vibrate

___46. Storing your scissors in your uniform pocket may result in

A. a severe cut
B. tarnishing of finish on the scissors
C. dulling of blades of the scissors
D. rust forming on the scissors

___47. The foundation for a good hairstyle is a correct hair

A. setting lotion
B. shaping
C. styling comb
D. brush

___48. Extra care must be taken when blow waving long hair because it

A. may become hard to manage and curl
B. may dry too quickly and become oily
C. may be drawn into the air intake of the dryer
D. could stick to the brush and become straight

___49. When doing a tint retouch, apply the tint only to the

A. hair root
B. hair ends
C. cold shaft
D. new growth

___50. A predisposition test is required before applying a(n)

A. vegetable derivative tint
B. animal derivative tint
C. metallic derivative tint
D. aniline derivative tint

___51. A client is now in the styling chair for a schedule virgin tint. After getting the coloring product fror the dispensary, the cosmetologist discovers there is no developer anywhere in the salon

A. use water for the developer and give the tint
B. use shampoo for developer
C. reschedule the appointment
D. ask the client to leave

___52. Synthetic/organic temporary hair colors are foun in

A. vegetable tints
B. aniline derivative tints
C. certified vegetable tints
D. metallic tints

___53. To prevent a line of demarcation during a tint retouch, it is important to avoid

A. rotating a bottle
B. overlapping the tint
C. mixing tint
D. rubbing the scalp

___54. Which of the following is the best definition of a permanent toner?

A. an aniline derivative tint in pastel colors
B. an aniline tint having a gold base
C. para-phenylene-diamine dyes
D. color that cannot be removed

___55. The lightest stage that hair can be bleached is

A. gold
B. pale yellow
C. pale red-gold
D. pale orange

___56. When the proper stage of streaking is reached, which shampoo is BEST to remove bleach?

A. mild
B. medicated (alkaline)
C. non-stripping (acid)
D. alkaline

___57. Before giving a lightener retouch, what should you do?

A. a predisposition test
B. brush the hair vigorously
C. examine the scalp for cuts and abrasions
D. give the client a strand test

___58. Full strength bleach on the scalp MAY cause

A. stinging
B. irritation
C. blistering
D. all of the above

___59. When giving a virgin bleach to medium brown hair, the cosmetologist should begin applying the lightener

A. 1/2" from scalp up through ends
B. from scalp to ends
C. from ends to scalp
D. center of hair shaft to ends

___60. Blocking and winding the hair at the beginning of a cold wave may begin in the

A. nape area
B. ear area
C. eye area
D. nose area

___61. To achieve a good curl when permanent waving, how much tension should be applied to the hair as it is wound?

A. very firm tension
B. very little tension
C. moderate-firm, even tension
D. no tension

___62. Before a cold wave is wrapped the hair is usually dried using a

A. blow comb
B. hand dryer
C. towel
D. rat-tail comb

___63. After processing a perm, what can you do to prevent the rods from being forced from the hair during rinsing ?

A. tighten them up
B. use low water pressure
C. put on a hair net
D. rinse with cool water

___64. In which of the following conditions should the cosmetologist REFUSE to give the client a cold wave?

A. a scar on the scalp
B. cranial surgical wound
C. a scalp freckle
D. an ulna surgical wound

___65. If a couple of small areas of the hair do not have enough curl one week after the wave process, you should give the client

A. a refund check
B. another cosmetologist
C. some pickup curls
D. another chemical wave

___66. The action of cold waving solution on the hair is one of

A. softening
B. hardening
C. shrinking
D. contracting

___67. During the winding process in cold waving, the physical bonds in the hair shaft that are broken are called

A. amino
B. cysteine
C. hydrogen
D. salt

___68. A self-timing permanent wave is one in which the manufacturer recommends that you

A. test curl every 3 minutes
B. towel blot each rod
C. process for a set period of time
D. place client under a dryer

___69. If cold waving hair that is bleached (lightened), it is best to select rods that are

A. large
B. small
C. midget
D. of any size

___70. A thio relaxer affects the hair shaft by causing it to

A. harden and swell
B. harden and shrink
C. soften and shrink
D. soften and swell

___71. If the client has a little spot on the scalp that is burning during a chemical hair relaxer, what should you do?

A. rinse all relaxer from hair immediately
B. apply an astringent to the spot
C. apply petrolatum to the spot
D. spray spot with cool water

___72. Before giving a retouch chemical relaxer, what should be applied to the previously relaxed hair first?

A. water
B. protective conditioner
C. presoftening rinse
D. prerelax shampoo

___73. Hair should be conditioned after a sodium hydroxide relaxer to prevent

A. breakage during combing and setting
B. dry, scaly scalp
C. red, irritated scalp
D. breakage during thermal pressing

___74. The neutralizing shampoo used in the chemical relaxing service is also called a

A. stabilizer
B. cleaner
C. conditioner
D. filler

___75. Chemical relaxers should be used carefully because the hair may

A. dissolve
B. stretch
C. become porous
D. become oily

___76. Before applying a chemical relaxer, analyze the hair for porosity, texture, and elasticity; then, examine the

A. relaxing kit
B. hairline
C. scalp
D. fingernails

___77. Before a chemical hair straightener, the cosmetologist would not

A. read label directions
B. examine the scalp
C. analyze the hair
D. brush the hair

___78. If the client has a little spot on the scalp that is burning during a chemical hair relaxer, what should you do?

A. rinse all relaxer from the hair immediately
B. apply an astringent to the spot
C. apply petrolatum to the spot
D. spray spot with cool water

___79. Hair is pressed only when it is

A. wet
B. towel dry
C. dryer dry
D. damp

___80. As the iron is rolled toward the scalp, what does the cosmetologist use to protect the client's scalp

A. cotton
B. towel
C. comb
D. an end paper

___81. What is the name for the service in which the ha
is pressed twice on the top of the strand, and onc
on the underside?

A. one press
B. light press
C. comb press
D. soft press

___82. What is one thing to watch out for when you are about to give a curl reformation?

A. too many test curls
B. client allergies
C. using too many rods
D. tangled hair

___83. Before applying the neutralizer to the rods when doing a curl reformation, the hair should be rins
with

A. conditioner
B. hot water
C. tepid water
D. cold water

___84. Before applying a curl reformation straightener, what should you do?

A. make a client record
B. apply the neutralizer to nape
C. apply a base to hairline
D. give a scalp treatment

___85. Before applying the neutralizer to the rods when doing a curl reformation, the hair should be

A. conditioned
B. rinsed with hot water
C. rinsed with tepid water
D. rinsed with cold water

___86. What is the one thing to watch out for when you are about to give a curl reformation?

A. too many test curls
B. client allergies
C. using too many rods
D. tangled hair

___87. Sweat and oil glands are alike in that they both move a fluid through a(n)

A. tube
B. duct
C. vessel
D. canal

___88. Another name for miliaria rubra is

A. prickly heat
B. sweat retention
C. anhidrosis
D. a cold sweat

___89. One way to penetrate unbroken skin is through the

A. adipose tissue
B. papilla
C. corium
D. follicle

___90. Ultra-violet rays are also called

A. red rays
B. gold rays
C. actinic rays
D. deep penetrating rays

___91. When tinting lashes and brows, petroleum jelly is used to protect the skin from

A. injury
B. abrasion
C. stain
D. scratches

___92. When the foundation makeup protrudes from the surface of the skin, what does this tell you about the skin's alkalinity?

A. high
B. low
C. neutral
D. zero

___93. What effect does the freshener have on the pores of the skin?

A. medicates
B. cleanses
C. opens
D. sanitizes

___94. Onychogryposis is the technical name for

A. ingrown nail
B. ringworm
C. claw nail
D. felon

___95. Once a nail becomes infected, it should be treated by a

A. barber
B. cosmetologist
C. manicurist
D. physician

___96. When selecting a hairpiece for a client, you will be able to match the color more easily by using a

A. pH color chart
B. color triangle
C. JL color ring
D. color comparison chart

___97. Given two students with identical training, what factors determine why one student will graduate from school and earn a lot more money than their classmate?

A. the greater money earner gives many free services
B. the one making more money treats their clients better
C. the student earning less money can't do the work
D. the student earning less didn't attend regularly

___98. What is the name for the establishment of a positive emotional relationship between you and your client?

A. caring
B. bonding
C. rapport
D. support

___99. What is the term used for describing the relationship between you and your client that keeps them coming back into the salon?

A. client retention
B. bonding
C. referral
D. client communications

___100. If the client's skin is mildly inflamed, which step of the shaving procedure should you skip?

A. lathering the beard
B. shaving
C. feathering the razor's edge
D. the steamer towel

DALTON'S STANDARDIZED FINAL TEST 11

Student Name ______________________________ Score _______ Date ___________

Instructions: Carefully read through each question, then read the answer choices. Write your choice of the word, or the phrase, that correctly completes the statement or answers the question, on the line provided.

___1. Cosmetology instructors are required to

A. complete a number of college courses
B. have worked in a beauty salon
C. participate annually in a hairstyling competition
D. all of the above

___2. The advantage(s) of being a manager-operator may include the opportunity to learn about

A. overhead expenses
B. accounts payable
C. inventory
D. all of the above

___3. Personal grooming relates to one's

A. daily appearance
B. daily cleanliness
C. hairstyle and voice
D. A and B.

___4. Personal hygiene relates to

A. promoting one's own health
B. preservation of one's health
C. oral care
D. A and B.

___5. Dental care for preserving healthy teeth starts with a daily mouthwash and

A. rinsing and flushing
B. rubbing and scratching
C. rinsing and rubbing
D. brushing and flossing

___6. Ethics is a system that measures human behavior that is

A. voluntary
B. involuntary
C. imposed by local police
D. imposed by the federal government

___7. A professional attitude is

A. natural
B. given when you are licensed
C. acquired in enrollment
D. learned

___8. To equal the strength of 6% hydrogen peroxide, you would have to use

A. 1 volume hydrogen peroxide
B. 2 volume hydrogen peroxide
C. 10 volume hydrogen peroxide
D. 20 volume hydrogen peroxide

___9. If cosmetology implements are aseptic, then they are

A. free from bacteria
B. unsanitary
C. soiled
D. covered

___10. Things that may be considered a health hazard are

A. forced air furnaces
B. impure air
C. clean body and clothes
D. hygienic salon practices

___11. The germicidal light used in some dry sanitizers is known as

A. fluorescent light
B. ultra-violet light
C. infrared light
D. incandescent light

___12. If the eye has been chemically burned, what should be done?

A. flush eye with cool water
B. flush eye with boric acid
C. apply alcohol
D. apply quats

___13. Which virus causes the AIDS disease?

A. Rhino virus
B. HIV virus
C. Influenza virus
D. Cold virus

___14. How is the AIDS disease transmitted from one person to another?

A. blood
B. semen
C. vaginal secretions
D. all of the above

___15. What route of transmission does the AIDS disease follow?

A. injection
B. blood transfusion
C. maternal
D. all of the above

___16. Soiled towels should be stored in a covered

A. linen hamper
B. metal container
C. plastic container
D. laundry basket

___17. A carrier is a person who has a disease that is

A. acute
B. contagious
C. occupational
D. common

___18. What common cosmetology chemical would kill the AIDS virus outside of the body?

A. household bleach
B. water
C. 1% hydrogen peroxide
D. 20% alcohol

___19. What strength hydrogen peroxide would destroy the AIDS virus outside of the body?

A. 1%
B. 2%
C. 3%
D. all of the above

___20. Hair-cutting implements are sanitized with

A. 30% alcohol
B. 30% formalin solution
C. 40% alcohol
D. 70% alcohol

___21. A 5 percent formalin solution is used mainly to sanitize a(n)

A. ultraviolet sanitizer
B. tweezers
C. cuticle scissors
D. styling chair

___22. The physical wrapping of the hair during cold wave breaks the

A. hydrogen bonds
B. cystine bonds
C. atomic bonds
D. molecular bonds

___23. Scalp hair usually grows at a monthly rate of

A. 1/4"
B. 1/2"
C. 3/4"
D. 1"

___24. Which of the following would a dermatologist prescribe for men for regular hair loss?

A. vitamin A
B. minoxidal
C. medicated shampoo
D. creme rinse

___25. Before applying a chemical depilatory, how should the cosmetologist protect the client?

A. buy only quality depilatories
B. apply gauze to the area to be worked on
C. give the client a skin test
D. ask client to remove jewelry

___26. The percentage of the hair shaft represented by the cortex layer is

A. 15%
B. 25%
C. 50%
D. 75%

___27. The technical term applied to the cyclical period when the hair begins to grow is the

A. anagen stage
B. terminal stage
C. telogen stage
D. origin stage

___28. When alopecia appears in the head, it looks like

A. red, circular bald patches
B. scaly, rectangular bald patches
C. non-inflamed, oval bald patches
D. oily scales and oval bald patches

___29. Using a short-wave electrical machine to stop the growth of a hair is called

A. electrolysis
B. trichosis
C. cometose
D. osmosis

___30. The skin and hair have a natural pH in a range of

A. 3.5 – 4.5.
B. 4.5 – 5.5.
C. 5.5 – 6.5.
D. 6.5 – 7.5.

___31. A mixed lightener would have a pH that is

A. acid
B. alkaline
C. neutral
D. none of the above

___32. When rinsing the client's hair with hot water, how should you detect temperature changes in the water?

A. watch for steam from the client's scalp
B. little finger of hand held under nozzle of hose
C. the color of the client's scalp turns bright pink
D. the shampoo changes color

___33. To prevent water from dripping onto the floor from the shampoo bowl, where should you leave the shampoo hose?

A. drain position
B. handle position
C. vacuum breaker position
D. none of the above

___34. Hair can be damaged by

A. brush rollers
B. heated rollers
C. thermal curling irons
D. all of the above

___35. When the hair is conditioned using strong chemicals, this is known as

A. pre-treating
B. preconditioning
C. duration conditioning
D. in-process conditioning

___36. Semicircular designs combed into the hair are called

A. waves
B. base direction
C. shapings
D. arcs

___37. Before combing out the finger wave, the hair should be

A. thoroughly dried
B. thoroughly lubricated
C. quite damp
D. sprayed with lacquer

___38. The main objective in finger waving the hair is to mold even

A. curls and softness
B. waves and ridges
C. shaping and direction
D. parts and shapes

___39. For the least amount of tightness when setting sculpture curls, you should use a

A. no-stem curl
B. half-stem curl
C. quarter-stem curl
D. long-stem curl

___40. Set sculpture curls within a shaping should

A. be separate
B. swing down
C. overlap
D. swing over

___41. To get the maximum amount of height or fullness, you should use a

A. no-stem curl
B. half-stem curl
C. long-stem curl
D. tight-stem curl

___42. When setting the hair with rollers, a curved form in the finished hairstyle is done by winding hair around the roller

A. 1 turn or less
B. 1-1/2 turns
C. 2 turns
D. none of the above

___43. The problem with a diamond-shaped face is that it is narrow at the chin and

A. eyebrows
B. cheekbones
C. jaws
D. forehead

___44. What draping supply is recommended for the client that is about to have a hair shaping only?

A. towel shampoo cape
B. shampoo cape
C. comb-out cape
D. chair cloth

___45. Super-curly hair should be cut with a

A. clipper
B. scissors
C. razor
D. thinning shears

___46. Proper storage of cutting implements is important to prevent

A. over-use of implements
B. injury to small children
C. rust from forming
D. the edge from becoming dull

___47. When cutting the hair with a shaper, it is important to

A. cut by using the guard
B. thin toward the scalp
C. use long, sliding strokes
D. blunt all hair

___48. If a razor is used to cut the hair, the hair should be

A. completely dry
B. slightly damp
C. completely wet
D. slightly moist

___49. During a razor cut, as the razor is cutting the hair, the comb is placed in the

A. pocket
B. drawer
C. other hand
D. other section

___50. The heat from the air waver should be directed

A. away from the scalp
B. toward the scalp
C. at the ends
D. toward the hair root

___51. A one-process permanent tint contains

A. aniline derivative dye
B. metallic dye
C. vegetable dye
D. henna dye

___52. Before applying an aniline derivative tint, the cosmetologist is required to give the client a

A. test curl
B. test wave
C. patch test
D. strand test

___53. The general term used to describe a lightener and toner is

A. separate application
B. single application
C. double application
D. triple application

___54. A predisposition test is required before applying a(n)

A. vegetable derivative tint
B. animal derivative tint
C. metallic derivative tint
D. aniline derivative tint

___55. When coloring the hair, terms such as cool, drab, and warm, describe

A. tones of a hair color
B. shades of a hair color
C. brightness of a hair color
D. depth of a hair color

___56. By law, a predisposition test must be given befor each

A. oxidation tint
B. bleach
C. temporary rinse
D. conditioning treatment

___57. How many stages does black hair go through to become pale blonde?

A. four
B. five
C. six
D. seven

___58. Decolorization takes place in which layer of the hair?

A. cuticle
B. cortex
C. medulla
D. all of the above

___59. Containers used for mixing bleach should be made of

A. iron
B. wood
C. metal
D. glass/plastic

___60. A retouch hair lightener is applied to the

A. new growth of hair
B. entire hair shaft
C. the ends only
D. cold shaft only

___61. Before applying a toner to gray or white hair, it is necessary to prelighten the hair in order to make the hair

A. resistant enough
B. porous enough
C. lower in pH.
D. lower in alkaline

___62. Pre-bleaching (lightening) is required before the application of a

A. semi-permanent rinse
B. one-process tint
C. permanent toner
D. temporary rinse

___63. When inspecting a wrapped cold wave, the smallest rods would usually be in the

A. crown section
B. nape section
C. eye section
D. ear section

___64. When giving a cold wave always read and follow the

A. manual's instructions
B. textbook's instructions
C. workbook's instructions
D. manufacturer's instructions

___65. When permanent waving the hair, how many turns must the hair be wound around the rod to achieve a curl pattern?

A. once
B. twice
C. four turns
D. five turns

___66. To remove dripping cold-waving solution, use a piece of cotton or the corner of a towel saturated with

A. cold water
B. warm water
C. tepid water
D. hot water

___67. When processing the cold wave, the hair tends to swell, or

A. expand
B. contract
C. harden
D. shrink

___68. The cold-waving solution is applied to the

A. rod, hair, and scalp
B. rod and hair
C. scalp and neutralizer
D. hair and scalp

___69. If cold waving hair that is bleached (lightened), it is best to select rods that are

A. large
B. small
C. midget
D. of any size

___70. The best shampoo to use after a chemical relaxer is a shampoo that has a(n)

A. oil base
B. acid pH.
C. alkaline pH.
D. neutral base

___71. As in cold waving, chemical relaxers work faster on hair that is

A. wiry
B. coarse
C. porous
D. non-porous

___72. Before giving a retouch chemical relaxer, what should be applied to the previously relaxed hair first?

A. water
B. protective conditioner
C. presoftening rinse
D. prerelax shampoo

___73. Hair should be conditioned after a sodium hydroxide relaxer to prevent

A. breakage during combing and setting
B. dry, scaly scalp
C. red, irritated scalp
D. breakage during thermal pressing

___74. After a chemical relaxer, a conditioner should be applied

A. after the hair is set
B. just before the comb-out
C. before the hair is styled with rollers
D. after the comb-out

___75. The chemical relaxer begins to work when what is applied?

A. hot water and shampoo
B. cold water and stabilizer
C. heat and friction
D. medium heat hair dryer

___76. Before a chemical hair straightener, the cosmetologist would not

A. read label directions
B. examine the scalp
C. analyze the hair
D. brush the hair

___77. One of the most important things to remember about the processing of a chemical relaxer is

A. apply it slowly and evenly
B. never leave the client unattended
C. never serve coffee during processing
D. brush the hair before neutralizing

___78. When pressing the hair, the hot comb is usually brought through the

A. top of the strand only
B. bottom of the strand only
C. top and bottom of each strand
D. center of each strand

___79. After a thermal wave, the hair is brushed and combed into a hairstyle

A. after the lanolin has been applied
B. while the hair is still hot
C. when the hair has been cooled
D. while the hair is lukewarm

___80. Before pressing the hair, it should be

A. combed and brushed
B. shampooed and dried
C. shampooed and marcelled
D. dried and curled

___81. Which type of hair will curl the fastest?

A. coarse hair
B. hair with elasticity
C. porous hair
D. fine hair

___82. During a curl reformation the rearranger has been applied, capped, and put under the dryer. When should it be checked?

A. every 5 minutes
B. every 10 minutes
C. every 15 minutes
D. it doesn't need to be checked

___83. During a permanent wave, how would the hair appear when the curl is properly formed around the rod?

A. dull, and slightly wet
B. foamy and resilient.
C. shiny, with the same shape as the rod
D. many small bubbles with some foam

___84. The double-application service in which super-curly hair is straightened, then curled, on permanent wave rods is called a(n)

A. recurl or soft curl
B. structuring or rebuilding
C. Afro-pick
D. none of the above

___85. When giving a curl reformation, it is very important to wear

A. a hair net
B. an operator apron
C. protective shoes
D. none of the above

___86. Sebum goes through a duct from the oil gland, and empties into the hair

A. papilla
B. root
C. follicle
D. cuticle

___87. The outermost (top) layer of the skin is the

A. epidermis
B. corium
C. subcutaneous tissue
D. adipose tissue

___88. An esthetician is a person who is mainly concerned with the promoting and preserving of health and beauty of the

A. fingernails
B. toenails
C. eyebrows
D. skin

____89. The largest and most efficient organ of the human body is the

A. heart
B. liver
C. pancreas
D. skin

____90. Of all the light from the sun, ultra-violet rays make up about

A. 8% of it
B. 12% of it
C. 24% of it
D. 36% of it

____91. What should be applied down the center of the nose to create an illusion that will make the nose appear longer?

A. corrective stick
B. rouge line
C. shadow
D. highlighter

____92. To blend in facial scars and blemishes, what kind of makeup stick should be used?

A. contour
B. rouge
C. corrective
D. powder

____93. After strip lashes are correctly positioned, the outside and inside ends are held in place for

A. one minute
B. two minutes
C. three minutes
D. four minutes

____94. Overgrowth or thickening of the nail is known as

A. hypertrophy
B. hypotrophy
C. tinea
D. agnails

____95. If hangnails are neglected, they may become

A. brittle
B. fragile
C. infected
D. loose

____96. The most expensive type of hair from which hairgoods are made is

A. synthetic hair
B. yak hair
C. angora hair
D. human hair

____97. When alopecia appears in the head, it looks like

A. red, circular bald patches
B. scaly, rectangular bald patches
C. non-inflamed, oval bald patches
D. oily scales and oval bald patches

____98. What can be done to make clients want to come into the salon?

A. make them feel good about their salon experience
B. sell them products they don't need
C. always call them by their first names
D. all of the above

____99. When you are asking the clients questions about their needs, what strategy are you using to provide services or products?

A. grilling
B. discovery
C. anticipation
D. all of the above

____100. If you use a straight razor, how do you protect yourself and your client from accidental cuts during the shaving service?

A. use of a guard
B. protective spray
C. use of an upward motion
D. being very careful

DALTON'S STANDARDIZED FINAL TEST 12

Student Name ______________________________ Score _______ Date __________

Instructions: Carefully read through each question, then read the answer choices. Write your choice of the word, or the phrase, that correctly completes the statement or answers the question, on the line provided.

___1. Personal hygiene includes

A. bathing or showering daily
B. oral and dental care
C. a well-balanced diet
D. all of the above

___2. The extra money paid to you for the sale of conditioners and shampoos is your

A. profit
B. retail commission
C. bonus
D. spiff

___3. A salon owner's income may vary according to the

A. number of salons owned
B. size of the salon
C. location of the salon
D. all of the above

___4. Which term fits the job description for a person who specializes in preserving the beauty of the client's face and neck?

A. facial expert
B. esthetician
C. electrologist
D. dermatologist

___5. To communicate, a thought or attitude is conveyed

A. verbally
B. nonverbally
C. person to person
D. all of the above

___6. Dental care for preserving healthy teeth starts with a daily mouthwash and

A. rinsing and flushing
B. rubbing and scratching
C. rinsing and rubbing
D. brushing and flossing

___7. The governing body in most states which is supposed to discipline members that violate professional ethics is the

A. bureau of ethics
B. state legislature
C. state association
D. state board

___8. It is your responsibility to

A. give as much service as needed
B. learn new methods of hairstyling
C. give services based on quality
D. all of the above

___9. A person immune to a disease, but who can infec others is known as a(n)

A. clinical
B. medical
C. agent
D. carrier

___10. Another name for public hygiene is

A. grooming
B. hair care
C. sanitation
D. community

___11. Practices in the beauty salon that help preserve t health of the public are called

A. fumigation-deodorization
B. salon grooming
C. cleaning-washing
D. sanitation-sterilization

___12. If the eye has been chemically burned, what should be done?

A. flush eye with cool water
B. flush eye with boric acid
C. apply alcohol
D. apply quats

___13. When removing implements from a wet sanitizer you should wear

A. an operator apron
B. a hair net
C. rubber gloves
D. neutralizing bib

___14. Hair-cutting implements are sanitized with

A. 70% alcohol
B. 40% alcohol
C. 30% formalin solution
D. 30% alcohol

___15. How is the AIDS disease transmitted from one person to another?

A. blood
B. semen
C. vaginal secretions
D. all of the above

___16. What route of transmission does the AIDS disease follow?

A. sexual contact
B. injection
C. touching
D. A and B only

___17. Metal electrodes should be sanitized with

A. 2% quats
B. 20% peroxide
C. 70% alcohol
D. 80% ammonium

___18. By law, which of the following must each beauty salon have available?

A. a fire blanket
B. a hot water dispenser
C. an emergency eye wash station
D. a fire extinguisher

___19. A carrier is a person who has a disease that is

A. acute
B. contagious
C. occupational
D. common

___20. Which of the following would destroy the AIDS virus outside the body?

A. water
B. 70% alcohol
C. shampoo
D. hand soap

___21. When giving a service, what should you do if you are exposed to blood?

A. see your doctor
B. wash exposed area with soap and water
C. apply a topical disinfectant
D. B and C only

___22. If you accidently cut your client's neck and it bleeds, what should you do?

A. put on disposable rubber gloves
B. wash area with soap and water
C. apply topical disinfectant to area
D. all of the above

___23. Hair is not found on the

A. forearm and wrists
B. forearm and nose
C. knuckles of the hands
D. soles of the feet

___24. When hair is in its resting cycle, and more likely to fall out, this stage is known as the

A. terminal stage
B. fall-out stage
C. hair loss stage
D. telogen stage

___25. What is the name for the male hair loss due to the aging process?

A. congenital alopecia
B. male-pattern baldness
C. hair thinning
D. routine hair loss

___26. Depilatories in the form of a cream, paste, or powder are chemical products used to

A. curl hair
B. remove hair
C. color hair
D. straighten hair

___27. The layer of the hair in which the coloring pigment is found is the

A. follicle
B. medulla
C. cortex
D. cuticle

____28. Before using a hot wax depilatory, the cosmetologist should

A. apply gauze to the work area
B. give the client instructions
C. check to be sure client is comfortable
D. check the temperature of the wax

____29. Hypertrichosis is a condition that is also called

A. supercilia hair
B. superfluous hair
C. ringed hair
D. twisted hair

____30. Shampoos with a pH greater than seven (7) are called

A. acid
B. alkaline
C. mild
D. neutral

____31. To equal the strength of 6% hydrogen peroxide, you would have to use

A. 1 volume hydrogen peroxide
B. 2 volume hydrogen peroxide
C. 10 volume hydrogen peroxide
D. 20 volume hydrogen peroxide

____32. An overly oily scalp is a disorder medically referred to as

A. steatoma
B. seborrhea
C. asteatosis
D. tinea

____33. How should you protect the client's clothing before shampooing the hair?

A. draping the cape over the back of the chair
B. cover all clothing with towels
C. place in plastic clothing protectors
D. place plastic towels across client's shoulder

____34. The natural lubricant that gives hair a beautiful luster or sheen is called

A. sebum
B. seborrhea
C. seconal
D. permanent color

____35. The extent that hair can be stretched without breaking is known as

A. pressure
B. tone
C. elasticity
D. texture

____36. The basic protein found in the hair shaft is

A. cuticle
B. medulla
C. sebum
D. keratin

____37. When the hair is conditioned using strong chemicals, this is known as

A. pre-treating
B. preconditioning
C. duration conditioning
D. in-process conditioning

____38. Scalp manipulations should not be given if the hair is going to be

A. cold waved
B. permanently colored
C. chemically lightened
D. all of the above

____39. The shaping between two finger-wave ridges is called the wave

A. direction
B. trough
C. arc
D. curl

____40. After the setting lotion has been applied, should the hair dry out during setting, spray more

A. filler on it
B. conditioner on it
C. water on it
D. setting lotion on it

____41. When putting a shaping into the hair, the hair should be

A. wet
B. damp
C. dry
D. moistened on the ends

____42. The standard or ideal facial shape is

A. oblong
B. round
C. oval
D. square

____43. What draping supply is recommended for the client that is about to have a hair shaping only?

A. towel shampoo cape
B. shampoo cape
C. comb-out cape
D. chair cloth

____44. When razor cutting, strokes that the cosmetologist should use are

A. firm and long
B. smooth and long
C. smooth and short
D. jerky and short

____45. To prevent the electric clipper blades from pulling the hair, what should you do?

A. apply oil to them
B. soak in alcohol
C. apply ammonia to them
D. dip them in peroxide

____46. What is the name given to one or more subsections of hair cut in the hairline or crown of the head that serve as a yardstick for cutting the rest of the hair?

A. trendline
B. radial line
C. bias line
D. guideline

____47. What will happen if you submerge your electric clipper in a wet sanitizer while it is plugged into an outlet?

A. the blades will slide
B. the clipper won't cut correctly
C. you will get an electric shock
D. your clipper will vibrate

____48. The hanging length cut around the hairline from which the rest of the hair is shaped is called the

A. high-sign
B. cutting length
C. guideline
D. form

____49. The foundation for a good hairstyle is a correct hair

A. setting lotion
B. shaping
C. styling comb
D. brush

____50. Extra care must be taken when blow waving long hair because it

A. may become hard to manage and curl
B. may dry too quickly and become oily
C. may be drawn into the air intake of the dryer
D. could stick to the brush and become straight

____51. Before applying an aniline derivative tint, omit the

A. hair brushing
B. patch test
C. strand test
D. metallic salt test

____52. Just before applying a hair tint, it would be a good safety precaution to

A. put cotton on the hairline
B. put cotton around the client's neck
C. check again for scalp abrasions
D. clean combs and brushes

____53. A single-application tint is prepared by mixing the required tint with

A. hard water
B. 10-volume peroxide
C. ammonia water
D. 20-volume peroxide

____54. To prevent overlapping on a tint retouch, the tint is applied from the scalp to about

A. 1/16" up to the tinted hair
B. 1/16" over the already tinted hair
C. 1/4" up to the tinted hair
D. 1/2" over the tinted hair

____55. The pH of a semi-permanent color falls in the range of

A. 4 to 6
B. 5 to 6
C. 7 to 9
D. 9 to 10.

____56. If you overlap bleach when doing a bleach retouch, it will result in

A. more elasticity
B. less elasticity
C. breakage
D. hair yellowing

___57. The lightest toner can only be applied to hair bleached to the

A. brown stage
B. red-gold stage
C. pale yellow stage
D. red stage

___58. When lightening and toning the hair, you should wear

A. protective shoes
B. a hair net
C. an operator apron
D. protective gloves

___59. Before giving a lightener retouch, what should you do?

A. a predisposition test
B. brush the hair vigorously
C. examine the scalp for cuts and abrasions
D. give the client a strand test

___60. A creme bleach continues to lighten because it remains

A. moist
B. thick
C. thin
D. dry

___61. The removal of a penetrating tint from the hair is called

A. relaxing
B. soap cap
C. stripping
D. tinting

___62. If the hair was vigorously brushed before a cold wave, the result could be

A. scalp irritations
B. alopecia areata
C. nail scratches
D. scalp tightening

___63. When sodium bromate fumes and ammonia fumes mix together in an open towel hamper, what could result?

A. a fire
B. a strong acid smell
C. discoloration of towels
D. stain in the hamper

___64. Before cold waving the entire head, the degree t which the hair will curl can be determined by using

A. concave curls
B. convex curls
C. test curls
D. pin curls

___65. Cotton is placed around the hairline before applying the cold-waving solution; it should be

A. removed after it is applied
B. allowed to remain until the neutralizer is applied
C. removed following the neutralizer
D. removed when the rods are taken out

___66. In which of the following conditions should the cosmetologist REFUSE to give the client a cold wave?

A. a scar on the scalp
B. cranial surgical wound
C. a scalp freckle
D. an ulna surgical wound

___67. If a couple of small areas of the hair do not hav enough curl one week after the wave process, y should give the client

A. a refund check
B. another cosmetologist
C. some pickup curls
D. another chemical wave

___68. When relaxing a permanent wave that is too cu where should you begin your application?

A. the nape section
B. the top section
C. the side section
D. the crown section

___69. When applying the waving solution as part of t permanent waving process, the cosmetologist s that there is a purple discoloration of the soluti on the client's towel What should the cosmetologist do?

A. stop and rinse the hair with water
B. apply neutralizer immediately
C. continue to give the permanent
D. apply a different waving solution

___70. The action of the cold waving solution is stopped, and the curl is fixed with a

A. developer
B. curler
C. shaper
D. neutralizer

___71. Before applying a chemical relaxer, the hair and scalp must be

A. shampooed
B. brushed
C. examined
D. tinted

___72. Before a chemical relaxer, the skin and scalp can be protected from chemical burns by applying a

A. neutralizer
B. stabilizer
C. base
D. jelly

___73. The difference between a base and no-base relaxer is that the no-base

A. does not require application of the base
B. always requires the use of protective gloves
C. is safer to use, but requires more time
D. is more dangerous to use, but requires more time

___74. If you use all of a particular relaxer, but are in need of more to complete the service, it is best to

A. add water to what is on the hair
B. add water to what is left in the jar, then apply to the hair
C. add a relaxer made by another company
D. neutralize the hair and continue when there is enough material to finish

___75. The neutralizing shampoo used in the chemical relaxing service is also called a

A. stabilizer
B. cleaner
C. conditioner
D. filler

___76. When relaxing virgin hair, the relaxer is always combed through the

A. scalp hair right away
B. ends of each strand right away
C. entire length of the strand
D. none of the above

___77. Before applying a chemical relaxer, analyze the hair for porosity, texture, and elasticity; then, examine the

A. relaxing kit
B. hairline
C. scalp
D. fingernails

___78. Before a chemical hair straightener, the cosmetologist would not

A. read label directions
B. examine the scalp
C. analyze the hair
D. brush the hair

___79. During the processing and neutralizing of a chemical relaxer service, what can be done to minimize neck irritation?

A. applying cotton coil
B. changing towel frequently
C. keeping the client's neck against the bowl
D. applying neutralizing cream

___80. Hair pressing is usually done using

A. 1/4" partings
B. 1/2" partings
C. 1" partings
D. 1-1/2" partings

___81. When thermal waving the hair, fine, short hairs around the hairline are best curled with

A. some pin curls
B. a smaller iron
C. a crimper
D. some perm rods

___82. The styling comb used in thermal waving should be made of

A. aluminum
B. steel
C. hard rubber
D. soft rubber

___83. Before applying a curl reformation straightener, what should you do?

A. make a client record
B. apply the neutralizer to the nape
C. apply a base to hairline
D. give a scalp treatment

___84. Before applying the neutralizer to the rods when doing a curl reformation, the hair should be rinsed with

A. conditioner
B. hot water
C. tepid water
D. cold water

___85. During a curl reformation, how much tension is used to wrap the hair on the rods?

A. no tension
B. moderate tension
C. slight tension
D. firm tension

___86. To be successful, what size rod subsections should the cosmetologist use when doing a curl reformation?

A. small subsections
B. medium subsections
C. large subsections
D. none of the above

___87. During a curl reformation, the hair dries out while you are wrapping the hair on the rods. What should you do?

A. apply more waving solution
B. apply water to dry strands
C. use spray-on conditioner
D. use two end wraps

___88. The outer layer of skin that contains 10 to 20 percent water is the

A. basal layer
B. granular layer
C. horny layer
D. lucid layer

___89. Another name for miliaria rubra is

A. prickly heat
B. sweat retention
C. anhidrosis
D. a cold sweat

___90. The thinnest layer of the skin is the

A. epidermis
B. corium
C. subcutaneous tissue
D. adipose tissue

___91. A clay pack is recommended for skin that is

A. dusty
B. oily
C. dry
D. flakey

___92. When tweezing the eyebrows, this should be do[ne] in which direction?

A. against the growth direction
B. with the growth direction
C. in an upward direction
D. downward toward the nose

___93. Small eyes can be made to appear larger. What type of makeup is applied to create this illusion?

A. contour
B. foundation
C. lip
D. white

___94. When applying semi-permanent lashes, dip the end of the lash in adhesive, stroke the client's lash, then

A. remove it
B. attach it
C. slip it over
D. slide it onto the lid

___95. When the skin around the nail is very sore, inflamed, swollen, and infectious, this disease is known as

A. onycholysis
B. onychophagy
C. paronychia
D. felon nails

___96. Once a nail becomes infected, it should be treat[ed] by a

A. barber
B. cosmetologist
C. manicurist
D. physician

___97. If a minor cut should occur during a manicure, apply powdered styptic, or a(n)

A. shampoo
B. antiseptic
C. creme rinse
D. disinfectant

___98. Today, salon stylists should think of themselves as

A. salespersons
B. helpers
C. educators
D. all of the above

___99. Talking with your clients about the possible solutions to some of their appearance problems is known as a

A. B. meeting
B. consultation
C. conversation
D. revelation

___100. What is the name for the stone used to sharpen a straight razor?

A. hone
B. whetstone
C. strop
D. crop

DALTON'S STANDARDIZED FINAL TEST 13

Student Name ________________________________ Score _______ Date __________

Instructions: Carefully read through each question, then read the answer choices. Write your choice of th word, or the phrase, that correctly completes the statement or answers the question, on the line provided.

___1. A newly licensed, full-time cosmetologist is usually paid

A. on a commission basis
B. on a part-time, hourly basis
C. hourly minimum wage
D. weekly

___2. The advantage(s) of being a manager-operator may include the opportunity to learn about

A. overhead expenses
B. accounts payable
C. inventory
D. all of the above

___3. Personal grooming relates to one's

A. daily appearance
B. daily cleanliness
C. hairstyle and voice
D. A and B.

___4. Personal hygiene relates to

A. promoting one's own health
B. preservation of one's health
C. oral care
D. A and B.

___5. Dental care for preserving healthy teeth starts with a daily mouthwash and

A. rinsing and flushing
B. rubbing and scratching
C. rinsing and rubbing
D. brushing and flossing

___6. Ethics is a system that measures human behavior that is

A. voluntary
B. involuntary
C. imposed by local police
D. imposed by the federal government

___7. A professional attitude is

A. natural
B. given when you are licensed
C. acquired in enrollment
D. learned

___8. To equal the strength of 6% hydrogen peroxide, you would have to use

A. 1 volume hydrogen peroxide
B. 2 volume hydrogen peroxide
C. 10 volume hydrogen peroxide
D. 20 volume hydrogen peroxide

___9. If cosmetology implements are aseptic, then they are

A. free from bacteria
B. unsanitary
C. soiled
D. covered

___10. The germicidal light used in some dry sanitizers i known as

A. fluorescent light
B. ultra-violet light
C. infrared light
D. incandescent light

___11. Uncleanliness can produce germs that cause

A. good health
B. local canities
C. disease
D. malnutrition

___12. Disease is caused mainly from the lack of

A. cleanliness
B. deodorizers
C. cold water
D. hairspray

___13. If the eye has been chemically burned, what should be done?

A. flush eye with cool water
B. flush eye with boric acid
C. apply alcohol
D. apply quats

___14. To be effective for sanitation, the strength of the quats to be used should be at least

A. 1:200
B. 1:200
C. 1:500
D. 1:1000

___15. How is the AIDS disease transmitted from one person to another?

A. blood
B. semen
C. vaginal secretions
D. all of the above

___16. What route of transmission does the AIDS disease follow?

A. injection
B. blood transfusion
C. maternal
D. all of the above

___17. Soiled towels should be stored in a covered

A. linen hamper
B. metal container
C. plastic container
D. laundry basket

___18. A carrier is a person who has a disease that is

A. acute
B. contagious
C. occupational
D. common

___19. What common cosmetology chemical would kill the AIDS virus outside of the body?

A. household bleach
B. water
C. 1% hydrogen peroxide
D. 20% alcohol

___20. What strength hydrogen peroxide would destroy the AIDS virus outside of the body?

A. 1%
B. 2%
C. 3%
D. all of the above

___21. Hair-cutting implements are sanitized with

A. 30% alcohol
B. 30% formalin solution
C. 40% alcohol
D. 70% alcohol

___22. A 5 percent formalin solution is used mainly to sanitize a(n)

A. ultraviolet sanitizer
B. tweezers
C. cuticle scissors
D. styling chair

___23. A soapy solution is used to remove foreign particles from

A. brushes
B. thinning shears
C. a razor
D. an ultraviolet sanitizer

___24. A common skin antiseptic would be

A. 3% hydrogen peroxide
B. 6% hydrogen peroxide
C. 9% hydrogen peroxide
D. 12% hydrogen peroxide

___25. The natural coloring pigment found in the hair is called

A. keratin
B. melanin
C. a tint
D. a dye

___26. Scalp hair usually grows at a monthly rate of

A. 1/4"
B. 1/2"
C. 3/4"
D. 1"

___27. Which of the following would a dermatologist prescribe for men for regular hair loss?

A. vitamin A
B. minoxidal
C. medicated shampoo
D. creme rinse

___28. Before applying a chemical depilatory, how should the cosmetologist protect the client?

A. buy only quality depilatories
B. apply gauze to the area to be worked on
C. give the client a skin test
D. ask client to remove jewelry

___29. The percentage of the hair shaft represented by the cortex layer is

A. 15%
B. 25%
C. 50%
D. 75%

___30. The technical term applied to the cyclical period when the hair begins to grow is the

A. anagen stage
B. terminal stage
C. telogen stage
D. origin stage

____31. What general prefix is used to describe most hair diseases?

A. tricho
B. tricko
C. trio
D. trigo

____32. The pH of a shampoo indicates the concentration of

A. hydrogen
B. oxygen
C. nitrogen
D. carbon

____33. Peroxide has a pH that is

A. acid
B. alkaline
C. neutral
D. none of the above

____34. When rinsing the client's hair with hot water, how should you detect temperature changes in the water?

A. watch for steam from the client's scalp
B. little finger of hand held under nozzle of hose
C. the color of the client's scalp turns bright pink
D. the shampoo changes color

____35. To prevent water from dripping onto the floor from the shampoo bowl, where should you leave the shampoo hose?

A. drain position
B. handle position
C. vacuum breaker position
D. none of the above

____36. To preserve the hairstyle against humidity in the air, the conditioner should contain a(n)

A. barrier coat
B. shield cover
C. wetting agent
D. antihumectant

____37. When the hair is conditioned using strong chemicals, this is known as

A. pre-treating
B. preconditioning
C. duration conditioning
D. in-process conditioning

____38. Hair can be damaged chemically by

A. improper bleaching
B. wave set
C. shampooing
D. hair cutting

____39. Semicircular designs combed into the hair are called

A. waves
B. base direction
C. shapings
D. arcs

____40. Before combing out the finger wave, the hair should be

A. thoroughly dried
B. thoroughly lubricated
C. quite damp
D. sprayed with lacquer

____41. The main objective in finger waving the hair is to mold even

A. curls and softness
B. waves and ridges
C. shaping and direction
D. parts and shapes

____42. Set sculpture curls within a shaping should

A. be separate
B. swing down
C. overlap
D. swing over

____43. To get the maximum amount of height or fullness, you should use a

A. no-stem curl
B. half-stem curl
C. long-stem curl
D. tight-stem curl

____44. When setting the hair with rollers, a curved form in the finished hairstyle is done by winding hair around the roller

A. 1 turn or less
B. 1-1/2 turns
C. 2 turns
D. none of the above

____45. The profile is the view of the head from the

A. front
B. back
C. side
D. face

___46. For a basic haircut, the cosmetologist would begin cutting the hair in the

A. top
B. side
C. crown
D. nape

___47. Super-curly hair should be cut with a

A. clipper
B. scissors
C. razor
D. thinning shears

___48. Proper storage of cutting implements is important to prevent

A. over-use of implements
B. injury to small children
C. rust from forming
D. the edge from becoming dull

___49. You should not use an electric clipper if

A. the client wants a trim
B. the set screw has been adjusted
C. it is noisy
D. any teeth are broken

___50. When cutting the hair with a shaper, it is important to

A. cut by using the guard
B. thin toward the scalp
C. use long, sliding strokes
D. blunt all hair

___51. If a razor is used to cut the hair, the hair should be

A. completely dry
B. slightly damp
C. completely wet
D. slightly moist

___52. The amount of bulk removed from the hair during a razor shaping is determined by the

A. pressure of the razor
B. weight of the razor
C. type of blade used
D. position of the razor guard

___53. Extra care must be taken when blow waving long hair because it

A. may become hard to manage and curl
B. may dry too quickly and become oily
C. may be drawn into the air intake of the dryer
D. could stick to the brush and become straight

___54. To prevent overlapping on a tint retouch, the tint is applied from the scalp to about

A. 1/16" up to the tinted hair
B. 1/16" over the already tinted hair
C. 1/4" up to the tinted hair
D. 1/2" over the tinted hair

___55. One of the main chemicals in aniline derivative tints is

A. sulfonated oils
B. ammonium thioglycolate
C. cystine disulfide
D. para-phenylene-diamine

___56. The name given to the process that explains the chemical reaction of mixing hydrogen peroxide and an aniline derivative tint is

A. hydrolization
B. oxidation
C. softening
D. filling

___57. A predisposition test is required before applying a(n)

A. vegetable derivative tint
B. animal derivative tint
C. metallic derivative tint
D. aniline derivative tint

___58. When coloring the hair terms such as cool, drab, and warm, describe

A. tones of a hair color
B. shades of a hair color
C. brightness of a hair color
D. depth of a hair color

___59. To prevent a line of demarcation during a tint retouch, it is important to avoid

A. rotating a bottle
B. overlapping the tint
C. mixing tint
D. rubbing the scalp

___60. When a cap is used, and strands of hair all over the head are lightened, this is known as

A. tinting
B. frosting
C. streaking
D. painting

___61. Lightening the hair begins with the application of a

A. stripping agent
B. toning agent
C. moisturizing agent
D. bleaching agent

___62. When lightening and toning the hair, you should wear

A. protective shoes
B. a hair net
C. an operator apron
D. protective gloves

___63. A retouch hair lightener is applied to the

A. new growth of hair
B. entire hair shaft
C. the ends only
D. cold shaft only

___64. When giving a lightener retouch, what would be the results if the mixture is overlapped?

A. nothing
B. a gold band
C. incomplete bleaching
D. breakage

___65. To equalize the porosity of the hair, use a

A. steamer
B. stripper
C. filler
D. equalizer

___66. Before a cold wave, gentle scalp manipulations follow the application of a

A. chemical relaxer
B. mild shampoo
C. strong shampoo
D. neutralizing shampoo

___67. Better saturation of the cold-waving solution into the hair is achieved when it is

A. wrapped correctly
B. analyzed accurately
C. curled properly
D. pressed thoroughly

___68. Before cold waving the entire head, the degree to which the hair will curl can be determined by using

A. concave curls
B. convex curls
C. test curls
D. pin curls

___69. During a wrapping procedure using waving solution, breakages can occur if too much tension is placed on the

A. hair
B. comb
C. end wrap
D. rod

___70. If a plastic cap is used to cover the permanent waving rods during processing, what should you be careful NOT to do?

A. allow too much heat to collect
B. tighten the cap too much
C. allow too much air to escape
D. clip the cap in the front section

___71. Cold waving hair involves a physical action, and

A. medical process
B. mineral process
C. chemical process
D. legal process

___72. A neck towel saturated with waving solution, and left around a client's neck may cause a chemical

A. burn
B. reaction
C. lesion
D. sore

___73. To stop the action of the sodium hydroxide and remove it from the hair, the cosmetologist

A. rinses and shampoos the hair
B. conditions, then rinses the hair
C. combs, then shampoos the hair
D. air neutralizes the hair

___74. As in cold waving, chemical relaxers work faster on hair that is

A. wiry
B. coarse
C. porous
D. non-porous

___75. Before giving a retouch chemical relaxer, what should be applied to the previously relaxed hair first?

A. water
B. protective conditioner
C. presoftening rinse
D. prerelax shampoo

___76. After chemically relaxing the hair for a client with super-curly hair, what service should NOT be given to the client?

A. roller set
B. regular electric curling iron set
C. pressing comb/thermal iron set
D. pick out style after hair has been dried

___77. After a chemical relaxer, a conditioner should be applied

A. after the hair is set
B. just before the comb-out
C. before the hair is styled with rollers
D. after the comb-out

___78. It is harmful to the hair to leave a chemical relaxer on it longer than

A. 10 minutes
B. 15 minutes
C. 20 minutes
D. 25 minutes

___79. The actions of chemical hair straightener cause the hair to

A. soften and swell
B. shape and curl
C. shift and mold
D. shrink and harden

___80. One of the most important things to remember about the processing of a chemical relaxer is

A. apply it slowly and evenly
B. never leave the client unattended
C. never serve coffee during processing
D. brush the hair before neutralizing

___81. In order to heat evenly, thermal irons should be made of high quality

A. brass
B. steel
C. aluminum
D. copper

___82. When thermal waving the hair, fine, short hairs around the hairline are best curled with

A. some pin curls
B. a smaller iron
C. a crimper
D. some perm rods

___83. What is the name for the service in which the hair is pressed twice on the top of the strand, and once on the underside?

A. one press
B. light press
C. comb press
D. soft press

___84. When applying the curl rearranger, you should wear

A. gloves
B. an operator apron
C. protective sleeves
D. all of the above

___85. During a curl reformation the rearranger has been applied, capped, and put under the dryer. When should it be checked?

A. every 5 minutes
B. every 10 minutes
C. every 15 minutes
D. it doesn't need to be checked

___86. Before applying the neutralizer to the rods when doing a curl reformation, the hair should be

A. conditioned
B. rinsed with hot water
C. rinsed with tepid water
D. rinsed with cold water

___87. What is the one thing to watch out for when you are about to give a curl reformation?

A. too many test curls
B. client allergies
C. using too many rods
D. tangled hair

___88. One way to penetrate unbroken skin is through the

A. adipose tissue
B. follicle
C. corium
D. subcutaneous tissue

___89. A sun block lotion would have what SPF rating number?

A. 5
B. 8
C. 12
D. 15

___90. The largest and most efficient organ of the human body is the

A. heart
B. liver
C. pancreas
D. skin

___91. After a blackhead has been removed, the cosmetologist should apply a(n)

A. hot towel
B. antiseptic
C. fumigant
D. deodorant

___92. The application of semi-permanent lashes is also referred to as

A. temporary lashes
B. permanent lashes
C. strip lashes
D. eye tabbing

___93. To blend in facial scars and blemishes, what kind of makeup stick should be used?

A. contour
B. rouge
C. corrective
D. powder

___94. What type of movement should be used when tweezing the eyebrows?

A. slow, sliding movement
B. quick movement
C. circular movement
D. zig-zag movement

___95. The inner part of the nail that affects its shape, size, and growth is known as the

A. plate
B. matrix
C. lunula
D. cuticle

___96. If hangnails are neglected, they may become

A. brittle
B. fragile
C. infected
D. loose

___97. To prevent a canvas block from becoming unsanitary and giving off an odor, it is advisable to cover it with a

A. nylon cap
B. synthetic fiber
C. plastic bag
D. rubber sheet

___98. What is the greatest fear faced by people in sales-related jobs?

A. which clothes to wear
B. what to do with the client's hair
C. what to do with the client's face
D. how to overcome rejection

___99. When a cosmetologist has so many appointments that it is difficult to fit in new clients, what is this called?

A. booked solid
B. full book
C. booked-up
D. booked to the hilt

___100. When shaving, what purpose does the application of lather serve?

A. softens the skin
B. smoothes the beard
C. softens the beard
D. feels soothing

DALTON'S STANDARDIZED FINAL TEST 14

Student Name ________________________ Score _______ Date ___________

Instructions: Carefully read through each question, then read the answer choices. Write your choice of the word, or the phrase, that correctly completes the statement or answers the question, on the line provided.

___1. Nonverbal communication refers to

A. listening to what is said
B. communicating with body movements
C. communicating with your hands
D. keeping steady eye contact during conversation

___2. Tonsorial is a term to describe a person who does what type of work?

A. the nails
B. the feet
C. hair coloring
D. barbering

___3. A salon owner's income may vary according to the

A. number of salons owned
B. size of the salon
C. location of the salon
D. all of the above

___4. Which term fits the job description for a person who specializes in preserving the beauty of the client's face and neck?

A. facial expert
B. esthetician
C. electrologist
D. dermatologist

___5. To communicate, a thought or attitude is conveyed

A. verbally
B. nonverbally
C. person to person
D. all of the above

___6. Dental care for preserving healthy teeth starts with a daily mouthwash and

A. rinsing and flushing
B. rubbing and scratching
C. rinsing and rubbing
D. brushing and flossing

___7. The governing body in most states which is supposed to discipline members that violate professional ethics is the

A. bureau of ethics
B. state legislature
C. state association
D. state board

___8. It is your responsibility to

A. give as much service as needed
B. learn new methods of hairstyling
C. give services based on quality
D. all of the above

___9. A person immune to a disease, but who can infect others is known as a(n)

A. clinical
B. medical
C. agent
D. carrier

___10. Things that may be considered a health hazard are

A. forced air furnaces
B. impure air
C. clean body and clothes
D. hygienic salon practices

___11. Another name for public hygiene is

A. grooming
B. hair care
C. sanitation
D. community

___12. Disease is caused mainly from the lack of

A. cleanliness
B. deodorizers
C. cold water
D. hairspray

___13. The electrical device that removes stale air from the salon is called a(n)

A. humidifier
B. ceiling fan
C. exhaust fan
D. de-humidifier

___14. Practices in the beauty salon that help preserve the health of the public are called

A. fumigation-deodorization
B. salon grooming
C. cleaning-washing
D. sanitation-sterilization

___15. If the eye has been chemically burned, what should be done?

A. flush eye with cool water
B. flush eye with boric acid
C. apply alcohol
D. apply quats

___16. Hair-cutting implements are sanitized with

A. 70% alcohol
B. 40% alcohol
C. 30% formalin solution
D. 30% alcohol

___17. How is the AIDS disease transmitted from one person to another?

A. blood
B. semen
C. vaginal secretions
D. all of the above

___18. What route of transmission does the AIDS disease follow?

A. sexual contact
B. injection
C. touching
D. A and B only

___19. Metal electrodes should be sanitized with

A. 2% quats
B. 20% peroxide
C. 70% alcohol
D. 80% ammonium

___20. By law, which of the following must each beauty salon have available?

A. a fire blanket
B. a hot water dispenser
C. an emergency eye wash station
D. a fire extinguisher

___21. A carrier is a person who has a disease that is

A. acute
B. contagious
C. occupational
D. common

___22. Which of the following would destroy the AIDS virus outside the body?

A. water
B. 70% alcohol
C. shampoo
D. hand soap

___23. When giving a service, what should you do if you are exposed to blood?

A. see your doctor
B. wash exposed area with soap and water
C. apply a topical disinfectant
D. B and C only

___24. A soapy solution is used to remove foreign particles from

A. brushes
B. thinning shears
C. a razor
D. an ultraviolet sanitizer

___25. The natural coloring pigment found in the hair is called

A. keratin
B. melanin
C. a tint
D. a dye

___26. When hair is in its resting cycle, and more likely to fall out, this stage is known as the

A. terminal stage
B. fall-out stage
C. hair loss stage
D. telogen stage

___27. What is the name for the male hair loss due to the aging process?

A. congenital alopecia
B. male-pattern baldness
C. hair thinning
D. routine hair loss

___28. What general term below is used to describe any diseased condition of the hair?

A. alopecia
B. hirsutism
C. trichosis
D. trichorrhexis nodosa

___29. Before applying a chemical depilatory, how should the cosmetologist protect the client?

A. buy only quality depilatories
B. apply gauze to the area to be worked on
C. give the client a skin test
D. ask client to remove jewelry

___30. The layer of the hair in which the coloring pigment is found is the

A. follicle
B. medulla
C. cortex
D. cuticle

___31. Before using a hot wax depilatory, the cosmetologist should

A. apply gauze to the work area
B. give the client instructions
C. check to be sure client is comfortable
D. check the temperature of the wax

___32. What general prefix is used to describe most hair diseases?

A. tricho
B. tricko
C. trio
D. trigo

___33. Shampoos with a pH greater than seven (7) are called

A. acid
B. alkaline
C. mild
D. neutral

___34. Peroxide has a pH that is

A. acid
B. alkaline
C. neutral
D. none of the above

___35. When rinsing the client's hair with hot water, how should you detect temperature changes in the water?

A. watch for steam from the client's scalp
B. little finger of hand held under nozzle of hose
C. the color of the client's scalp turns bright pink
D. the shampoo changes color

___36. Hair can be damaged by

A. brush rollers
B. heated rollers
C. thermal curling irons
D. all of the above

___37. When the hair is conditioned using strong chemicals, this is known as

A. pre-treating
B. preconditioning
C. duration conditioning
D. in-process conditioning

___38. Hair can be damaged chemically by

A. improper bleaching
B. wave set
C. shampooing
D. hair cutting

___39. Scalp manipulations should not be given if the hair is going to be

A. cold waved
B. permanently colored
C. chemically lightened
D. all of the above

___40. The shaping between two finger-wave ridges is called the wave

A. direction
B. trough
C. arc
D. curl

___41. For the least amount of tightness when setting sculpture curls, you should use a

A. no-stem curl
B. half-stem curl
C. quarter-stem curl
D. long-stem curl

___42. A large stand-up curl could also be called a barrel curl or

A. skip-curl
B. cascade curl
C. closed-end curl
D. clockwise curl

___43. When putting a shaping into the hair, the hair should be

A. wet
B. damp
C. dry
D. moistened on the ends

____44. The standard or ideal facial shape is

A. oblong
B. round
C. oval
D. square

____45. If too much bulk is removed from coarse hair, it tends to

A. look smooth and natural
B. stick out from the head
C. be super curly
D. set more easily

____46. When razor cutting, strokes that the cosmetologist should use are

A. firm and long
B. smooth and long
C. smooth and short
D. jerky and short

____47. To prevent the electric clipper blades from pulling the hair, what should you do?

A. apply oil to them
B. soak in alcohol
C. apply ammonia to them
D. dip them in peroxide

____48. What is the name given to one or more subsections of hair cut in the hairline or crown of the head that serve as a yardstick for cutting the rest of the hair?

A. trendline
B. radial line
C. bias line
D. guideline

____49. What will happen if you submerge your electric clipper in a wet sanitizer while it is plugged into an outlet?

A. the blades will slide
B. the clipper won't cut correctly
C. you will get an electric shock
D. your clipper will vibrate

____50. Storing your scissors in your uniform pocket may result in

A. a severe cut
B. tarnishing of finish on the scissors
C. dulling of blades of the scissors
D. rust forming on the scissors

____51. To thin hair during a shaping means to

A. shorten it
B. add to its length
C. increase its bulk
D. decrease its bulk

____52. The heat from the air waver should be directed

A. away from the scalp
B. toward the scalp
C. at the ends
D. toward the hair root

____53. A one-process permanent tint contains

A. aniline derivative dye
B. metallic dye
C. vegetable dye
D. henna dye

____54. Before applying an aniline derivative tint, the cosmetologist is required to give the client a

A. test curl
B. test wave
C. patch test
D. strand test

____55. A client is now in the styling chair for a scheduled virgin tint. After getting the coloring product from the dispensary, you discover there is no developer anywhere in the salon

A. use water for the developer, and tint
B. use shampoo for developer
C. reschedule the appointment
D. ask the client to leave

____56. Synthetic/organic temporary hair colors are found in

A. vegetable tints
B. aniline derivative tints
C. certified vegetable tints
D. metallic tints

____57. By law, a predisposition test must be given before each

A. oxidation tint
B. bleach
C. temporary rinse
D. conditioning treatment

___58. How many stages does black hair go through to become pale blonde?

A. four
B. five
C. six
D. seven

___59. Decolorization takes place in which layer of the hair?

A. cuticle
B. cortex
C. medulla
D. all of the above

___60. Containers used for mixing bleach should be made of

A. iron
B. wood
C. metal
D. glass/plastic

___61. The client has received a frosting and complains it's too "heavy". How could you reduce the amount of frosted hair?

A. apply tint all over the head
B. give client a tintback
C. apply a filler
D. give client a reverse frosting

___62. A drastic color change from dark to very light hair color requires

A. pre-toning
B. pre-lightening
C. pre-tipping
D. pre-frosting

___63. Pre-bleaching (lightening) is required before the application of a

A. semi-permanent rinse
B. one-process tint
C. permanent toner
D. temporary rinse

___64. Where should soiled facial linens be stored

A. on the station
B. on the facial chair
C. in a closed container
D. with the facial supplies

___65. Before a cold wave is wrapped the hair is usually dried using a

A. blow comb
B. hand dryer
C. towel
D. rat-tail comb

___66. When permanent waving the hair, how many turns must the hair be wound around the rod to achieve a curl pattern?

A. once
B. twice
C. four turns
D. five turns

___67. In which of the following conditions should the cosmetologist REFUSE to give the client a cold wave?

A. a scar on the scalp
B. cranial surgical wound
C. a scalp freckle
D. an ulna surgical wound

___68. If a couple of small areas of the hair do not have enough curl one week after the wave process, you should give the client

A. a refund check
B. another cosmetologist
C. some pickup curls
D. another chemical wave

___69. Cold waving resistant hair would usually require a

A. longer processing time
B. shorter processing time
C. conditioner
D. toner

___70. Two basic chemicals used in cold-waving solution are

A. ammonia and formalin
B. sulfuric acid and ammonia
C. carbolic acid and formalin
D. thioglycolic acid and ammonia

___71. A neck towel saturated with waving solution, and left around a client's neck may cause a chemical

A. burn
B. reaction
C. lesion
D. sore

____72. If unsure which strength chemical relaxer should be used, the cosmetologist should take a(n)

A. patch test
B. strand test
C. skin test
D. allergy test

____73. If the client has a little spot on the scalp that is burning during a chemical hair relaxer, what should you do?

A. rinse all relaxer from hair immediately
B. apply an astringent to the spot
C. apply petrolatum to the spot
D. spray spot with cool water

____74. Should a chemical relaxer accidently drip into the client's eye, what should you do?

A. stop action by applying neutralizer to eye
B. flush eye with lots of water
C. blot chemical and apply hot water
D. mist eye with bottle of warm water

____75. After a sodium hydroxide relaxer has processed, but before it is shampooed, the hair should be thoroughly

A. combed
B. conditioned
C. rinsed
D. brushed

____76. The neutralizing shampoo used in the chemical relaxing service is also called a

A. stabilizer
B. cleaner
C. conditioner
D. filler

____77. When giving a chemical relaxer, which areas of the head are the most fragile and most likely to be damaged?

A. crown and top sections
B. front hairline and nape sections
C. crown and front hairline sections
D. crown and nape sections

____78. When applying a chemical relaxer, it is important that you AVOID

A. misting the hair with water
B. using small sections
C. tugging on the hair
D. timing your application

____79. One of the most important things to remember about the processing of a chemical relaxer is

A. apply it slowly and evenly
B. never leave the client unattended
C. never serve coffee during processing
D. brush the hair before neutralizing

____80. Once heated for use, the temperature of thermal irons is tested on

A. the touch of the hand
B. a piece of white tissue
C. a damp sponge
D. the client's hair

____81. As the iron is rolled toward the scalp, what does the cosmetologist use to protect the client's scalp?

A. cotton
B. towel
C. comb
D. an end paper

____82. Before thermal waving super-curly hair, the cosmetologist should

A. color it
B. press it
C. shape it
D. comb it

____83. Before pressing the hair, it should be

A. combed and brushed
B. shampooed and dried
C. shampooed and marcelled
D. dried and curled

____84. When doing a curl reformation, how often should the rearranger be tested?

A. 1 – 2 minutes
B. 3 – 5 minutes
C. 6 – 8 minutes
D. 9 – 10 minutes

____85. Before applying the neutralizer to the rods when doing a curl reformation, the hair should be rinsed with

A. conditioner
B. hot water
C. tepid water
D. cold water

___86. During a curl reformation, how much tension is used to wrap the hair on the rods?

A. no tension
B. moderate tension
C. slight tension
D. firm tension

___87. What is the name for the product that straightens the hair in the curl reformation service?

A. chemical relaxer
B. chemical rearranger
C. hair straightener
D. hair filler

___88. When giving a curl reformation, it is very important to wear

A. a hair net
B. an operator apron
C. protective shoes
D. none of the above

___89. The normal temperature of the human body is

A. 97.3 degrees
B. 97.6 degrees
C. 98.4 degrees
D. 98.6 degrees

___90. The outermost (top) layer of the skin is the

A. epidermis
B. corium
C. subcutaneous tissue
D. adipose tissue

___91. The word used to describe a kneading or rolling facial movement is

A. effleurage
B. petrissage
C. friction
D. tapotement

___92. If strip eyelashes are to fit correctly, what must be done before the lashes are put on the client?

A. measuring
B. weighing
C. cleansing
D. arching

___93. Small eyes can be made to appear larger. What type of makeup is applied to create this illusion?

A. contour
B. foundation
C. lip
D. white

___94. After strip lashes are correctly positioned, the outside and inside ends are held in place for

A. one minute
B. two minutes
C. three minutes
D. four minutes

___95. When the cuticle sticks to the base of the nail as it grows out, this condition is known as

A. agnails
B. tinea
C. blue nails
D. pterygium

___96. Once a nail becomes infected, it should be treated by a

A. barber
B. cosmetologist
C. manicurist
D. physician

___97. To prevent a canvas block from becoming unsanitary and giving off an odor, it is advisable to cover it with a

A. nylon cap
B. synthetic fiber
C. plastic bag
D. rubber sheet

___98. What is the first step in becoming a successful cosmetologist?

A. styling the hair well
B. answering the phone well
C. realizing you are a salesperson
D. knowing that you can help all clients

___99. If a client is booked for a permanent wave, which of the following would be classified as an extra service?

A. haircut
B. frosting
C. protein conditioner
D. all of the above

___100. If you should accidently draw blood when giving the client a shave, what should you do first?

A. apply pressure to stop the bleeding
B. put on rubber gloves
C. apply antiseptic
D. put styptic on wound

DALTON'S STANDARDIZED FINAL TEST 15

Student Name ______________________ Score ______ Date ________

Instructions: Carefully read through each question, then read the answer choices. Write your choice of th word, or the phrase, that correctly completes the statement or answers the question, on the line provided.

___1. A student who has a positive attitude

A. is reliable
B. gets along with other people
C. learns when convenient
D. A and B.

___2. Regular physical examination by a doctor may lead to discovery of a

A. physical exercise
B. prophylaxis
C. public hygiene
D. disease

___3. The advantage(s) of being a manager-operator may include the opportunity to learn about

A. overhead expenses
B. accounts payable
C. inventory
D. all of the above

___4. Personal grooming relates to one's

A. daily appearance
B. daily cleanliness
C. hairstyle and voice
D. A and B.

___5. Personal hygiene relates to

A. promoting one's own health
B. preservation of one's health
C. oral care
D. A and B.

___6. Dental care for preserving healthy teeth starts with a daily mouthwash and

A. rinsing and flushing
B. rubbing and scratching
C. rinsing and rubbing
D. brushing and flossing

___7. Ethics is a system that measures human behavior that is

A. voluntary
B. involuntary
C. imposed by local police
D. imposed by the federal government

___8. A professional attitude is

A. natural
B. given when you are licensed
C. acquired in enrollment
D. learned

___9. To equal the strength of 70% ethyl alcohol, you would have to use

A. 20% isopropyl alcohol
B. 39%isopropyl alcohol
C. 85% isopropyl alcohol
D. 99% isopropyl alcohol

___10. If cosmetology implements are aseptic, then they are

A. free from bacteria
B. unsanitary
C. soiled
D. covered

___11. A person immune to a disease, but who can infect others is known as a(n)

A. clinical
B. medical
C. agent
D. carrier

___12. Another name for public hygiene is

A. grooming
B. hair care
C. sanitation
D. community

___13. If the eye has been chemically burned, what should be done?

A. flush eye with cool water
B. flush eye with boric acid
C. apply alcohol
D. apply quats

___14. When removing implements from a wet sanitizer you should wear

A. an operator apron
B. a hair net
C. rubber gloves
D. neutralizing bib

___15. How is the AIDS disease transmitted from one person to another?

A. blood
B. semen
C. vaginal secretions
D. all of the above

___16. What route of transmission does the AIDS disease follow?

A. injection
B. blood transfusion
C. maternal
D. all of the above

___17. Soiled towels should be stored in a covered

A. linen hamper
B. metal container
C. plastic container
D. laundry basket

___18. A carrier is a person who has a disease that is

A. acute
B. contagious
C. occupational
D. common

___19. What common cosmetology chemical would kill the AIDS virus outside of the body?

A. household bleach
B. water
C. 1% hydrogen peroxide
D. 20% alcohol

___20. What strength hydrogen peroxide would destroy the AIDS virus outside of the body?

A. 1%
B. 2%
C. 3%
D. all of the above

___21. If you accidently cut your client's neck and it bleeds, what should you do?

A. put on disposable rubber gloves
B. wash area with soap and water
C. apply topical disinfectant to area
D. all of the above

___22. The function of the hair is to

A. adorn the body
B. protect the skin
C. adorn the head
D. all of the above

___23. Hair is an example of

A. hard keratin
B. soft keratin
C. Henle's layer
D. Huxley's layer

___24. The glands in the scalp that naturally lubricate the hair during brushing are called

A. apocrine
B. sebaceous
C. sudoriferous
D. eccrine

___25. Depilatories in the form of a cream, paste, or powder are chemical products used to

A. curl hair
B. remove hair
C. color hair
D. straighten hair

___26. The percentage of the hair shaft represented by the cortex layer is

A. 15%
B. 25%
C. 50%
D. 75%

___27. The technical term applied to the cyclical period when the hair begins to grow is the

A. anagen stage
B. terminal stage
C. telogen stage
D. origin stage

___28. Hypertrichosis is a condition that is also called

A. supercilia hair
B. superfluous hair
C. ringed hair
D. twisted hair

___29. The skin and hair have a natural pH in a range of

A. 3.5 – 4.5.
B. 4.5 – 5.5.
C. 5.5 – 6.5.
D. 6.5 – 7.5.

___30. Peroxide has a pH that is

A. acid
B. alkaline
C. neutral
D. none of the above

___31. Scabies is an infestation of the scalp by

A. the itch mite
B. head lice
C. ringworm
D. tinea

___32. An overly oily scalp is a disorder medically referred to as

A. steatoma
B. seborrhea
C. asteatosis
D. tinea

___33. To prevent water from dripping onto the floor from the shampoo bowl, where should you leave the shampoo hose?

A. drain position
B. handle position
C. vacuum breaker position
D. none of the above

___34. To preserve the hairstyle against humidity in the air, the conditioner should contain a(n)

A. barrier coat
B. shield cover
C. wetting agent
D. antihumectant

___35. The basic protein found in the hair shaft is

A. cuticle
B. medulla
C. sebum
D. keratin

___36. If damaged hair is going to be given a service that uses strong chemicals the cosmetologist should recommend

A. preconditioning
B. prelightening
C. pre-filling
D. preneutralizing

___37. Semicircular designs combed into the hair are called

A. waves
B. base direction
C. shapings
D. arcs

___38. The main objective in finger waving the hair is to mold even

A. curls and softness
B. waves and ridges
C. shaping and direction
D. parts and shapes

___39. After the setting lotion has been applied, should the hair dry out during setting, spray more

A. filler on it
B. conditioner on it
C. water on it
D. setting lotion on it

___40. To get the maximum amount of height or fullness you should use a

A. no-stem curl
B. half-stem curl
C. long-stem curl
D. tight-stem curl

___41. When setting the hair with rollers, a curved form in the finished hairstyle is done by winding hair around the roller

A. 1 turn or less
B. 1-1/2 turns
C. 2 turns
D. none of the above

___42. To correct a diamond-shaped face, fullness is needed everywhere, except at the

A. cheekbones
B. eyebrows
C. forehead
D. jaw

___43. For a basic haircut, the cosmetologist would begin cutting the hair in the

A. top
B. side
C. crown
D. nape

___44. When dry, super-curly hair should be shortened using a

A. clipper
B. scissors
C. razor
D. thinning shears

___45. Proper storage of cutting implements is important to prevent

A. over-use of implements
B. injury to small children
C. rust from forming
D. the edge from becoming dull

___46. The technique of holding the hair upward toward the crown or top of the head during a hair shaping is called

A. low-elevation
B. high-elevation
C. feather edging
D. stepping

___47. When cutting the hair with a shaper, it is important to

A. cut by using the guard
B. thin toward the scalp
C. use long, sliding strokes
D. blunt all hair

___48. The hanging length cut around the hairline from which the rest of the hair is shaped is called the

A. high-sign
B. cutting length
C. guideline
D. form

___49. The amount of bulk removed from the hair during a razor shaping is determined by the

A. pressure of the razor
B. weight of the razor
C. type of blade used
D. position of the razor guard

___50. Extra care must be taken when blow waving long hair because it

A. may become hard to manage and curl
B. may dry too quickly and become oily
C. may be drawn into the air intake of the dryer
D. could stick to the brush and become straight

___51. When doing a tint retouch, apply the tint only to the

A. hair root
B. hair ends
C. cold shaft
D. new growth

___52. Aniline derivative tints color the hair because they are

A. penetrating tints
B. metallic dyes
C. henna dyes
D. vegetable tints

___53. The general term used to describe a lightener and toner is

A. separate application
B. single application
C. double application
D. triple application

___54. A predisposition test is required before applying a(n)

A. vegetable derivative tint
B. animal derivative tint
C. metallic derivative tint
D. aniline derivative tint

___55. When coloring, terms such as cool, drab, and warm, describe

A. tones of a hair color
B. shades of a hair color
C. brightness of a hair color
D. depth of a hair color

___56. The pH of a semi-permanent color falls in the range of

A. 4 to 6
B. 5 to 6
C. 7 to 9
D. 9 to 10.

___57. Which of the following is the best definition of a permanent toner?

A. an aniline derivative tint in pastel colors
B. an aniline tint having a gold base
C. para-phenylene-diamine dyes
D. color that cannot be removed

___58. The lightest stage that hair can be bleached is

A. gold
B. pale yellow
C. pale red-gold
D. pale orange

___59. When the proper stage of streaking is reached, which shampoo is BEST to remove bleach?

A. mild
B. medicated (alkaline)
C. non-stripping (acid)
D. alkaline

___60. Removing artificial color from the hair requires the use of a

A. stripper
B. steamer
C. dye solvent
D. bleach

___61. If bleach drips onto the skin, the bleach should be removed using

A. cold-cool water
B. tepid-hot water
C. hot water only
D. very hot water

___62. When giving a virgin bleach to medium brown normal hair, the cosmetologist should begin applying the lightener

A. 1/2" from scalp up through ends
B. from scalp to ends
C. from ends to scalp
D. center of hair shaft to ends

___63. To achieve a good curl when permanent waving, how much tension should be applied to the hair during wrapping?

A. very firm tension
B. very little tension
C. moderate-firm, even tension
D. no tension

___64. The greatest risk of hair damage during cold waving is presented by hair that is

A. conditioned
B. retouched
C. over lighted
D. tinted

___65. When giving a cold wave always read and follow the

A. manual's instructions
B. textbook's instructions
C. workbook's instructions
D. manufacturer's instructions

___66. After processing a perm, what can you do to prevent the rods from being forced from the hair during rinsing ?

A. tighten them up
B. use low water pressure
C. put on a hair net
D. rinse with cool water

___67. Cotton is placed around the hairline before applying the cold-waving solution; it should be

A. removed after it is applied
B. allowed to remain until the neutralizer is applied
C. removed following the neutralizer
D. removed when the rods are taken out

___68. To remove dripping cold-waving solution, use a piece of cotton or the corner of a towel saturated with

A. cold water
B. warm water
C. tepid water
D. hot water

___69. When wrapping a ponytail cold wave, it is better to begin wrapping in the

A. bottom section
B. top section
C. middle section
D. front section

___70. If a neutralizing bib is used for neutralizing the permanent, where should you place a small piece of cotton?

A. by the ears
B. across the forehead
C. under the eye hook
D. around the nape

___71. A neck towel saturated with waving solution, and left around a client's neck may cause a chemical

A. burn
B. reaction
C. lesion
D. sore

___72. If super-curly hair has been thermal pressed, or is otherwise very damaged, the cosmetologist should

A. use the mild strength relaxer
B. advise a tint to even the hair porosity
C. refuse the chemical relaxer
D. refer the person to another salon

___73. As in cold waving, chemical relaxers work faster on hair that is

A. wiry
B. coarse
C. porous
D. non-porous

___74. The difference between a base and no-base relaxer is that the no-base

A. does not require application of the base
B. always requires the use of protective gloves
C. is safer to use, but requires more time
D. is more dangerous to use, but requires more time

___75. The application of a base or no-base relaxer would begin in the

A. front hairline section
B. left-side section
C. right-side section
D. crown or nape section(s)

___76. After a chemical relaxer, a conditioner should be applied

A. after the hair is set
B. just before the comb-out
C. before the hair is styled with rollers
D. after the comb-out

___77. After instruction and practice, what is the ideal amount of time for applying and processing a chemical relaxer?

A. 4 minutes
B. 6 minutes
C. 15 minutes
D. 20 minutes

___78. When rinsing the chemical relaxer from the hair, to avoid tangling, it is important to use

A. low to medium water pressure
B. high water pressure
C. hot water at all times
D. an alkaline shampoo

___79. If the client has a little spot on the scalp that is burning during a chemical hair relaxer, what should you do?

A. rinse all relaxer from the hair immediately
B. apply an astringent to the spot
C. apply petrolatum to the spot
D. spray spot with cool water

___80. When thermal pressing the hair, which area of the head is usually the hair the most fragile and subject to breakage?

A. hairline
B. crown
C. top-crown sections
D. crown into the side sections

___81. After the hair is pressed, the thermal iron forms the curl by rotating the iron using a(n)

A. clicking action
B. sliding actions
C. oval action
D. back and forth action

___82. The styling comb used in thermal waving should be made of

A. aluminum
B. steel
C. hard rubber
D. soft rubber

___83. During a curl reformation, the hair dries out while you are wrapping the hair on the rods. What should you do?

A. apply more waving solution
B. apply water to dry strands
C. use spray-on conditioner
D. use two end wraps

___84. During a curl reformation the rearranger has been applied, capped, and put under the dryer. When should it be checked?

A. every 5 minutes
B. every 10 minutes
C. every 15 minutes
D. it doesn't need to be checked

___85. Before applying a curl reformation straightener, what should you do?

A. make a client record
B. apply the neutralizer to nape
C. apply a base to hairline
D. give a scalp treatment

___86. The double-application service in which super-curly hair is straightened, then curled, on permanent wave rods is called a(n)

A. recurl or soft curl
B. structuring or rebuilding
C. Afro-pick
D. none of the above

___87. During a curl reformation, the hair dries out while you are wrapping the hair on the rods. What should you do?

A. apply more waving solution
B. apply water to dry strands
C. use spray-on conditioner
D. use two end wraps

___88. Adipose tissue is also referred to as

A. cuticle
B. fatty
C. epidermis
D. dermis

___89. Another name for miliaria rubra is

A. prickly heat
B. sweat retention
C. anhidrosis
D. a cold sweat

___90. One way to penetrate unbroken skin is through the

A. adipose tissue
B. papilla
C. corium
D. follicle

___91. What percentage of the sunlight is represented by infrared rays?

A. 40 %
B. 60 %
C. 80 %
D. 90 %

___92. In terms of the client's natural eyelashes, where are the strip lashes placed?

A. below
B. above
C. even with
D. on

___93. When the foundation makeup protrudes from the surface of the skin, what does this tell you about the skin's alkalinity?

A. high
B. low
C. neutral
D. zero

___94. What effect does the freshener have on the pores of the skin?

A. medicates
B. cleanses
C. opens
D. sanitizes

___95. Trimming or filing nails too deeply into corners can cause

A. hangnails
B. ingrown nails
C. nail thickening
D. brittle nails

___96. If hangnails are neglected, they may become

A. brittle
B. fragile
C. infected
D. loose

___97. To prevent a canvas block from becoming unsanitary and giving off an odor, it is advisable to cover it with a

A. nylon cap
B. synthetic fiber
C. plastic bag
D. rubber sheet

___98. What is the name for the establishment of a positive emotional relationship between you and your client?

A. caring
B. bonding
C. rapport
D. support

___99. How is a stylist usually paid for the sale of retail products in the salon to their clients?

A. $2.00 per item
B. $3.00 per item
C. $5.00 per item
D. a commission

___100. Which of the following should be used to put a finishing edge on your straight razor?

A. towel
B. strop
C. hone
D. comb

Answers – Final Test Questions

DALTON'S FINAL TEST 1

1. A	26. B	51. C	76. C
2. D	27. A	52. D	77. D
3. D	28. A	53. A	78. A
4. D	29. A	54. C	79. A
5. D	30. A	55. A	80. C
6. A	31. A	56. C	81. A
7. D	32. A	57. A and D	82. B
8. D	33. C	58. A	83. C
9. D	34. A	59. A	84. B
10. B	35. C	60. C	85. B
11. A	36. B	61. C	86. C
12. D	37. A	62. C	87. C
13. B	38. C	63. A	88. A
14. D	39. A	64. C	89. D
15. B	40. A	65. A	90. B
16. B	41. C	66. A	91. C
17. A	42. D	67. A	92. A
18. C	43. A or B	68. C	93. B
19. A	44. B	69. A	94. C
20. D	45. B	70. B	95. D
21. A	46. A	71. C	96. C
22. B	47. C	72. B	97. B
23. B	48. C	73. A or D	98. B
24. D	49. B	74. C	99. B
25. A	50. D	75. C	100. D

DALTON'S FINAL TEST 2

1. C	26. B	51. A	76. A
2. B	27. C	52. A	77. A
3. D	28. C	53. D	78. B
4. B	29. D	54. C	79. B
5. D	30. A	55. B	80. C
6. D	31. B	56. A	81. B
7. D	32. A	57. D	82. A
8. D	33. B	58. D	83. C
9. B	34. A	59. C	84. D
10. B	35. D	60. C	85. A
11. D	36. D	61. A	86. D
12. A	37. A	62. A	87. A
13. A	38. D	63. A	88. A
14. B	39. A	64. C	89. A
15. D	40. D	65. B	90. D
16. C	41. C	66. B	91. B
17. D	42. A	67. A	92. A
18. B	43. A	68. A	93. B
19. B	44. B	69. D	94. C
20. D	45. C	70. A	95. C
21. D	46. A	71. C	96. B
22. A	47. D	72. C	97. A
23. A	48. C	73. A	98. B
24. D	49. A	74. C	99. A
25. D	50. B	75. A	100. A

DALTON'S FINAL TEST 3

1. B	26. B	51. C	76. C
2. D	27. C	52. C	77. B
3. D	28. D	53. A	78. A
4. D	29. A	54. D	79. B
5. D	30. B	55. B	80. C
6. A	31. B	56. A	81. C
7. D	32. A	57. B	82. D
8. D	33. B	58. A	83. D
9. D	34. A	59. B	84. A
10. C	35. A	60. D	85. A
11. A	36. D	61. A	86. C
12. C	37. D	62. A	87. A
13. B	38. C	63. C	88. D
14. D	39. B	64. C	89. A
15. B	40. A	65. A	90. B
16. B	41. B	66. C	91. B
17. A	42. A	67. A	92. A
18. C	43. A	68. A	93. B
19. D	44. C	69. A	94. B
20. D	45. D	70. C	95. D
21. D	46. A or B	71. A	96. D
22. A	47. B	72. B	97. C
23. D	48. D	73. D	98. B
24. A	49. A	74. B	99. C
25. B	50. C	75. D	100. C

DALTON'S FINAL TEST 4

1. D	26. B	51. A	76. C
2. D	27. C	52. C	77. B
3. B	28. D	53. C	78. A
4. D	29. C	54. B	79. B
5. D	30. A	55. C	80. C
6. D	31. A	56. C	81. B
7. D	32. A	57. C	82. C
8. A	33. B	58. A and D	83. D
9. B	34. A	59. C	84. C
10. B	35. D	60. B	85. D
11. D	36. C	61. C	86. D
12. A	37. D	62. D	87. D
13. D	38. D	63. A	88. D
14. A	39. B	64. C	89. A
15. B	40. C	65. B	90. D
16. D	41. A	66. C	91. C
17. C	42. C	67. A	92. A
18. D	43. D	68. C	93. D
19. B	44. C	69. A	94. D
20. B	45. A	70. C	95. C
21. D	46. D	71. B	96. C
22. A	47. C	72. B	97. A
23. D	48. A	73. C	98. D
24. D	49. B	74. A	99. C
25. B	50. B	75. C	100. B

DALTON'S FINAL TEST 5

1. B	26. D	51. A	76. B
2. D	27. A	52. D	77. D
3. D	28. A	53. D	78. D
4. D	29. B	54. B	79. D
5. D	30. A	55. D	80. A
6. A	31. A	56. A	81. B
7. D	32. A	57. A	82. D
8. D	33. A	58. D	83. A
9. B	34. A	59. B	84. C
10. C	35. A	60. C	85. A
11. A	36. C	61. A	86. B
12. A	37. A	62. D	87. D
13. B	38. B	63. A	88. A
14. D	39. D	64. B	89. A
15. B	40. C	65. C	90. C
16. B	41. A	66. C	91. A
17. A	42. A	67. B	92. A
18. C	43. D	68. A	93. B
19. D	44. D	69. B	94. A
20. D	45. A or B	70. D	95. C
21. D	46. B	71. B	96. C
22. D	47. B	72. C	97. B
23. A	48. A	73. A	98. D
24. B	49. C	74. A	99. A
25. C	50. C	75. C	100. B

DALTON'S FINAL TEST 6

1. D	26. C	51. A	76. A
2. B	27. C	52. D	77. D
3. D	28. D	53. D	78. A
4. B	29. B	54. C	79. B
5. D	30. B	55. A	80. D
6. D	31. A	56. B	81. C
7. D	32. B	57. C	82. D
8. D	33. A	58. D	83. D
9. D	34. D	59. A and D	84. C
10. C	35. D	60. C	85. D
11. D	36. D	61. B	86. A
12. A	37. D	62. C	87. C
13. C	38. B	63. C	88. D
14. A	39. A	64. A	89. D
15. B	40. B	65. C	90. D
16. D	41. A	66. A	91. A
17. C	42. C	67. B	92. A
18. D	43. B	68. C	93. B
19. B	44. C	69. A	94. D
20. B	45. A	70. B	95. D
21. D	46. D	71. A	96. B
22. D	47. C	72. C	97. B
23. D	48. C	73. D	98. A
24. D	49. B	74. D	99. B
25. B	50. C	75. A or D	100. C

DALTON'S FINAL TEST 7

1. D	26. D	51. A	76. C
2. D	27. A	52. D	77. B
3. D	28. C	53. C	78. A
4. D	29. A	54. D	79. C
5. D	30. A	55. C	80. B
6. A	31. B	56. A	81. D
7. D	32. A	57. B	82. A
8. D	33. A	58. D	83. A
9. A	34. D	59. A	84. B
10. B	35. A	60. C	85. D
11. A	36. C	61. C	86. B
12. D	37. B	62. C	87. A
13. B	38. A	63. C	88. A
14. D	39. C	64. C	89. C
15. B	40. A	65. A	90. B
16. B	41. A	66. C	91. C
17. A	42. A	67. C	92. B
18. C	43. D	68. A	93. B
19. D	44. A or B	69. C	94. D
20. A	45. B	70. B	95. C
21. A	46. D	71. B	96. C
22. A	47. A	72. B	97. A
23. B	48. C	73. C	98. D
24. B	49. C	74. C	99. A
25. C	50. C	75. A	100. A

DALTON'S FINAL TEST 8

1. A	26. B	51. C	76. B
2. A	27. C	52. C	77. A
3. D	28. D	53. B	78. B
4. B	29. A	54. B	79. C
5. D	30. B	55. D	80. B
6. D	31. A	56. C	81. C
7. D	32. B	57. A and D	82. D
8. D	33. A	58. C	83. A
9. B	34. D	59. C	84. B
10. C	35. C	60. C	85. A
11. A	36. D	61. B	86. A
12. D	37. D	62. A	87. D
13. D	38. A	63. B	88. A
14. A	39. D	64. B	89. A
15. A	40. C	65. C	90. B
16. B	41. A	66. C	91. B
17. D	42. D	67. A	92. A
18. C	43. C	68. C	93. B
19. D	44. A	69. C	94. C
20. B	45. D	70. C	95. D
21. B	46. C	71. A	96. C
22. D	47. A	72. A	97. C
23. A	48. B	73. A	98. D
24. D	49. A	74. D	99. C
25. B	50. A	75. D	100. C

DALTON'S FINAL TEST 9

1. D	26. D	51. D	76. A
2. D	27. A	52. C	77. A
3. D	28. B	53. A	78. B
4. A	29. B	54. C	79. A
5. D	30. A	55. C	80. A
6. D	31. B	56. D	81. B
7. A	32. A	57. D	82. A
8. D	33. A	58. A	83. A
9. B	34. D	59. D	84. A
10. C	35. D	60. C	85. A
11. A	36. C	61. B	86. A
12. C	37. B	62. A	87. D
13. D	38. B	63. C	88. D
14. D	39. A	64. A	89. A
15. B	40. A	65. A	90. D
16. B	41. C	66. C	91. A
17. A	42. B	67. C	92. A
18. C	43. A or B	68. D	93. B
19. D	44. B	69. A	94. C
20. D	45. D	70. C	95. D
21. A	46. A	71. A	96. B
22. B	47. C	72. C	97. A
23. B	48. C	73. B	98. C
24. B	49. C	74. C	99. C
25. C	50. A	75. C	100. A

DALTON'S FINAL TEST 10

1. D	26. C	51. C	76. C
2. D	27. D	52. B	77. D
3. B	28. A	53. B	78. D
4. D	29. A	54. A	79. C
5. D	30. A	55. B	80. C
6. D	31. A	56. C	81. D
7. D	32. A	57. C	82. B
8. D	33. A	58. D	83. C
9. A	34. A	59. A	84. C
10. D	35. A	60. A	85. C
11. A	36. D	61. C	86. B
12. D	37. B	62. C	87. B
13. D	38. C	63. C	88. A
14. C	39. A	64. B	89. D
15. D	40. A	65. C	90. C
16. B	41. D	66. A	91. C
17. B	42. C	67. C	92. A
18. D	43. A	68. C	93. B
19. D	44. B	69. A	94. C
20. A	45. C	70. D	95. D
21. A	46. A	71. D	96. C
22. D	47. B	72. B	97. B
23. B	48. C	73. A	98. C
24. B	49. D	74. A	99. A
25. C	50. D	75. A	100. D

DALTON'S FINAL TEST 11

1. D	26. D	51. A	76. D
2. D	27. A	52. C	77. B
3. D	28. C	53. C	78. C
4. D	29. A	54. D	79. C
5. D	30. B	55. A	80. B
6. A	31. B	56. A	81. C
7. D	32. B	57. D	82. A
8. D	33. A	58. B	83. C
9. A	34. D	59. D	84. A
10. B	35. D	60. A	85. D
11. B	36. C	61. B	86. C
12. A	37. A	62. C	87. A
13. B	38. B	63. B	88. D
14. D	39. D	64. D	89. D
15. D	40. C	65. B	90. A
16. B	41. A	66. A	91. D
17. B	42. A	67. A	92. C
18. A	43. D	68. B	93. A
19. C	44. D	69. A	94. A
20. D	45. A or B	70. B	95. C
21. D	46. B	71. C	96. D
22. A	47. A	72. B	97. C
23. B	48. C	73. A	98. A
24. B	49. C	74. C	99. B
25. C	50. A	75. C	100. D

DALTON'S FINAL TEST 12

1. D	26. B	51. A	76. D
2. B	27. C	52. C	77. C
3. D	28. D	53. D	78. D
4. B	29. B	54. A	79. B
5. D	30. B	55. C	80. A
6. D	31. D	56. C	81. B
7. D	32. B	57. C	82. C
8. D	33. A	58. D	83. C
9. D	34. A	59. C	84. C
10. C	35. C	60. A	85. D
11. D	36. D	61. C	86. A
12. A	37. D	62. A	87. A
13. C	38. D	63. A	88. C
14. A	39. B	64. C	89. A
15. D	40. C	65. A	90. A
16. D	41. A	66. B	91. B
17. C	42. C	67. C	92. B
18. D	43. D	68. A	93. A
19. B	44. C	69. C	94. B
20. B	45. A	70. D	95. C
21. D	46. D	71. C	96. D
22. D	47. C	72. C	97. B
23. D	48. C	73. A	98. D
24. D	49. B	74. D	99. B
25. B	50. C	75. A	100. A

DALTON'S FINAL TEST 13

1. C	26. B	51. C	76. C
2. D	27. B	52. A	77. C
3. D	28. C	53. C	78. B
4. D	29. D	54. A	79. A
5. D	30. A	55. D	80. B
6. A	31. A	56. B	81. B
7. D	32. A	57. D	82. B
8. D	33. A	58. A	83. D
9. A	34. B	59. B	84. A
10. B	35. A	60. B	85. A
11. C	36. D	61. D	86. C
12. A	37. D	62. D	87. B
13. A	38. A	63. A	88. B
14. D	39. C	64. D	89. D
15. D	40. A	65. C	90. D
16. D	41. B	66. B	91. B
17. B	42. C	67. A	92. D
18. B	43. A	68. C	93. C
19. A	44. A	69. A	94. B
20. C	45. C	70. B	95. B
21. D	46. D	71. C	96. C
22. D	47. A or B	72. A	97. C
23. A	48. B	73. A	98. D
24. A	49. D	74. C	99. B
25. B	50. A	75. B	100. C

DALTON'S FINAL TEST 14

1. B	26. D	51. D	76. A
2. D	27. B	52. A	77. B
3. D	28. C	53. A	78. C
4. B	29. C	54. C	79. B
5. D	30. C	55. C	80. B
6. D	31. D	56. B	81. C
7. D	32. A	57. A	82. B
8. D	33. B	58. D	83. B
9. D	34. A	59. B	84. B
10. B	35. B	60. A and D	85. C
11. C	36. D	61. D	86. D
12. A	37. D	62. B	87. B
13. D	38. A	63. C	88. D
14. D	39. D	64. C	89. D
15. A	40. B	65. C	90. A
16. A	41. D	66. B	91. B
17. D	42. B	67. B	92. A
18. D	43. A	68. C	93. A
19. C	44. C	69. A	94. A
20. D	45. B	70. D	95. D
21. B	46. C	71. A	96. D
22. B	47. A	72. B	97. C
23. D	48. D	73. D	98. C
24. A	49. C	74. B	99. D
25. B	50. A	75. C	100. B

DALTON'S FINAL TEST 15

1. D	26. D	51. D	76. C
2. D	27. A	52. A	77. C
3. D	28. B	53. C	78. A
4. D	29. B	54. D	79. D
5. D	30. A	55. A	80. A
6. D	31. A	56. C	81. A
7. A	32. B	57. A	82. C
8. D	33. A	58. B	83. A
9. D	34. D	59. C	84. A
10. A	35. D	60. C	85. C
11. D	36. A	61. A	86. A
12. C	37. C	62. A	87. A
13. A	38. B	63. C	88. B
14. C	39. C	64. C	89. A
15. D	40. A	65. D	90. D
16. D	41. A	66. C	91. C
17. B	42. A	67. A	92. B
18. B	43. D	68. A	93. A
19. A	44. A or B	69. A	94. B
20. C	45. B	70. C	95. B
21. D	46. B	71. A	96. C
22. D	47. A	72. C	97. C
23. A	48. C	73. C	98. C
24. B	49. A	74. A	99. D
25. B	50. C	75. D	100. B